Cancer of Unknown Primary

Alwin Krämer • Harald Löffler
Editors

Cancer of Unknown Primary

Springer

Editors
Alwin Krämer
Clinical Cooperation Unit Molecular Hematology/Oncology
German Cancer Research Center (DKFZ) and University of Heidelberg
Heidelberg
Germany

Harald Löffler
Clinical Cooperation Unit Molecular Hematology/Oncology
German Cancer Research Center (DKFZ) and University of Heidelberg
Heidelberg
Germany

ISBN 978-3-319-22580-7 ISBN 978-3-319-22581-4 (eBook)
DOI 10.1007/978-3-319-22581-4

Library of Congress Control Number: 2015952541

Springer Cham Heidelberg New York Dordrecht London

Printed on acid-free paper

Springer International Publishing AG Switzerland is part of Springer Science+Business Media (www.springer.com)

Contents

Chapter 1
Introduction

Harald Löffler and Alwin Krämer

1.1 Defining Cancer of Unknown Primary

Cancer of unknown primary (CUP) usually refers to histologically proven cancer where no primary lesion has been detected although the initial diagnostic work-up has been completed. The label "CUP" should not be used when a metastatic lesion has been found but an appropriate search for a primary origin has not yet been done. This is already the first problem with the definition of CUP, since it is not exactly defined what the minimum requirements with respect to an appropriate staging are. Indeed, CUP nowadays accounts for 2–3 % of all cancer-related deaths in Germany [1], while older publications state the proportion of CUP to be 5–10 % of all cancers [2], with this likely being the result of improved diagnostic possibilities to identify the primary.

Malignant lesions of non-epithelial origin such as lymphomas and sarcomas must not be categorized as CUP, meaning that CUP usually refers to an epithelial origin. On the other hand, undifferentiated tumors with unknown primary and no signs of any differentiation – neither epithelial nor non-epithelial – are compatible with the definition of CUP, simply because there is no other meaningful category. This delineation is also somewhat problematic, since the assignment of epithelial versus non-epithelial origin depends on the diagnostic methodology used: It can safely be assumed that the "undifferentiated tumor" category has lost ground over the past, say, 30 years due to the improved repertoire of immunohistochemistry, and site-of-origin assignment by gene expression profiling and related techniques may bring this category on the verge of extinction.

Thirdly, the definition of "no primary" is far from being always clear. There are CUP cases with multiple, more or less equally advanced metastases, but others

H. Löffler (✉) • A. Krämer
Clinical Cooperation Unit Molecular Hematology/Oncology, German Cancer Research Center (DKFZ) and University of Heidelberg, Heidelberg, Germany
e-mail: h.loeffler@Dkfz-Heidelberg.de; a.kraemer@Dkfz-Heidelberg.de

A. Krämer, H. Löffler (eds.), *Cancer of Unknown Primary*,
DOI 10.1007/978-3-319-22581-4_1

show a leading lesion or a solitary one, and here the question may arise whether the leading or solitary lesion is in fact the primary. Arguments against the notion of the leading lesion being the primary (which, of course, should be default) may include the presence of more than one possible assignment, e.g., an adenocarcinoma within the liver which could be intrahepatic cholangiocarcinoma as well as a metastasis from an unknown primary [3], or a histology clearly arguing against the clinically suspected origin, e.g., if a CT scan suggests nodal-positive lung cancer but histology suggests intestinal adenocarcinoma in the absence of an intestinal lesion. In such cases, primary lesions showing atypical or rare histologic features should be always considered. For example, when a solitary skin lesion with a histology suggestive of adenocarcinoma but no systemic involvement is found, primary adnexal carcinoma of the skin must be considered [4].

Finally, it has to be mentioned that some authors have extended the definition of CUP also to cases where metastases without a primary were diagnosed solely based on clinical findings without histological confirmation [5, 6]. We do not think that this approach is useful, since even if we are quite sure from a clinical perspective that lesions are malignant, they could still be lymphoma or sarcoma. Hence, cases without histological confirmation should rather be called "suspected malignoma, not otherwise specified," and of course, a histological confirmation is nowadays nearly always recommended – the only exception being cases where the general condition or comorbidities clearly preclude any cancer-specific intervention.

In summary, there is some inconsistency regarding the definition of CUP both in clinical practice and in the literature. Within this book, we would like to adhere to the definition of histologically proven cancer with no primary despite completed staging, excluding non-epithelial malignancies.

1.2 Some Thoughts About History and Present

Though not being historians, we think we are on the safe side stating that CUP has been known for longer than cytostatic drug therapy to treat it: A database search with the combination "cancer" and "unknown primary" retrieved a paper from 1946 as earliest search result [7]. The earliest registry data on CUP we are aware of cover the period 1921–1981; in this series, less than 20 % of patients received cytostatic drugs or hormones [5]. In 1993, Hainsworth and Greco, the authors of Chap. 11 of this book, stated [8]: "The majority of patients with cancer of an unknown primary site do not benefit from other than supportive treatment. A minority, however, do benefit from palliative treatment, and a few are candidates for curative treatment." This minority was defined by the presence of a clear working hypothesis warranting site-specific therapy [8].

Although this view is unfortunately not completely outdated yet, it has shifted quite significantly since then because of two reasons: Firstly, drug therapy for the abovementioned majority of CUP patients has been improved as combinations containing platinum derivatives and third-generation cytostatics have been successfully established due to promising results in phase II trials. Moreover, the advent of molecularly targeted drugs, although not widely established in CUP yet, offers a clear perspective for further improvements of which the majority of CUP patients may benefit. Secondly, our possibilities toward finding a working hypothesis have clearly improved due to immunohistochemistry, which was introduced in the 1980s and has been further advanced since then, and gene expression profiling, which has been made available in recent years.

Today, we face the problem of how to handle these new possibilities since there is still a shortage of evidence-based data. In this book, we will repeatedly be confronted with the contrast between currently established standards and novel possibilities. We think that there is no definitive answer to the question how much evidence is needed in order to integrate these novel possibilities into standard of care. Regarding this, we hope that our book will be helpful in ongoing discussions by offering a balanced view on current evidence.

1.3 Our Approach Toward CUP

When a patient is labeled as having CUP, it should be avoided to perform endless diagnostic studies which may be triggered by the reluctance to accept the fact that we cannot find the primary. Likewise, we should stop believing that, when we have finally come to the conclusion that we really cannot find the primary, there is more or less nothing we can do for the patient anymore. Instead, we should keep in mind that at present, the median overall survival of CUP patients lies in the range of 1 year. Therefore, taking a rapid decision about how to help our patient best might be preferable over spending several months of this remaining lifetime performing diagnostics. On the other hand, we must keep in mind that there are subgroups of CUP with a clearly better prognosis. Hence, diagnostics should focus on identifying these subgroups while avoiding procedures from which no therapeutic consequences are expected.

This book is intended to give some advice on how to handle these complex challenges in the management of CUP patients. First of all, we would like to equip the reader with in-depth knowledge about both current evidence and novel approaches in the diagnostics and therapy of CUP. Based on this, we advocate a structured approach toward the management of CUP patients. We will start with some fundamentals about epidemiology, biology, and prognostic factors, and then look at our diagnostic repertoire and its rational use in detail. Next, the reader will find details about current therapeutic strategies for both the "standard case" and important subgroups to be treated differently. Finally, we will turn to emerging novel diagnostic and therapeutic strategies, which are subject to current research activities and will lead us to possible future directions.

References

1. Löffler H, Neben K, Krämer A. Cancer of unknown primary: epidemiology and pathogenesis. Radiologe. 2014;54(2):107–11. PubMed CUP-Syndrom : Epidemiologie und Pathogenese.
2. Stewart JF, Tattersall MH, Woods RL, Fox RM. Unknown primary adenocarcinoma: incidence of over investigation and natural history. Br Med J. 1979;1(6177):1530–3. PubMed Pubmed Central PMCID: 1599694.
3. Länger F, von Wasielewski R, Kreipe HH. Bedeutung der Immunhistochemie für die Diagnose des Cholangiokarzinoms. Pathologe. 2006;27(4):244–50. PubMed Bedeutung der Immunhistochemie fur die Diagnose des Cholangiokarzinoms.
4. Wick MR, Goellner JR, Wolfe 3rd JT, Su WP. Adnexal carcinomas of the skin. I. Eccrine carcinomas. Cancer. 1985;56(5):1147–62. PubMed.
5. Altman E, Cadman E. An analysis of 1539 patients with cancer of unknown primary site. Cancer. 1986;57(1):120–4. PubMed.
6. Levi F, Te VC, Erler G, Randimbison L, La Vecchia C. Epidemiology of unknown primary tumours. Eur J Cancer. 2002;38(13):1810–2. PubMed.
7. Lampe I, Santin G. Metastatic carcinoma in neck of unknown primary site; salvage by radiation treatment. Univ Hosp Bull. 1946;12(11):106. PubMed.
8. Hainsworth JD, Greco FA. Treatment of patients with cancer of an unknown primary site. N Engl J Med. 1993;329(4):257–63. PubMed.

Chapter 2
Epidemiology, Risk Factors, and Survival in CUP: Pointers to Disease Mechanisms

Kari Hemminki

2.1 Introduction

The focus of my epidemiological studies has been on familial cancer, based on the Swedish "Family-Cancer Database" (FCD), initially assembled from various national registers in 1994 and updated thereafter approximately biannually ten times. FCD covers essentially the whole Swedish population organized in families over the past 100 years with cancers obtained from the Swedish Cancer Registry which started in year 1958 [1]. With a population base of close to 15 million and close to 2 million cancers, it is the largest database of its kind in the world. Having assessed the familial risks for all primary cancers, we realized a few years ago that the cancer registry had an entry "cancer of unknown primary" which we did not know much of and had never analyzed it. According to the first background reading, CUP did not appear interesting because it was described as a heterogeneous disease without known risk factors. However, once we ventured to start analyses, interesting results emerged on familial risks and these encouraged us to characterize epidemiology and survival in CUP on various aspects which will be described here, together with the sparse global literature on the topic [2].

Population-based epidemiology on CUP is limited to a handful of papers before about 2010. The reason has been that the diagnostic codes for CUP have not been well defined and, for example, Cancer Incidence in Five Continents, published by International Agency for Research on Cancer (IARC), has included CUP in diagnostic category "other and unspecified" which has been interpreted in various ways in national cancer registration guidelines. The World Cancer Report 2008, published by IARC, does not recognize search words for CUP [3]. Even on the clinical side

K. Hemminki
Division of Molecular Genetic Epidemiology, German Cancer Research Center (DKFZ), Heidelberg, Germany

Lund University, Malmö, Sweden
e-mail: k.hemminki@dkfz.de

A. Krämer, H. Löffler (eds.), *Cancer of Unknown Primary*,
DOI 10.1007/978-3-319-22581-4_2

CUP has been a neglected condition, diagnosis is time-consuming and difficult, patients are feeble and desperate about vague information, and no specific treatment can be offered.

The International Classification of Diseases (ICD) codes for CUP have changed over time. In ICD-7 (used in Sweden 1958–1986), the code was 199 while in ICD-9 (used in Sweden 1987–1992), the codes were 195–199 and in ICD-O and subsequent versions, it has been C80. However, different authors have defined their codes slightly differently and there is no agreed international definition of CUP as described [4]. From ICD-9 onward, the code has specified the location where metastases were found, distinguishing lymph nodal metastases and those in internal organs, such as liver, respiratory system, abdominal cavity, bone, brain, etc. A nonspecific code CUP is also listed which is often used for patients with multiple metastatic locations. The Swedish Cancer Registry gives the cause of death using ICD codes and for CUP, the cause of death is in most cases the cancer that, according to the death registrar, killed the patient [5]. Thus, these data allow analysis of mortality depending on the location of metastases as will be discussed later. This is different from primary cancers for which the cause of death is given as the primary cancer instead of the metastasis that caused the death. Results on survival studies relating to location of fatal metastases will be discussed later under Sect. 2.6.

Histological distribution of CUP in the Swedish Cancer Registry includes four main types: adenocarcinoma, undifferentiated "cancer," squamous cell carcinoma (SCC), and melanoma. The code for undifferentiated "cancer" is ambiguous, but in the context of CUP, it refers to epithelial tumors and should be "carcinoma." The first 2 ones are by far the most common ones and show many similar clinical features. Histology is an important predictor of survival and it may be used to infer about the hidden primary cancer.

2.2 Population-Based Versus Hospital-Based Studies

CUP is a fatal disease and the reader should take note that for fatal diseases, many aspects of disease characteristics depend on the time point in the disease process when these were observed. For fatal diseases, it is particularly important to understand the distinction between the concepts "at diagnosis" and "at referral," frequently overlooked, resulting in false conclusions [6]. Thus, one has to be cautious in interpreting results from case–control- or hospital-based studies because the "case" population is selected to be the surviving population from the "at diagnosis" population, and the selection is likely to affect, for example, the histological distribution of cancers in favor of the more benign histological types. In the case of CUP, the selection may include enrichment of, e.g., young patients with metastases in lymph nodes. The selection tends to be most severe in tertiary/quaternary referral centers. When judging the superior treatment results from such centers, one needs first to question how representative the patient clientele is. At the extreme of selection, survival rates from clinical trials specify the survival in patients selected on certain entrance criteria into a specific treatment. Cancer registries collect in principle "at diagnosis" data, but even high-quality registries may have underpresentation of, for example, very old patients or borderline or difficult diagnoses [7].

CUP, being among the most fatal cancers, is very sensitive to the selection of the patient population, as discussed elsewhere [8]. Greco and Pavlidis cited nine studies on median survival time for CUP patients; for three cancer registry-based studies, the survival ranged from 2.75 to 4 months and for hospital-based studies, it ranged from 3 to 11 months [9]. In population-based studies, the median survival is 3 months or shorter and 1-year survival around 20 % (www.nice.ong.uk/cg104) [4, 10–12]. Survival kinetics show a steep time-dependent monotonous decline making clear that a large proportion of very frail patients would not survive a referral to tertiary/quaternary centers.

To illustrate the effect of deleting early fatalities from a survival study, I used, for Table 2.1, the empirical Swedish data on adenocarcinoma of CUP affecting only lymph nodes (axilla, head, and neck sites specified) or with metastatic spread to extranodal visceral organs (liver, bone, and mediastinum) [11]. Follow-up of patients was started at time 0 ("at diagnosis"), at month 3, or at month 7 ("at referral"). All median survival times improved once the early fatal cases were excluded. For CUP with metastasis at extranodal sites, the median survival was 7 months when the follow-up was started at month 3. This is somewhat less favorable than the 8–12 months cited by a recent expert review [13]. Another consequence of starting follow-up late is that the patient population becomes enriched in favorable histologies and subtypes, shown by increasing proportions of lymph node metastasis (axillary nodes increasing from 3.7 to 10.0 %) in populations for which the first months were omitted in Table 2.1. Conversely, the proportion of the fatal sites decreased, liver cases from 74.1 to 58.4 %.

These kinds of selections are also the likely reason for the apparent discourse between the autopsy-verified primary sites of CUP and those assigned by molecular methods (gene expression analysis) [14]. The latter tissue-of-origin assignments score much higher proportions of relatively benign cancers, particularly breast cancers, compared to autopsy data for which the lung and the pancreas dominate [15]. Many of the studies applying molecular methods used patient samples from referral hospitals.

2.3 Incidence

The CUP incidence variation may reflect the diagnostic trend, the completeness and validity of cancer registration, or the real variation in incidence in a group of heterogeneous cancers. CUP incidence rates ranging from 5 to 10 per 100,000 have been reported in Nordic countries during 1998–2002 when the incidence has been at its maximum [16, 17]. Van de Wouw et al. reported that approximately 2500 new patients were diagnosed annually in the Netherlands from 1984 to 1992, giving an age-standardized incidence rate of 6.7 per 100,000 for males and 5.3 per 100,000

Table 2.1 Follow-up information on CUP patients

	Start of follow-up								
	0 months+			3 months+			7 months+		
Metastatic sites	Cases (%)	Cancer deaths	Median survival	Cases (%)	Cancer deaths	Median survival	Cases (%)	Cancer deaths	Median survival
Lymph nodes	576	434	8	405	286	15	292	185	28
Axilla	131 (3.7 %)	67	74	107 (6.2 %)	46	119	92 (10.0 %)	33	.
Head and neck	202 (5.7 %)	167	7	136 (7.8 %)	111	12	97 (10.5 %)	77	16
Extranodal	5576	4934	3	2824	2479	7	1523	1288	11
Liver	2650 (74.1 %)	2407	2	1121 (64.5 %)	1014	7	540 (58.4 %)	476	10
Bone	552 (15.4 %)	475	5	344 (19.8 %)	296	7	174 (18.8 %)	147	14
Mediastinum	40 (1.1 %)	33	7	31 (1.8 %)	25	14	21 (2.3 %)	16	19

for females [10]. The incidence of CUP is identical for men and women in Sweden, but in some countries, there is a small male or female excess [4, 12, 17]. Cases of CUP are diagnosed from age 30 onward with the peak age at diagnosis being in the 70s [17]. Brewster and coworkers discuss the sensitivity of the apparent incidence to the definition of CUP [4].

In the Nordic countries, CUP incidence increased until about 1995–2000, followed by a sharp decline which seems to be continuing [16, 17]. In the USA, the decline in incidence started already in around 1980 [12]. The decline in CUP incidence, which has been opposite to the incidence of all cancers, has implied that the proportion of CUP cases of all cancer has dropped from about 4–2 % [12, 16, 17]. Because of high fatality, CUP ranks the third or fourth among cancer deaths [4, 12]. In Sweden, the decrease in incidence has been noted for most metastatic locations but particularly for the liver [18]. The reasons for the decline are not known, but it is likely that new detection methods, including imaging techniques, have facilitated the detection of small dormant primary tumors. Diagnostic procedures have also become better defined and a CUP nowadays is really a CUP and not just an unspecified cancer. Another suggested possibility is that the decrease is the consequence of the declining incidence trends for some underlying primary sites of CUP, such as lung cancer [19]. However, the rate of decline in CUP incidence has been so fast that this latter contribution can only be a minor factor. CUP incidence trends were analyzed by birth cohort to detect differences among diagnostic periods [17]. The overall incidence trends were replicated in each birth cohort, suggesting minor birth cohort effects. The curves were similar for both sexes, providing further evidence, in view of the opposite lung cancer trends for men and women, for the overwhelming contribution of diagnostic methods to the recent decline in incidence.

2.3.1 *Incidence in Immigrants to Sweden*

Migrant studies comparing cancer incidence among immigrants to that in the native population are of great value in identifying environmental and genetic factors in cancer etiology [20]. The classical migrant studies on Japanese immigrants to the USA and on European immigrants to Australia have provided strong arguments for the predominant environmental etiology of cancer. Immigrant studies may also provide supplementary and confirmatory data on the incidence of cancer in indigenous populations, especially in countries with no reliable cancer registration [21]. Previous immigrant studies showed that cancer incidence among immigrants tended to approach that in the native population during the process of acculturation [21].

The incidence of CUP varies worldwide, even within ethnically homogeneous populations. The underlying reasons for these differences may include both genetic and environmental effects. Alternatively, the possible influence of differences in clinical and diagnostic performance, the frequency of autopsies, or the completeness and validity of cancer registration cannot be overlooked. The only identified immigrant study on CUP was conducted in Sweden, a country of a relatively high incidence of CUP [22]. Sweden has a covering cancer registration and a publicly funded health-care system. Immigrants account for 15 % of the population. All of this mark Sweden as an excellent place for immigrant studies. The authors hypothesized that exposure to risk factors early in life could impact on the occurrence of CUP, similar to experience with other cancers [21]. As all cancers are recorded in the nationwide cancer registry, differences in registration and coding practice can be minimized. The authors used a population-based cohort design to evaluate relative risks of CUP among first-generation immigrants, with a secondary aim being to estimate CUP incidence rates in the indigenous population.

The Swedish FCD was used to identify the study population, containing information on 1110 male and 1230 female CUP cases in immigrants compared with 13,949 male and 16,558 female CUP cases in native Swedes [22]. The median age at immigration was 28 for male CUP patients, 27 for female CUP patients, and 27 and 25, respectively, for all male and female immigrants. The median age at diagnosis of CUP was 64 for male immigrants and 67 for female immigrants, compared with 70 and 71, respectively, for male and female native Swedes. The average difference between age at immigration and age at diagnosis was over three decades for both sexes. Finns constituted the largest immigrant population. Standardized incidence ratios (SIRs) for CUP among immigrants varied considerably, probably reflecting the risk in the country of origin. The overall risk was significantly decreased (SIR = 0.88), especially in females (0.82 [22]). Reduced risks were observed in immigrants from a number of countries, including Finland (SIR = 0.89), Turkey (0.53), Iraq (0.51), Iran (0.33), Asian Arab countries (0.39), India (0.41), and East Asia (0.38) (both sexes analyzed together). Significant risk reductions were also observed among female immigrants from Germany (SIR = 0.76) and Greece (0.31). Conversely, risk of CUP was significantly increased among Danish immigrants. Increased risk was additionally observed among male immigrants from the Benelux countries (SIR = 1.67) and the former Yugoslavia (1.26). The increased or decreased CUP risks observed were concluded to suggest that early life environmental risk factors or genetic factors influence the development of CUP. A further resolution of the questions about causation awaits the second generation to be old enough to allow assessment of risks. The observed differences may give clues about incidence rates in countries of origin for which incidence data are lacking.

2.4 Risk Factors

Information on etiological factors and risk factors that contribute to the pathogenesis of CUP is extremely scarce. Smoking is the only established environmental risk factor for CUP [23, 24]. The risk of smoking in the Swedish CUP patients was 1.82-fold, substantially higher for CUP with respiratory system metastases (4.90) than for CUP with liver metastases (2.03) [23]. There was also evidence that body mass index was inversely related to CUP with liver metastases which the authors speculated might be due to alcohol abuse. In the European Prospective Investigation into Cancer and Nutrition (EPIC) cohort, a total of 651 incident CUP patients were detected [24]. Risk of being diagnosed with CUP was strongly related to smoking, with a relative risk of 3.66 for current, heavy smokers (26+ cigarettes/day) compared to never smokers. The data were adjusted for alcohol consumption, body mass index, waist circumference, and level of education. For alcohol consumption and level of education, weaker associations were observed but they were no longer statistically significant after adjusting for smoking and indices of obesity. The risk of CUP was increased by approximately 30 % for subjects in the highest versus lowest quartiles of waist circumference [24].

Low socioeconomic status and tobacco smoking-correlated occupations are risk factors for CUP; medical doctors had the lowest risk according to a Nordic occupational cancer study [25]. Poverty, race, and low educational level have been reported as risk factors in the USA [12]. In Scotland, the index of multiple deprivation almost doubled the risk [4]. This index is a weighted combination of data for income, employment, health, education, and access to services. The socioeconomic gradient is likely to be confounded by smoking at least to a certain degree.

We have unpublished data showing the association of both type 1 and type 2 diabetes with CUP. Familial risk is another established risk factor, discussed below.

2.5 Familial Risk

Family history has been fundamental to the understanding of heritable components in cancer and the discovery of cancer-predisposing genes. Even though high-risk cancer syndromes are rare, they have been important for the understanding of overall genetic mechanisms of cancer. We aimed, first, to estimate the occurrence of CUP in two or more family members, which would suggest a shared etiology for concordant disease. Then, familial clustering of CUP with any cancer was studied, with the hypothesis being that discordant associations may be informative for the site of the unknown primary tumor. A high discordant familial association between CUP and, say, lung cancer would suggest that lung cancer was the unknown primary site in the CUP patient.

Data from the Swedish FCD showed that 191 offspring diagnosed with CUP had family members who were also diagnosed with CUP [2]. Since a total of 6844 offspring were diagnosed with CUP, the familial cases of CUP accounted for 2.8 % of all cases. Altogether, offspring CUP patients had 5332 parents or siblings diagnosed with any cancer. Lung cancer was diagnosed in 512 offspring whose family members were diagnosed with CUP, these cases accounting for 3.1 % of lung cancer cases in the offspring generation, the highest proportion of all cancers. For any cancer, the proportion was 2.4 %. Age at diagnosis did not differ between familial and nonfamilial cases, with the exception of nervous system cancer and leukemia, the age differences for which were explained by the inclusion of more childhood cancers in the nonfamilial group. The total number of CUP patients was 35,168.

Familial risks were analyzed in three mutually exclusive proband groups defined by family history: parent only, sibling only, and parent and sibling [2]. The last group was referred to as multiplex families as multiple individuals were affected.

As an example, a familial relative risk (SIR) of 2.00 for CUP would indicate that offspring of parents with CUP were twice as likely to be diagnosed with CUP compared to offspring whose parents were not diagnosed with CUP. Each of the proband types allowed an independent set of comparisons. When an increased SIR was seen in more than one comparison, a chance association was deemed to be unlikely. The SIR for CUP was 1.08 when only parents were diagnosed with CUP but was 1.69 when only siblings were diagnosed with CUP ($p<0.01$). With regard to discordant associations, CUP incidence was increased in families with lung cancer cases: parent only SIR = 1.22, sibling only SIR = 1.76, and parent and sibling SIR = 3.29 (all $p<0.01$). CUP incidence was also increased in families with liver cancer (SIR = 1.31 for parent only cases and 1.61 for sibling probands) and kidney cancer (SIR = 1.62 for siblings and 4.83 for multiplex families). The remaining CUP associations were found in only a single proband group: colorectal cancer in multiplex families (SIR = 1.86), when parents were diagnosed with upper aerodigestive tract (1.28) and bladder cancers (1.17), and when siblings presented with rectal (1.40) and breast (1.15) cancers. The essential results are illustrated in Fig. 2.1 by each proband type.

Analyses were also carried out in reverse order, i.e., of cancer in offspring whose family members were diagnosed with CUP [2]. For parent–offspring relationships, the analyses were completely independent of the above data. For siblings, the SIRs for colorectal (1.26) and kidney cancers (1.82) increased. The SIRs for colon (1.12),

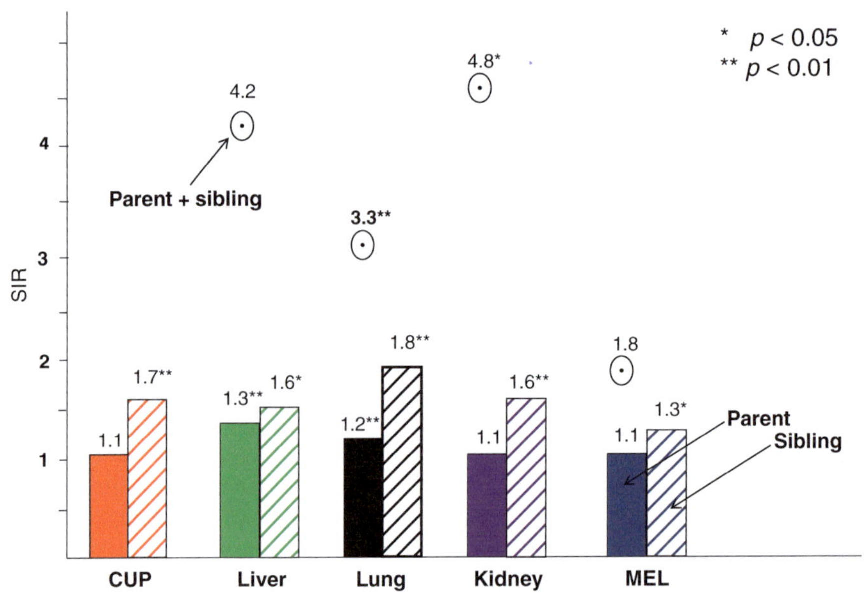

Fig. 2.1 Familial risk (*SIR*) for CUP when a parent (*left bars*), a sibling (*right bars*), or a parent and a sibling (*round symbol*) were diagnosed with the indicated cancers. The SIRs and their significances are shown on *top* of the *bars* or *symbols*. CUP patients had no affected parents + siblings (The source is Hemminki et al. [2])

pancreatic (1.26), ovarian (1.18), and prostate cancers (1.08) were significantly increased when the parents were diagnosed with CUP.

The results had several implications. In previous studies on discordant familial cancers, it has been consistently found that discordant familial risks are always lower, usually much lower, than concordant risks, implying that the genetic or environmental risk factors of familial clustering are strongest for a defined type of cancer [26]. The present results did not follow the established pattern. CUP showed no concordant familial clustering between parents and offspring, whereas many associations between CUP and discordant sites were significant between parents and offspring. A second inconsistency was that, even though the SIR for CUP among siblings was elevated to 1.69, it was lower than or equal to the associations between siblings for CUP–lung (1.76, 1.87), CUP–kidney (1.62, 1.82), and CUP–liver (1.61, 1.67) cancer pairs. A third deviation from the established pattern was that CUP was associated with high SIRs for multiplex families of colorectal (1.86), lung (3.29), and kidney cancers (4.83) in which a parent and at least one offspring were diagnosed with these cancers. Such high risks are best explained by CUP being highly related to these cancers, suggesting that the primary tumors originated from these organ sites. This reasoning should also explain the high risks among siblings in CUP–lung and CUP–kidney cancer pairs.

The familial associations suggest that the lungs, kidney, and colorectum are common but not exclusive sites of primary tumors, in line with the findings of autopsy studies [15, 27]. Interestingly, although molecular methods used in tissue-of-origin assignment studies have largely confirmed the autopsy results, they appeared to show increased frequencies for breast and bladder as sites of the primary tumors. In the present analysis, breast and bladder cancers were associated with CUP but each only in a single analysis.

Taken together, the family data have several implications. First, CUP is not a randomly occurring metastatic cancer; instead, it shows defined familial clustering. Second, familial clustering occurs between many cancer sites, the number of which may be limited by the statistical power of the present study. Third, the strong association of CUP with families of kidney, lung, and colorectal cancers suggests a marked genetic basis. Fourth, the involvement of many organ sites suggests that some mechanisms controlling defense against primary tumors and metastatic growth are shared by many cancer types. Fifth, the familial sites shared by CUP are likely to suggest sites of origin for CUP. Finally, a mechanistic exploration of CUP is a challenge, but it potentially offers rewarding insights into both host defense against primary tumors and the metastatic process in general.

2.6 Survival

The probability of survival after diagnosis of CUP was over 20 % at 12 months [17]. Survival by sex, tumor type, period of diagnosis, lymph node involvement, and age at diagnosis was explored separately. No sex difference was noted. Survival was worse in cases of adenocarcinoma and undifferentiated carcinoma compared with SCC and other histological types. Analysis of survival by period of diagnosis showed that those diagnosed in the 1960s had better survival compared to the other cohorts, which may reflect the low incidence of adenocarcinoma during the early part of the study period. Patients with nodal CUP persistently experienced a better prognosis than extranodal CUP cases: the probability of survival at 12 months in these two patient groups was around 70 % and less than 20 %, respectively. Age at diagnosis was significantly associated CUP patient mortality, with older patients showing worse survival. The recent data from Sweden and Scotland show minor improvements in survival, while the US data show none [4, 12, 28]. The Swedish data showed significant improvements for CUP with metastatic locations in the pelvis, peritoneum, and nervous system which were suggested to be due to therapeutic gains [28].

A detailed survival study of all Swedish CUP patients showed a large difference between histological types (Fig. 2.2) [11]. The survival curves for adenocarcinoma (8276 deaths) and undifferentiated carcinoma (2404 deaths) were almost superimposable, with a 12-month survival (shown by a vertical line) of 17 and 16 %, respectively. Half of the observed deaths occurred within the first 3 months after diagnosis, i.e., the median survival time was 3 months. The 12-month survival for squamous cell carcinoma (384 deaths) was 36 % and for melanoma (460 deaths), it was 51 %; the median survival times were 6 and 13 months. For CUP overall, the 12-month survival was 19 % and the median survival was 3 months.

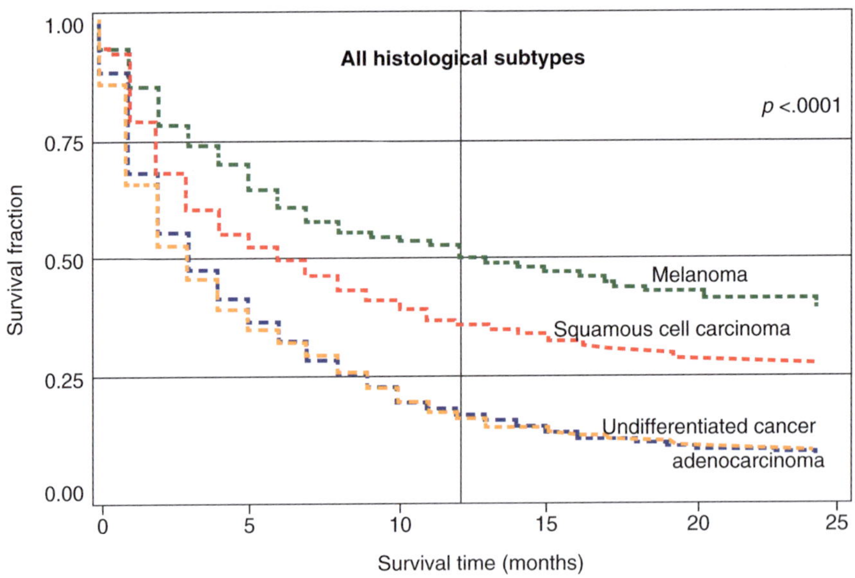

Fig. 2.2 Kaplan–Meier survival curves for CUP patients with extranodal metastasis by histology. The p-value in the *top right corner* refers heterogeneity of the survival kinetics (log-rank test) (Source Hemminki et al. [11])

In the same study, data for survival in adenocarcinoma and in undifferentiated carcinoma at extranodal sites were shown by location of metastases in the left and right panels of Fig. 2.3 [11]. Graphs for adenocarcinoma patients (left panel) show

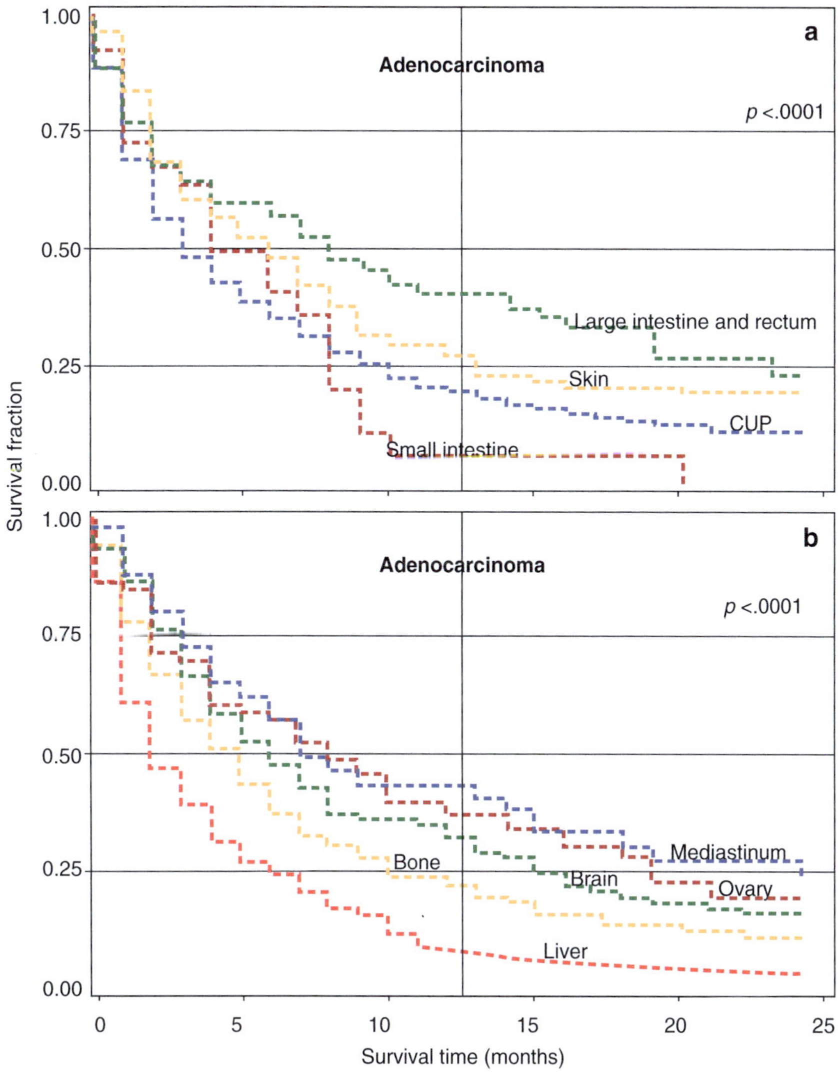

Fig. 2.3 *Panels*: (**a**, **b**) Kaplan–Meier survival curves for CUP patients with adenocarcinoma histology by metastatic location. Survival curves for cancer in the peritoneum, other digestive organ and spleen, lung, and pleura are not shown, but they are almost superimposable with unspecified CUP (shown by "CUP," i.e., no specific location given). *Panels*: (**c**, **d**) Kaplan–Meier survival curves for CUP patient with undifferentiated carcinoma by metastatic location. The *p*-value in the top right corner of each panel refers heterogeneity of the survival kinetics (log-rank test) (Source Hemminki et al. [11])

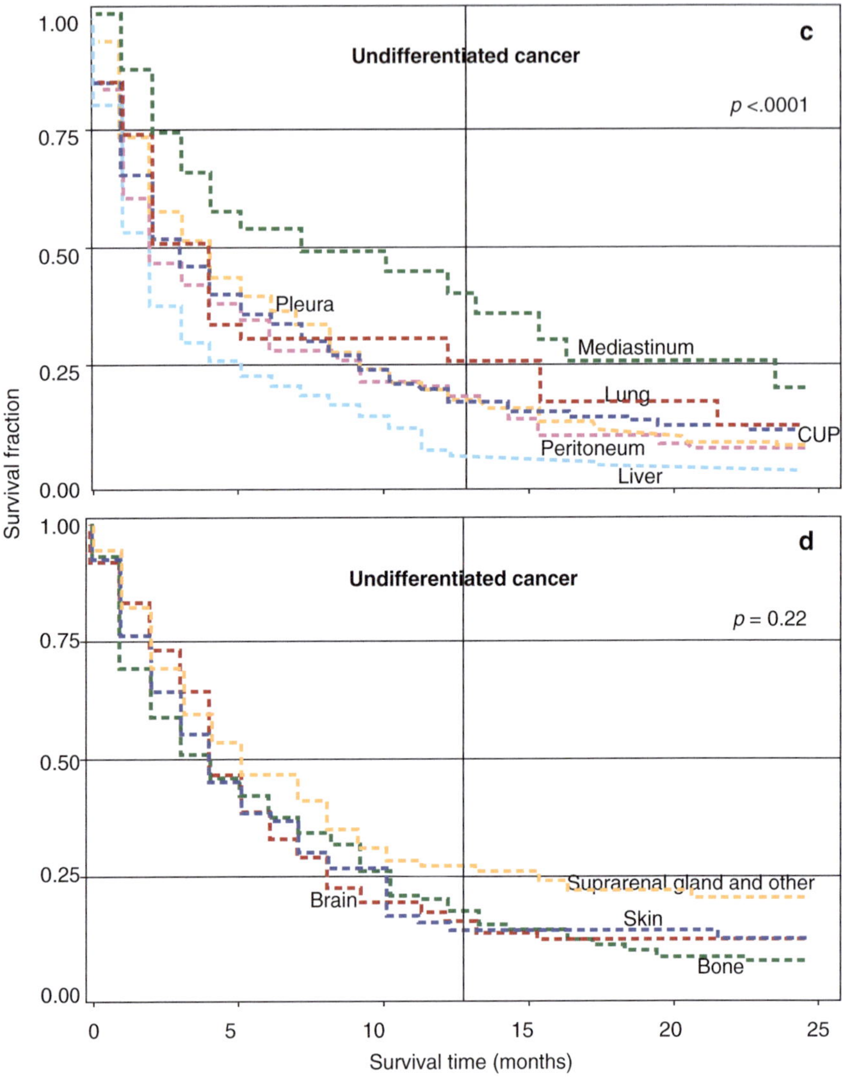

Fig. 2.3 (continued)

that the 12-month survival was lowest for patients with small intestinal (5 %) and liver (7 %) metastases. The 12-month survival for unspecified CUP (i.e., no location given) was 19 %; the survival curves for metastases in the peritoneum (12-month survival 17 %), other digestive organs and spleen (19 %), lung (20 %), and pleura (21 %) were almost superimposable with unspecified CUP and they were not shown. Bone adenocarcinoma showed also a 21 % survival fraction, skin 27 %, suprarenal gland and other sites 28 % (not shown), and brain 32 %. Patients with metastases in the ovaries (36 %), colorectum (40 %), and mediastinum (43 %) had the most favorable survival. For undifferentiated carcinoma (right panel), the survival was at least as poor as for adenocarcinoma for most metastatic locations; patients with mediastinal tumor masses survived best.

When metastases were limited to lymph nodes, the 12-month survival was 41 % and median survival was 8 months [11]. Patients affected in the head and neck, axillary, and inguinal regions had the best prognosis and those with abdominal and intrapelvic metastases the worst prognosis. The published data underline the importance of histology and location of metastasis in assisting clinical decision-making: hazard ratios differed by a factor of five among extranodal and nodal metastases [11].

As no population-based survival data were available on CUP linking the location with the cause of death, we decided to investigate the issue [29]. However, basing analysis on the cause of death may be confusing because normally, the cause of cancer-related death in cancer patients is the primary cancer. However, CUP is an exception at least in Sweden because it is the only cancer for which death certificates give the site of fatal organ metastasis, as judged by the death registrar, as the cause of death. Death certificates are of high quality in Sweden because 85 % of cancer patients die in hospitals and, for over 90 % of cancer deaths, the related hospital records have been the basis on which the death certificate was issued [5, 29].

A total of 9300 CUP patients with extranodal metastases of adenocarcinoma and undifferentiated carcinoma were identified from the Swedish Cancer Registry. Lung cancer was the most common cause of death in patients with CUP metastasis in the respiratory system, nervous system, bone, and skin, with a median survival of 3 months. Patients with peritoneal/retroperitoneal and pelvical metastasis died of ovarian cancer, with a favorable median survival of 8 months. Patients with pancreatic, liver, biliary, and colorectal cancers with liver metastasis succumbed quickly. The data showed that the location of metastases predicts site-specific cancer deaths which may point to the hidden primary tumor. The diagnostic arsenal should be used to find lung tumors when metastases are diagnosed in the respiratory or nervous system, bone, or skin; ovarian tumors should be suspected after diagnosis of pelvical metastases [29].

A similar study on site-specific cancer deaths was carried out in 1500 CUP patients diagnosed only with lymph node metastasis [30]. Among the patients with head and neck metastasis, 59 % died of lung cancer, as above defined in the death certificate. Patients with axillary metastasis died of lung and breast cancer in equal proportions. Over half of head and neck SCCs were associated with lung cancer deaths. With a few exceptions, survival in CUP patients with lymph node metastasis in site-specific cancer (e.g., lung cancer) was indistinguishable from survival in patients with metastatic primary cancer at that site (e.g., primary lung cancer). The association between lymph node metastases with cancer deaths in the draining organ and the often superimposable survival kinetics in CUP patients with primary metastatic cancers at the related site suggested that draining organs host the hidden primaries. Lung cancer was the main cause of death after lymph node metastases, and efforts should be intensified to find tumors in that organ [30].

In another study, survival kinetics of CUP was compared to primary cancers that had metastasized to the same organ where CUP metastases were found. In general, CUP patients had poorer survival than patients with known primaries [31]. The exceptions were CUP with brain and respiratory system metastases. Of CUP sites, liver metastases had the worst prognosis. Survival in CUP was comparable to that in metastatic lung cancer. These data showed large survival differences in organ-defined metastases depending on the original cancer [31]. We speculate that the aggressive behavior of CUP may be due to initial immunosuppression and immunoediting which may allow accumulation of mutations. Upon escape from the suppressed state, an unstoppable tumor spread ensues.

2.7 Risk of Subsequent Cancer

Subsequent cancer is defined as the second- or higher-order primary malignancy that occurs after the first primary cancer. The reasons for subsequent primary cancers may be the same environmental and genetic factors that predispose to the first cancer, but they additionally include treatment- and surveillance-related factors [32]. Many known cancer syndromes, including BRCA-related breast cancers, Lynch syndrome, and Li–Fraumeni syndrome, are characterized by an increased risk of multiple primary cancers. Regression or dormancy of the primary tumor, resistance to therapy, and the development of early, systemic metastases are hallmarks of CUP. Subsequent cancers could turn out to be reemerging hidden primaries of CUP. We thus hypothesized that CUP may impact on the occurrence of subsequent cancers due to its aggressive behavior and immunological disturbances.

Adenocarcinomas account for over 50 % of all CUP cases and nearly 40 % of subsequent cancers after CUP [33]. The kappa test was applied to assess the histological concordance between CUP and subsequent cancers. The overall value of kappa was 0.23, indicating that the association was not entirely random. Around 40 % of subsequent cancers were identified during the first follow-up year. Among the 32 most common cancers, significantly elevated risks were noted for 16 sites. The overall SIR was 1.69 ($p<0.01$) [33]. The highest SIRs were observed for cancers in the small intestine (7.91), followed by male genital organs (6.78), aerodigestive tract (4.75), and the thyroid gland (4.35). The observed risk increases for non-Hodgkin's lymphoma and skin SCC, two hallmarks of dysregulated immunity, support the role of suppressed immune function in the present study. This was consistent with previous reports that iatrogenic immunosuppression was a risk factor for cancer development, particularly for skin SCC and non-Hodgkin's lymphoma. Increased risk was even found in reverse analyses (CUP as the second cancer). Impaired immune function among CUP patients may predispose to virus-related cancers such as female vulvar cancer, male penile cancer, and anal cancer, all of which are highly related to human papillomavirus.

2.7.1 *Detection of Subsequent Cancers after CUP Diagnosis: Assessment of Performance of Diagnostic Tests*

As for CUP no diagnostic effort is spared to find the primary cancer, we thought of testing the success of the diagnostic work-up by analyzing cancer risk following diagnosis of CUP. The hypothesis was that with perfect diagnostic success, no second cancers would be diagnosed shortly after CUP diagnosis. The study would be informative of the efficiency of the modern diagnostic modalities in finding tumors and CUP patients would appear an optimal choice of study [34]. The standard diagnostic work-up includes, among others, computed tomography (CT) of the thorax, abdomen, and pelvis, and in selected cases mammography and endoscopic examinations [35]. CT is a key diagnostic tool which was introduced about 50 years ago and is detecting a large proportion of the found primaries [36, 37]. In Sweden, the first CT instruments were acquired in the early 1970s, and the cumulative number of instruments reached 15 by 1979, 85 by 1989, and 125 by 1999 [38]. This implies that it is important to consider the time axis and tumors generally diagnosable by CT in such a study.

A total of 28,000 CUP patients were identified in the nationwide Swedish FCD [34]. We recorded the age-standardized incidence (ASR) and the relative risk (RR) for subsequent cancers diagnosed in CUP patients in various periods from year 1980 to 2008. We focused on the first 6 months as the diagnostic work-up for CUP and a later follow-up. Among second cancers following CUP, diagnosable by CT, there was a large 6.80-fold increase in RR in follow-up 0–0.4 years from period 1980–1989 to 2000–2008. For follow-up 0.5–2.9 years, the RR was 0.60. The ASR for second cancer after CUP decreased by some 85 % from the follow-up 0–0.4 years to the subsequent follow up times. Cancers that apparently escaped detection in the work-up for CUP included kidney, colorectal, bladder, ovarian, small intestinal, endometrial, and male genital cancers. In the setting of CUP, the data suggest that modern diagnostic methods can detect many more tumors than were detected earlier but all tumors were not detected and the patients did not become completely tumor-free [34]. Essentially similar results were reached in a joint Swedish–German study on a much larger population of CUP patients [39].

2.8 Epidemiology Suggesting Hidden Primaries?

In Sect. 2.4, we implied that family history of CUP with discordant sites may suggest that the discordant site could be the hidden primary site. We continued these efforts by considering the cause of death in CUP patients because this is often coded as the cancer in the organ which the death registrar considered having killed the patient, a practice different from primary cancers. There usually is a correlation between the site of CUP metastases and cause of death or that these could be deduced from known metastatic pathways [29]. Metastases in the respiratory

Table 2.2 Familial risks in CUP with a site-specific cancer death

Site	A. Cases	RR (95 % CI)	B. Cases	RR (95 % CI)
Liver	13	**1.84** (1.15–2.94)	20	**2.07** (1.22–3.51)
Pancreas	13	**2.03** (1.23–3.34)	22	**2.07** (1.16–3.67)
Lung	96	**1.85** (1.49–2.28)	108	**2.22** (1.65–2.98)
Breast	19	**1.71** (1.06–2.75)	9	1.26 (0.71–2.23)
Ovary	17	**2.35** (1.69–3.26)	8	1.65 (0.68–3.99)
Prostate	12	**1.57** (1.06–2.33)	3	1.91 (0.70-5.22)
Kidney	3	1.18 (0.44–3.19)	5	**3.01** (1.37–6.63)
Melanoma	21	**2.28** (1.28–4.06)	17	**2.53** (1.46–4.38)

A RR for offspring cancer X when family member was diagnosed with CUP and died of cancer X. *B* RR for offspring CUP and death in cancer X when family member was diagnosed with cancer X from Hemminki et al. [11]. The 95 % CIs of bolded RRs do not overlap with 1.00

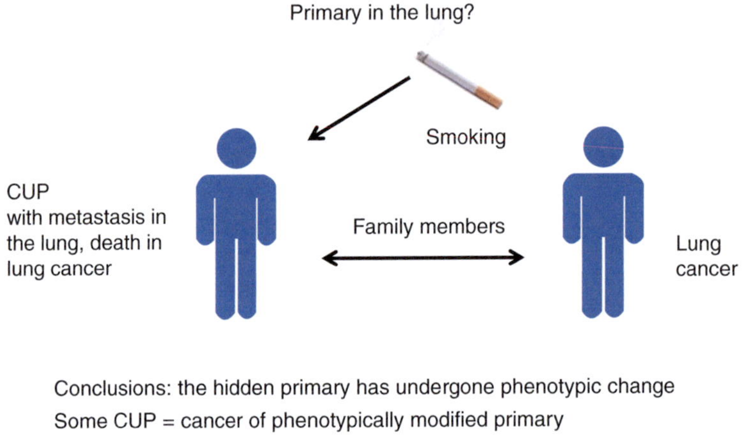

Fig. 2.4 The present favored interpretation of the results on CUP related to smoking or family history. The example is on lung cancer, but the familial parts apply to any cancer with which CUP associated. The conclusion is presented in the *bottom* of the figure (The data are derived from Hemminki et al. [5])

system resulted in death with lung cancer and those in the liver with death in liver cancer [5]. A total of 41,500 CUP patients were identified, and relative risks (RRs) were calculated for cancer X when a family member was diagnosed with CUP and died of cancer X (Table 2.2; [5]). The RR for lung cancer in offspring was 1.85 when a parent or sibling was diagnosed with CUP and died of lung cancer according to death certificates. Significant increases for familial associations were found for 7 other cancers, the highest RRs being for thyroid (8.85) and ovarian cancers (2.35), melanoma (2.28), and pancreatic cancer (2.02). Many familial associations were also significant when offspring CUP patients died of cancer X that had been diagnosed in family members. The cause of death after being diagnosed with CUP frequently matched the cancer found in a family member, suggesting that the CUP had originated in that tissue. The findings on familial risk are summarized in Fig. 2.4, together with data on the effects of smoking described in Sect. 2.3.

How could we mechanistically rationalize the above data summarized in Table 2.2? The assumed metastatic tissue had probably undergone extensive immunoediting complicating pathological tissue-of-origin assignment [40]. The immune system eradicates recognizable tumor clones and edits out immunogenic features eventually resulting in a poorly immunogenic or immunosuppressive "stealth clone" capable of rapid expansion. The editing process may have destroyed the features recognized by the immunohistochemical (IHC) arsenal used in tissue identification [41]. In addition to the immunological and apoptotic mechanisms of halting tumor growth, data have accumulated on roles of epithelial–mesenchymal transition, senescence, microenvironment, and tumor stem cells in the process of metastasis [42–46]. We speculated that some CUP cases are phenotypically modified primary cancers, rather than metastases of unknown primaries [5]. Such data provide substance to statements about CUP by some authors: "unknown primary or unknown biology" [47].

How can we reconcile the above findings in terms of modern tissue-of-origin determinations, based on gene expression profiling and IHC, which report success rates of the order of 70 % [48, 49]? The accumulating gene expression profiling and IHC data often report that primaries may reside in organs other than those biopsied for metastasis [13–15, 50, 51]. However, the large majority of these studies are probably focused on CUP populations with relatively good survival, because tissue-of-origin identification may not benefit patients with a survival prognosis of only a few months, including those with pancreatic, liver, and lung metastases [11]. Many gene expression studies thus have large numbers of patients with nodal metastasis, with relatively favorable survival times of 1 year or more [52–56]. For all CUP patients, the median survival is about 3 months in population-based studies catching all patients [10, 11]. The bottom line is that gene expression profiling and IHC techniques correctly diagnosed primary sites in about 80 % of cases when metastases of known primary sites were analyzed [57]. The performance of IHC dropped when tumors were poorly differentiated. In some tissue-of-origin studies which have included patients with metastatic liver, pancreatic, and lung cancers, the tissue identification at these sites has often failed because of assumed dedifferentiation and phenotypic changes [50, 52, 58, 59]. The conclusion from the cited literature is that many of the published tissue-of-origin identification studies have recruited CUP patients with a relatively benign disease, for which the primary tumor may reside in organ other than the one where metastases were found. In such cases, our family studies would not show familial risks.

In another study by us, data on the causes of death were used and survival in CUP was compared with metastatic cancer with a known primary tumor [60]. An organ-specific cancer was identified as a cause of death in approximately 60 % of all CUP patients. For adenocarcinoma, lung cancer was the most frequent cause of death (20 %), followed by pancreatic cancer (14 %) and ovarian cancer (11 %). Lung cancer was the most common cause of death in patients with CUP metastases diagnosed in the nervous system (69 %), respiratory system (53 %), and bone (47 %), whereas ovarian cancer was the most common cause of death when CUP was diagnosed in the pelvis (47 %) or the peritoneum (32 %). In CUP diagnosed in the liver, liver and pancreatic cancer deaths accounted for 26 and 22 %, respectively. Also in squamous cell CUP, lung cancer was the most common cause of death (45 %). The data suggested that the primary site appeared frequently to be either the organ where CUP metastases were diagnosed or an organ which may be traced through the known metastatic patterns of different cancer types [60].

2.9 Conclusions

The basic epidemiological studies by us and others have shown that the incidence of CUP is decreasing but the survival remains dismal in spite of small improvements. Evidence on risk factors has also emerged, including, with various levels of evidence, tobacco smoking, alcohol, body mass index, diabetes, and family history. The evidence appears to suggest that CUP is a heterogeneous disease. The effect of tobacco smoking is strongest on CUP with metastases in the respiratory system and alcohol may influence CUP with liver metastases. The most likely explanation is that the primary tumor resides in these organs but cannot be recognized because of phenotypic changes or that these exposures facilitate metastases in these organs through an unknown mechanism (see Fig. 2.4). The family data on incident and fatal cancers is difficult to explain by any other means but that the assumed metastases originate from primary cancers in the same organs after a phenotypic change (Fig. 2.4). The smoking and family data appear to distinguish a type of assumed CUP which is a phenotypically modified primary cancer, rather than an unknown primary [5]. These are rare examples that epidemiology is able to propose disease mechanisms which molecular pathology has not been able to resolve. If our present results turn out to be verified by tissue-of-origin determinations, the currently defined CUP would present in two forms, one truly a CUP and the other a phenotypically modified primary. What the relative proportion of the two forms is remains currently unknown.

Acknowledgments Jan Sundquist, Kristina Sundquist, Jianguang Ji, Hao Liu, Akseli Hemminki, Matias Riihimäki, Melanie Bevier, and Xiaochen Shu contributed to various stages of the reported studies.

Financial Support KH received support to these studies by Deutsche Krebshilfe and the Swedish Council for Working Life and Social Research.

References

1. Hemminki K, Ji J, Brandt A, Mousavi SM, Sundquist J. The Swedish Family-Cancer Database 2009: prospects for histology-specific and immigrant studies. Int J Cancer. 2010;126:2259–67. PubMed Epub 2009/07/31. Eng.
2. Hemminki K, Ji J, Sundquist J, Shu X. Familial risks in cancer of unknown primary: tracking the primary sites. J Clin Oncol. 2011;29:435–40.
3. Boyle P, Levin B, editors. World cancer report 2008. Lyon: IARC; 2008.

4. Brewster DH, Lang J, Bhatti LA, Thomson CS, Oien KA. Descriptive epidemiology of cancer of unknown primary site in Scotland, 1961–2010. Cancer Epidemiol. 2014;38(3):227–34. PubMed Epub 2014/04/15. Eng.
5. Hemminki K, Bevier M, Sundquist J, Hemminki A. Cancer of unknown primary (CUP): does cause of death and family history implicate hidden phenotypically changed primaries? Ann Oncol. 2012;23:2720–4. PubMed Epub 2012/04/05. Eng.
6. Vajdic C, Wyld L, Symons J. The challenge of attributing causality in cancer of unknown primary. Int J Cancer. 2013;133(5):1266–7.
7. Ji J, Sundquist K, Sundquist J, Hemminki K. Comparability of cancer identification among Death Registry, Cancer Registry and Hospital Discharge Registry. Int J Cancer. 2012;131(9):2085–93. PubMed Epub 2012/02/07. Eng.
8. Hemminki K, Riihimaki M, Sundquist K, Hemminki A. The challenges of understanding cancer of unknown primary. Int J Cancer. 2013;133(5):1268–9. PubMed Epub 2013/02/13. Eng.
9. Greco FA, Pavlidis N. Treatment for patients with unknown primary carcinoma and unfavorable prognostic factors. Semin Oncol. 2009;36:65–74. PubMed Epub 2009/01/31. Eng.
10. van de Wouw AJ, Janssen-Heijnen ML, Coebergh JW, Hillen HF. Epidemiology of unknown primary tumours; incidence and population-based survival of 1285 patients in Southeast Netherlands, 1984–1992. Eur J Cancer. 2002;38:409–13. PubMed Epub 2002/01/31. Eng.
11. Hemminki K, Bevier M, Hemminki A, Sundquist J. Survival in cancer of unknown primary site: population-based analysis by site and histology. Ann Oncol. 2012;23:1854–63.
12. Urban D, Rao A, Bressel M, Lawrence YR, Mileshkin L. Cancer of unknown primary: a population-based analysis of temporal change and socioeconomic disparities. Br J Cancer. 2013;109(5):1318–24. PubMed Pubmed Central PMCID: Pmc3778275. Epub 2013/07/19. Eng.
13. Greco FA, Oien K, Erlander M, Osborne R, Varadhachary G, Bridgewater J, et al. Cancer of unknown primary: progress in the search for improved and rapid diagnosis leading toward superior patient outcomes. Ann Oncol. 2012;23:298–304. PubMed Epub 2011/06/29. Eng.
14. Greco F, Hainsworth J. Cancer of unknown primary site. In: DeVita VJ, Hellman S, Rosenberg S, editors. Cancer: principles and practice of oncology. 9th ed. Philadelphia: Lippincott; 2011. p. 2033–51.
15. Pentheroudakis G, Greco FA, Pavlidis N. Molecular assignment of tissue of origin in cancer of unknown primary may not predict response to therapy or outcome: a systematic literature review. Cancer Treat Rev. 2009;35:221–7. PubMed Epub 2008/12/03. Eng.
16. Brustugun OT, Helland A. Rapid reduction in the incidence of cancer of unknown primary. A population-based study. Acta Oncol. 2014;53(1):134–7. PubMed Epub 2013/04/05. Eng.
17. Shu X, Sundquist K, Sundquist J, Hemminki K. Time trends in incidence, causes of death, and survival of cancer of unknown primary in Sweden. Eur J Cancer Prev. 2012;21:281–8. PubMed Epub 2011/10/05. Eng.
18. Bevier M, Sundquist J, Hemminki K. Incidence of cancer of unknown primary in Sweden: analysis by location of metastasis. Eur J Cancer Prev. 2012;21:596–601. PubMed Epub 2012/03/06. Eng.
19. Randen M, Rutqvist LE, Johansson H. Cancer patients without a known primary: incidence and survival trends in Sweden 1960–2007. Acta Oncol. 2009;48:915–20. PubMed Epub 2009/04/14.Eng.
20. Parkin DM, Iscovich J. Risk of cancer in migrants and their descendants in Israel: II. Carcinomas and germ-cell tumours. Int J Cancer. 1997;70:654–60.
21. Hemminki K, Forsti A, Khyatti M, Anwar WA, Mousavi M. Cancer in immigrants as a pointer to the causes of cancer. Eur J Public Health. 2014;24 Suppl 1:64–71. PubMed Epub 2014/08/12. Eng.
22. Shu X, Sundquist K, Sundquist J, Hemminki K. Risk of cancer of unknown primary among immigrants to Sweden. Eur J Cancer Prev. 2012;21(1):10–4. PubMed Epub 2011/11/03. Eng.
23. Hemminki K, Chen B, Melander O, Manjer J, Hallmans G, Hemminki A. Smoking and body-mass-index as risk factors for subtypes of cancer of unknown primary. Int J Cancer. 2015;136(1):246–7. PubMed Epub 2014/05/16. Eng.

24. Kaaks R, Sookthai D, Hemminki K, Krämer A, Boeing H, Wirfält E, et al. Risk factors for cancers of unknown primary site (CUP) – results from the prospective EPIC cohort. Int J Cancer. 2014;135(10):2475–81.
25. Pukkala E, Martinsen JI, Lynge E, Gunnarsdottir HK, Sparen P, Tryggvadottir L, et al. Occupation and cancer – follow-up of 15 million people in five Nordic countries. Acta Oncol. 2009;48:646–790. PubMed Epub 2009/11/21. Eng.
26. Hemminki K, Sundquist J, Brandt A. Do discordant cancers share familial susceptibility? Eur J Cancer. 2012;48:1200–7. PubMed Epub 2011/10/29. Eng.
27. Blaszyk H, Hartmann A, Bjornsson J. Cancer of unknown primary: clinicopathologic correlations. APMIS. 2003;111:1089–94. PubMed Epub 2003/12/18. Eng.
28. Riihimaki M, Hemminki A, Sundquist K, Hemminki K. Time trends in survival from cancer of unknown primary: small steps forward. Eur J Cancer. 2013;49(10):2403–10. PubMed Epub 2013/03/23. Eng.
29. Hemminki K, Riihimaki M, Sundquist K, Hemminki A. Site-specific survival rates for cancer of unknown primary according to location of metastases. Int J Cancer. 2013;133(1):182–9. PubMed Epub 2012/12/13. Eng.
30. Hemminki K, Bevier M, Sundquist J, Hemminki A. Site-specific cancer deaths in cancer of unknown primary diagnosed with lymph node metastasis may reveal hidden primaries. Int J Cancer. 2013;132:944–50. PubMed Epub 2012/06/26. Eng.
31. Riihimaki M, Thomsen H, Hemminki A, Sundquist K, Hemminki K. Comparison of survival of patients with metastases from known versus unknown primaries: survival in metastatic cancer. BMC Cancer. 2013;13:36. PubMed Pubmed Central PMCID: Pmc3565900. Epub 2013/01/30. Eng.
32. Travis LB. The epidemiology of second primary cancers. Cancer Epidemiol Biomarkers Prev. 2006;15:2020–6.
33. Shu X, Liu H, Ji J, Sundquist K, Forsti A, Sundquist J, et al. Subsequent cancers in patients diagnosed with cancer of unknown primary (CUP): etiological insights? Ann Oncol. 2012;23:269–75. PubMed Epub 2011/04/01. Eng.
34. Hemminki K, Liu H, Hemminki A, Sundquist J. Power and limits of modern cancer diagnostics: cancer of unknown primary. Ann Oncol. 2012;23:760–4. PubMed Epub 2011/08/09. Eng.
35. Pavlidis N, Briasoulis E, Pentheroudakis G. Cancers of unknown primary site: ESMO Clinical Practice Guidelines for diagnosis, treatment and follow-up. Ann Oncol. 2010;21 Suppl 5:v228–31. PubMed Epub 2010/06/29. Eng.
36. Abbruzzese JL, Abbruzzese MC, Lenzi R, Hess KR, Raber MN. Analysis of a diagnostic strategy for patients with suspected tumors of unknown origin. J Clin Oncol. 1995;13:2094–103. PubMed Epub 1995/08/01. Eng.
37. Varadhachary GR, Abbruzzese JL, Lenzi R. Diagnostic strategies for unknown primary cancer. Cancer. 2004;100:1776–85. PubMed Epub 2004/04/28. Eng.
38. Jonsson E, Banta HD. Health care technology in Sweden. Health Policy. 1994;30:257–94. PubMed Epub 1994/09/05. Eng.
39. Liu H, Hemminki K, Sundquist J, Holleczek B, Katalinic A, Emrich K, et al. Second primary cancers after cancer of unknown primary in Sweden and Germany: efficacy of the modern work-up. Eur J Cancer Prev. 2013;22(3):210–4. PubMed Epub 2012/09/11. Eng.
40. Schreiber RD, Old LJ, Smyth MJ. Cancer immunoediting: integrating immunity's roles in cancer suppression and promotion. Science. 2011;331:1565–70. PubMed Epub 2011/03/26. Eng.
41. Oien K. Pathologic evaluation of unknown primary cancer. Semin Oncol. 2009;36:8–37.
42. Bissell MJ, Labarge MA. Context, tissue plasticity, and cancer: are tumor stem cells also regulated by the microenvironment? Cancer Cell. 2005;7:17–23. PubMed Epub 2005/01/18. Eng.
43. Eccles SA, Welch DR. Metastasis: recent discoveries and novel treatment strategies. Lancet. 2007;369:1742–57. PubMed Epub 2007/05/22. Eng.
44. Udagawa T. Tumor dormancy of primary and secondary cancers. APMIS. 2008;116:615–28.
45. Collado M, Serrano M. Senescence in tumours: evidence from mice and humans. Nat Rev Cancer. 2010;10:51–7. PubMed Epub 2009/12/24. Eng.

46. Bissell MJ, Hines WC. Why don't we get more cancer? A proposed role of the microenvironment in restraining cancer progression. Nat Med. 2011;17(2011):320–9. PubMed Epub 2011/03/09. Eng.
47. Stella GM, Senetta R, Cassenti A, Ronco M, Cassoni P. Cancers of unknown primary origin: current perspectives and future therapeutic strategies. J Transl Med. 2012;10:12. PubMed Epub 2012/01/26. Eng.
48. Greco FA, Lennington WJ, Spigel DR, Hainsworth JD. Molecular profiling diagnosis in unknown primary cancer: accuracy and ability to complement standard pathology. J Natl Cancer Inst. 2013;105(11):782–90. PubMed Epub 2013/05/04. Eng.
49. Varadhachary GR, Raber MN. Cancer of unknown primary site. N Engl J Med. 2014;371(8):757–65. PubMed Epub 2014/08/21. Eng.
50. Monzon FA, Koen TJ. Diagnosis of metastatic neoplasms: molecular approaches for identification of tissue of origin. Arch Pathol Lab Med. 2010;134:216–24. PubMed Epub 2010/02/04. Eng.
51. Hainsworth JD, Rubin MS, Spigel DR, Boccia RV, Raby S, Quinn R, et al. Molecular gene expression profiling to predict the tissue of origin and direct site-specific therapy in patients with carcinoma of unknown primary site: a prospective trial of the Sarah Cannon Research Institute. J Clin Oncol. 2013;31(2):217–23. PubMed.
52. Tothill RW, Kowalczyk A, Rischin D, Bousioutas A, Haviv I, van Laar RK, et al. An expression-based site of origin diagnostic method designed for clinical application to cancer of unknown origin. Cancer Res. 2005;65:4031–40. PubMed Epub 2005/05/19. Eng.
53. Varadhachary GR, Talantov D, Raber MN, Meng C, Hess KR, Jatkoe T, et al. Molecular profiling of carcinoma of unknown primary and correlation with clinical evaluation. J Clin Oncol. 2008;26:4442–8. PubMed Epub 2008/09/20. Eng.
54. Varadhachary GR, Spector Y, Abbruzzese JL, Rosenwald S, Wang H, Aharonov R, et al. Prospective gene signature study using microRNA to identify the tissue of origin in patients with carcinoma of unknown primary. Clin Cancer Res. 2011;17:4063–70. PubMed Epub 2011/05/03. Eng.
55. Bridgewater J, van Laar R, Floore A, Van TVL. Gene expression profiling may improve diagnosis in patients with carcinoma of unknown primary. Br J Cancer. 2008;98:1425–30. PubMed Epub 2008/04/17. Eng.
56. Greco FA, Spigel DR, Yardley DA, Erlander MG, Ma XJ, Hainsworth JD. Molecular profiling in unknown primary cancer: accuracy of tissue of origin prediction. Oncologist. 2010;15:500–6. PubMed Epub 2010/04/30. Eng.
57. Handorf CR, Kulkarni A, Grenert JP, Weiss LM, Rogers WM, Kim OS, et al. A multicenter study directly comparing the diagnostic accuracy of gene expression profiling and immunohistochemistry for primary site identification in metastatic tumors. Am J Surg Pathol. 2013;37(7):1067–75. PubMed Epub 2013/05/08. Eng.
58. Horlings HM, van Laar RK, Kerst JM, Helgason HH, Wesseling J, van der Hoeven JJ, et al. Gene expression profiling to identify the histogenetic origin of metastatic adenocarcinomas of unknown primary. J Clin Oncol. 2008;26:4435–41. PubMed Epub 2008/09/20. Eng.
59. Monzon FA, Medeiros F, Lyons-Weiler M, Henner WD. Identification of tissue of origin in carcinoma of unknown primary with a microarray-based gene expression test. Diagn Pathol. 2010;5:3. PubMed Epub 2010/03/09. Eng.
60. Riihimaki M, Hemminki A, Sundquist K, Hemminki K. Causes of death in patients with extranodal cancer of unknown primary: searching for the primary site. BMC Cancer. 2014;14:439. PubMed Pubmed Central PMCID: Pmc4077560. Epub 2014/06/16. Eng.

Chapter 3
Biologic Features of CUP

Harald Löffler and Alwin Krämer

3.1 Introduction

Ideally, the biology of a given tumor entity is described by one or several genetic aberrations inducing functional changes which finally lead to the acquisition of typical hallmarks of cancer like evasion of apoptosis or independence from growth signals [1]. At first sight, this does not seem to be applicable to CUP since its naming might not be more than a convention: We call all cancers "CUP" where we cannot find a primary, which is probably due to technical limitations in most cases as, in fact, this group might comprise many biologically different types of cancers. Hence, the biology of each of these types might be defined by the hidden primary. This view would imply that a CUP originating from a given organ, e.g., the lung, is expected to display the same mutation spectrum, phenotype, prognosis, and response to a given therapy as a cancer originating from the same organ but showing an overt primary, e.g., lung cancer. Moreover, this would imply that the choice of therapy must always be dictated by the site of origin (and sometimes, of course, additionally the histological subtype, as exemplified by the differences between small cell and non-small cell lung cancer), and, therefore, every effort has to be made to find this site of origin. Last but not least, this would also imply that the only important point regarding the biology of CUP is where its origins are and how the frequencies of sites of origin are distributed in patient populations assigned to the CUP category.

However, there is a contrasting view, which is based on the fact that there is something which at least the majority of CUPs have in common, namely, the absence of a primary lesion. So what if there is a common biological mechanism responsible for this obviously unusual selective growth advantage of metastases over the primary tumor? This might be relevant since this common mechanism

H. Löffler (✉) • A. Krämer
Clinical Cooperation Unit Molecular Hematology/Oncology, German Cancer Research Center (DKFZ) and University of Heidelberg, Heidelberg, Germany
e-mail: h.loeffler@Dkfz-Heidelberg.de; a.kraemer@Dkfz-Heidelberg.de

A. Krämer, H. Löffler (eds.), *Cancer of Unknown Primary*,
DOI 10.1007/978-3-319-22581-4_3

might be of prognostic relevance and sensitive to specific therapies or might even confer resistance to the usual site-specific therapies. Such a common mechanism would define CUP as a true entity which is independent from other organ cancer entities. Pentheroudakis et al. have therefore proposed the term "primary metastatic disease" as a designation possibly better suited to describe the true nature of CUP [2].

Of course, the two views – CUP as an umbrella term for different tumor types versus CUP as a true entity with genuine features – are not completely mutually exclusive. Actually, we tend to believe that a given CUP shares some features with typical organ tumors from its site of origin, but also has some "typical CUP" features in common with other CUPs from other organs.

With this chapter, we aim to summarize the existing evidence regarding the biology of CUP. Most work on this subject is based on the hypothesis that there must be some "genuine CUP" features. On the other hand, we feel that this chapter would be incomplete without covering the current knowledge regarding common sites of origin and their identification. We will start with two sections intended to equip the reader with some background, beginning with some theoretical considerations why there might be no identifiable primary lesion, followed by an overview of methods on how to elucidate the biology of CUP. The next sections will be dedicated to the actual evidence we have, starting with work on identification of sites of origin and followed by studies dedicated to "genuine CUP" features, which we tried to group according to specific regulators, involved pathways, and affected phenotypes.

3.2 Why Is There No Primary Tumor?

The diagnosis of CUP implies the assumption that there is a primary tumor though it cannot be found. It is generally believed that this is based on a selective growth advantage of metastases (or a growth disadvantage of the primary). Before discussing mechanisms underlying this reasonable pathogenetic model, we would like to highlight some alternative explanations.

Noteworthily, a review of autopsy data revealed that in 27 % of cases, the primary remained undetected even after autopsy [3]. Hence, there may be a subset of CUP cases where a primary lesion does not exist. Several unrelated reasons may explain this phenomenon (Fig. 3.1):

- The primary tumor is present, but not recognized as being the primary because of atypical histologic features, e.g., a lung lesion with features of gastrointestinal adenocarcinoma. Quite frequently, the distinction between CUP and a defined primary is arbitrary, as, for example, in case of CK7-positive adenocarcinoma with one prominent liver lesion, which could be intrahepatic cholangiocarcinoma as well as a metastasis from a primary somewhere else within the upper gastrointestinal tract; these possibilities cannot be reliably distinguished from each other by immunohistochemistry [5]. Sometimes, rare cancer types are missed to consider. An example is adenocarcinomas presenting as solitary skin

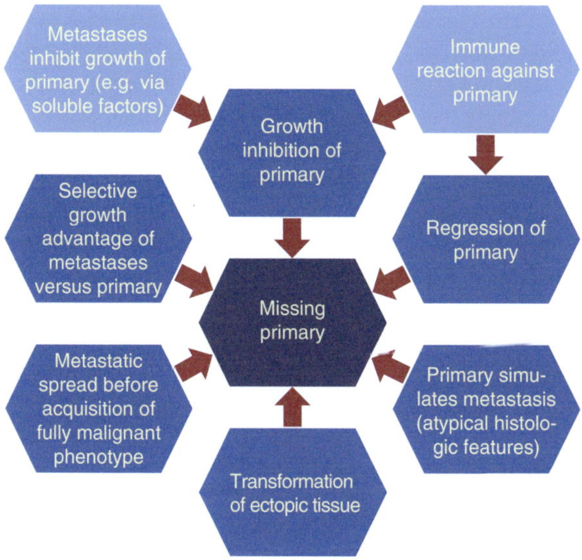

Fig. 3.1 Hypothetical explanations why there is no primary lesion detectable in CUP. See text for details (Figure adapted from Löffler et al. [4])

lesion, which are quite frequently classified as CUP but could as well be primary adnexal carcinomas of the skin [6]. In such cases, it is advisable to perform a thorough search for primary lesions located somewhere else and, whenever there is no distant primary detected, to drop the CUP diagnosis in favor of the assumption that the solitary (or leading) lesion is in fact the primary.

- A related situation is the malignant transformation of ectopic tissue which is usually not present at the site of origin. This seems to be a major underlying cause of extragonadal germ cell tumors, which are therefore classified as germ cell tumors and not as CUP if the germ cell phenotype is obvious [7]. This assumption is largely based on the fact that there are benign counterparts – teratomas – which are known to occur also at extragonadal sites [8]. If the germ cell phenotype of a malignant tumor is not obvious, a germ cell tumor might be misclassified as CUP. Hence, CUPs with midline distribution and germ cell features are to be treated as germ cell tumors, as discussed in greater detail in later chapters.
- The primary tumor has been accidentally removed before it became evident, but after having seeded metastases. For example, we have noticed that patients with CUP compatible with genitourinary tract primaries quite often present with a history of genitourinary tract surgery or related interventions such as hysterectomy or cervical conization, which sometimes had revealed suspicious findings such as in situ neoplasms. One might object that such interventions are performed very frequently in general, so in order to prove an association between CUP and preceding resections of occult primary lesions, it would be necessary to investigate this correlation in a systematic study, which has however, to our knowledge, not been performed yet.

- The primary tumor has disappeared. This may be the extreme variant of what will be discussed later on, namely, a growth inhibition of the primary lesion, which in this case not only has stopped growing but even shrinked until extinction. For example, it has been reported that testicular cancers can present as metastases with a "burned-out" primary tumor, consisting of a fibrous scar, often associated with intratubular germ cell neoplasia [9]. Some authors believe that "burned-out" primary tumors are the mechanism underlying extragonadal germ cell tumors [9], thereby providing an alternative hypothesis to the above-discussed model of malignant transformation of ectopic tissue.
- The primary lesion has spread to one or several metastatic sites before becoming malignant. This conclusion may be drawn from a study of squamous cell CUPs involving cervical lymph nodes, which used microsatellite analysis to search for the primary site [10]. In 10 of 18 patients studied, a histologically benign mucosal biopsy specimen showing a pattern of genetic alterations identical to that present in the lymph node metastases was found [10]. This is a somewhat counterintuitive finding since it indicates that a clonal population can metastasize before it acquires other features of malignancy such as invasive growth, thereby inverting the traditional model of the adenoma-carcinoma sequence placing metastatic spread at the end of tumor evolution.

Having listed these possible exceptions, we come back to the general view that most CUPs likely reflect a selective growth advantage of metastases or a growth inhibition of the primary. These two possibilities may not be exactly identical, since the former assumes that the metastases simply grow faster than the primary, which might grow slowly or not at all but is not actively inhibited, while the latter possibility might include active inhibition of the growth of the primary, which might eventually even be eradicated, as discussed above. We will discuss possible underlying mechanisms later in this chapter, but first have a look at some basic facts that may help us understand the biology of CUP.

3.3 A Short Overview of Methodology Used in Studies on CUP Biology

Here, we cannot provide a comprehensive coverage of all methods used in the context of tumor biology research. Instead, we would like to point out how research on the biology of CUP has evolved historically.

The oldest approach toward CUP biology were autopsy studies, some of which were published in the 1970s, with the oldest autopsy dating back to 1944 [3]. The same approach – to search for the primary lesion by histomorphologic examination of the putative site of origin – was later also applied to living patients, e.g., by examining resected testicles in cases with extragonadal germ cell tumors [9]. Other methods with longer tradition include cytogenetic studies, Southern blot, and fluorescence in situ hybridization [11]. Finally, the first relevant experiments using model organisms such as mice also date back to the 1970s [12].

The description of oncogenes and tumor suppressor genes in the 1970s and the clinical implementation of immunohistochemistry in the 1980s prompted the use of this method to study the tumor cell-specific expression of relevant genes since the 1990s [13]. Also starting in the 1990s, mutations of relevant genes were investigated by sequencing [14]. In the era of Sanger sequencing, this implied not only selection of genes but typically also selection of relevant exons to be examined, hence requiring educated guesses on where relevant mutations might be found.

The general limitation that not more than a few genes at a time could be examined was overcome by array-based technologies such as gene expression and array comparative genomic hybridization, enabling researchers to study large numbers or even all relevant genes concomitantly. The first studies utilizing these methods to study CUP were published shortly after 2000 [15]. During the following decade, gene expression profiling was established as a method to assign likely sites of origin to CUP specimens by comparing their gene expression profiles with the profiles of tumors of defined origin. Hence, gene expression profiling is nowadays regarded as a promising clinical tool which may be useful to guide therapeutic decisions. This will be discussed in greater detail in Chap. 11. On the other hand, these studies so far have not contributed to our understanding of CUP biology, partly because they were not designed for that purpose and partly because mRNA expression data alone are not sufficient to explain pathogenetic mechanisms.

The latest improvement of the repertoire of methods to study CUP biology is massively parallel sequencing, also referred to as next-generation sequencing, which can be applied in two variants: Either the whole genome or exome of a tumor specimen is sequenced, which requires parallel analysis of healthy tissue to distinguish tumor-specific somatic mutations from germline variants, or sequencing is restricted to a panel of relevant genes, which reduces the complexity of analysis. A pioneering study applying next-generation sequencing to CUP cases was published in 2013 [16]. Since several meeting abstracts on this topic have been published, it is safe to assume that more publications can be expected over the next few years, which will clearly scale up our knowledge about the genetic basis of CUP. It remains to be seen what this will tell us about the biology of CUP.

3.4 Sites of Origin of CUP

Once the diagnosis of CUP has been established, it is very unlikely that a primary tumor becomes evident during lifetime. According to own experience, this is the case in less than 10 % of patients – provided that the diagnosis of CUP has been based on an appropriate staging. Interestingly, we failed to find any systematic evidence (i.e., a prospective study) regarding this relationship. It seems that if the growth of a primary lesion is inhibited or has stopped, it usually does not resume growth during the course of the disease. Hence, one is left with autopsy data. A review of existing studies revealed 12 studies comprising 884 autopsies performed within the period from 1944 to 2000 [3]. The most frequently identified site of origin was the lung (20 %), followed by the pancreas (17 %). Other gastrointestinal sites were identified in 15 % of cases. Interestingly, in total a primary was identified in 73 % of cases, while it remained undetected even after autopsy in 27 % of cases (Fig. 3.2), raising some doubts about whether there is always a primary lesion, as discussed above in this chapter already. This study also included a comparison between autopsies performed before and after 1980, which did not reveal major differences, neither regarding the frequencies of specified primary sites nor with regard to the overall rate of identified versus unidentified primaries [3].

The same publication also investigated the frequency distribution of primary sites assigned by gene expression profiling and related methods, taking into account four studies with more than 500 cases published between 2001 and 2007 [3]. Surprisingly, this revealed major differences to the autopsy data (Fig. 3.2): With gene expression profiling, the breast was the most frequent primary organ (13 %), while a breast primary was a rare finding in autopsies (less than 1 %). Other frequent molecularly assigned primary sites were the pancreas (11 %), bowel (11 %), and lung (10 %), which was more similar to what was expected from the autopsy data. To further complicate matters, a large study was published in 2013 which included 252 patients where gene expression profiling was successfully performed to direct site-specific therapy [17]. Within that cohort, the most frequently assigned primary site was the biliary tract (21 %), which contradicted both the autopsy findings (liver or bile duct identified as primary sites in 6 % of cases) and the older gene expression data published between 2001 and 2007 (liver or bile duct assigned as primary site in 7 % of cases; Fig. 3.2). The second most frequent primary site according to the 2013 data was the urothelium (12 %), which was in agreement with the 2001–2007 gene

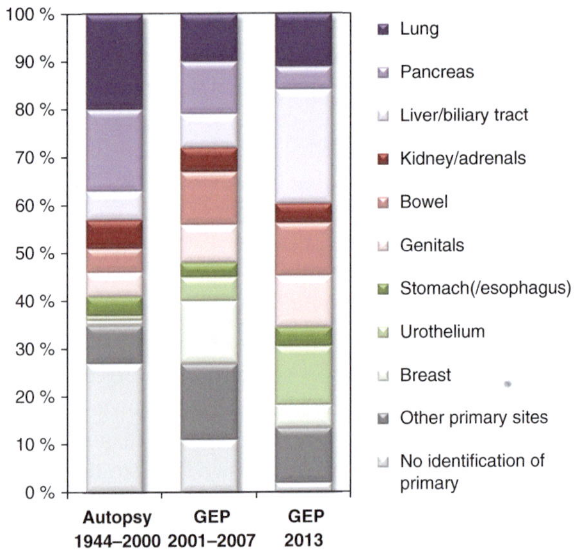

Fig. 3.2 Relative distribution of sites of origin of CUP assigned by different methods. *Left*: Pooled data from 844 autopsies performed between 1944 and 2000 [3]. *Middle*: Pooled data from gene expression profiling (GEP) of more than 500 cases from four studies published in the years 2001–2007 [3]. *Right*: GEP data of 252 patients from a study published in 2013 [17] (Figure adapted from Löffler et al. [4])

expression data (5 % bladder/ureter) but not with the autopsy findings (1 % bladder/ ureter). Other frequent primary sites in the 2013 series were the colorectum (11 %) and non-small cell lung cancer (11 %), while the pancreas accounted for only 5 % of molecularly assigned primary sites in this latest series [17].

How can these discrepancies be explained? One point that needs to be considered is that the distribution of primary sites might have changed in recent years due to changed epidemiology and due to the fact that improved diagnostic possibilities might have reduced the overall fraction of cancers classified as CUP. One might object that changes in epidemiology were not apparent in the comparison between older and newer autopsy data. Another confounder may be differences in definitions such as the fact that in the autopsy series, primary sites were defined as physical organs (e.g., liver comprising different histologies such as hepatocellular and cholangiocellular carcinoma), while gene expression profiling assigns histological types (e.g., urothelium comprising different physical sites such as bladder, ureter, renal pelvis), but a closer look at the data seems to indicate that this cannot explain all discrepancies, e.g., regarding the breast as primary site. A third confounder may be patient selection, since gene expression profiles have been mostly studied in the setting of tertiary/quaternary referral centers, as detailed in Sect. 2.2 of this book. Also taking into account this, we still doubt that all discrepancies regarding frequencies of primary sites can be readily explained. We therefore should keep in mind that gene expression-based site of origin assignment has never been verified by autopsy data. Instead, its verification was based on its ability to correctly classify tumors with known primary origin on one hand and the concordance with immunohistochemical and clinical suspicions on the other hand. With regard to the biology of CUP, an interesting alternative to explain these discrepancies would be molecular and phenotypic mimicry, i.e., tumors originating from a given organ change their phenotype (and the corresponding gene expression profile) in a way resembling the profile of another organ. This might also explain why sometimes histologic types obviously contradicting the clinical distribution pattern of metastatic spread are found. Of course, this mimicry hypothesis is speculative, but the methods described above used to verify gene expression-based assignment would be blind toward such mimicry. After all, it would be highly desirable to systematically verify molecularly assigned sites of origin in autopsied patients.

3.5 Chromosomal Aberrations, Aneuploidy, and Tumor Evolution in CUP

A classical hallmark of cancer is chromosomal instability facilitating tumor evolution [18]. Chromosomal instability leads to aneuploidy, and hence aneuploidy is often taken as an indicator of underlying chromosomal instability [19], although it has to be mentioned that aneuploidy is defined as a state (a numerical deviation from the diploid karyotype), while chromosomal instability is defined as a rate (the frequency of changes of chromosome content per cell division, often measured as variation of the number of chromosomes in a given population). Indeed, aneuploidy is found in the majority of solid cancers [19, 20]. As early as 1985, it was published that among 152 patients with metastatic adenocarcinoma of unknown primary site, 70 % showed aneuploidy detected by flow cytometric measurement of DNA content [21]. Although there were no major differences in overall survival, the authors pointed out that 18 % of patients with diploid tumors but only 9 % of patients with aneuploid tumors survived for more than 2 years [21].

A more recent study [22] combined microsatellite analysis with immunohistochemistry to compare different metastatic lesions from 14 CUP patients. In four of these cases, this was complemented by comparative genomic hybridization (CGH). The authors could not only verify a clonal relationship between multiple lesions present in each patient, but also presented evidence for clonal evolution at least in a subset of cases [22].

Several groups have characterized CUP on the chromosomal level by classical cytogenetics, CGH, or fluorescence in situ hybridization (FISH) [23, 24]. Apparently, CUP is a cytogenetically heterogeneous disease without high percentages of recurrent chromosomal aberrations. As possible application, it has been demonstrated that the cytogenetic profile is suitable to pinpoint to an organ of origin in a fraction of cases: One study published in 2003 demonstrated that 5 out of 20 patients originally classified as CUP could be reclassified by means of G-banding, CGH, and FISH, 5 of whom had lymphoma [24]. However, it should be noted that with current immunohistochemical methodology, it might be less likely that lymphomas are misclassified as CUP. Another interesting finding of this study was that a lower number of chromosomal changes (up to five versus more than five) were associated with a significantly better survival [24].

A more specific role has been established for gains of the short arm of chromosome 12, most typically as isochromosome i(12p), which is a typical aberration of testicular germ cell cancer [25]. In 1995, Motzer et al. [11] published a series of 40 CUP cases, of whom 12 (30 %) displayed an i(12p), an increased 12p copy number, or a deletion of the long arm of chromosome 12. This patient group likely suffering from germ cell tumors showed a response rate of 75 % to cisplatin-based therapy, whereas in patients without these cytogenetic findings, the response rate to cisplatin was only 18 % [11]. Similar results were published by others [26]. Hence, tumors with i(12p) or equivalent findings should be treated as germ cell tumors, and cytogenetic studies are suited for identification of such cases. We will come back to CUP with germ cell features in later chapters since this is one of the established prognostically favorable subgroups.

3.6 Genetic Aberrations in CUP Tumors

Several publications addressed genetic aberrations in CUP in the era before the advance of high-throughput technologies. This implied the directed investigation of known oncogenes and tumor suppressors, thereby aiming to reproduce the findings in larger entities such as lung or colorectal cancer. Compared to these entities, study populations of CUP patients were typically small and heterogeneous, with different publications being less well comparable to each other due to differing standards for definition of CUP. In addition, the applied methods vary from study to study, as do the proteins and genes examined, making it difficult to systematize results. In the following, we have tried to arrange the discussed publications mainly according to protein(s) and pathway(s) involved.

One of the first studies of oncogene expression in CUP samples was published in 1995 [13]. Among 26 patients, 96 % were judged positive for MYC, 92 % for RAS, and 65 % for HER-2/neu expression. This was based on immunohistochemistry staining, which impedes reliable conclusions about a true overexpression resulting from genetic changes. Hainsworth et al. [27] used the standardized DAKO score to investigate HER-2/neu expression in 94 CUP samples, among which 10 cases (11 %) showed HER-2/neu overexpression (at least 2+ according to DAKO score). Similar results were obtained in another independent investigation [28], reporting HER-2/neu overexpression in 16 out of 45 patients (36 %). It may be concluded that HER-2/neu is overexpressed in a substantial minority of CUP cases.

Massard et al. reported expression of EGF receptor (EGFR), which is important as a therapeutic target, in 66 % among 54 cases, while the proportion of c-KIT expression and HER-2/neu overexpression were 10 % and 4 % in this study, respectively [29]. Furthermore, the authors reported that EGFR expression was significantly correlated with response to cisplatin-based chemotherapy [29]. Dova et al. investigated 50 CUP cases and found EGFR expression in 74 % and strong expression in 12 % of cases [30]. From a clinical perspective, a more relevant finding would be activating EGFR mutations at the genetic level since they are regarded as predictor for response to anti-EGFR therapy, while immunohistochemical detection of EGFR expression is a poor predictor regarding this, although the absence of mutations does not preclude response to drugs targeting EGFR [31]. In this regard, the mentioned study by Dova et al. included genetic analyses of EGFR, but disappointingly, activating EGFR mutations were not found [30]. Another publication, which will be discussed in detail further below [32], reported EGFR positivity in 15 out of 69 cases (22 %). In conclusion, it seems that methodological differences impede comparisons between these studies and preclude any firm conclusions.

Another group of therapeutic targets are type III receptor tyrosine kinases including c-KIT (CD117) and the platelet-derived growth factor receptors PDGFRα and PDGFRβ, which can be targeted by imatinib and some of its derivatives [33]. As already mentioned, the percentage of cases positive for c-KIT reported by Massard et al. was only 10 % [29]. Dova and coworkers found c-KIT expression by immunohistochemistry in 30 out of 37 CUP specimens (81 %), 5 of which (13 %) exhibited strong positivity [34]. PDGFRα was positive in 15 (50 %) and strongly positive in 1 (3 %) out of 30 cases in this analysis [34]. As with EGFR, screening for mutations within exon 11 of c-KIT and exons 12 and 18 of PDGFRα did not reveal any mutations [34]. Even less data exist regarding PDGFRβ, which was positive in 17 out of 69 cases (25 %) in one study [32]. We conclude that data regarding type III receptor tyrosine kinases in CUP are sparse. Nevertheless, it might be assumed that these kinases do not play a major role in this disease.

More than 50 % of human cancers carry mutations in the TP53 gene, which is therefore regarded as the most important tumor suppressor [35]. Regarding its role in CUP, an early study was published in 1993, which comprised a screening for

TP53 mutations within the exons 5–9 (which are most frequently affected by TP53 mutations) in a small series of 15 CUP biopsy specimens and eight cell lines established from CUP samples [14]. With this approach, TP53 mutations were detected in 26 % of cases, a proportion lower than usually found in other solid tumors. In contrast, a later study of 47 CUP cases using immunohistochemistry revealed expression of TP53 and BCL-2 in 70 % and 65 % and overexpression of these proteins in 53 % and 40 % of tumors, respectively [36]. Since TP53 overexpression correlates well with p53 mutation, these data suggest a frequency of mutant TP53 in the magnitude of 50 %, which would be closer to the percentages reported for other cancers. This finding was independently confirmed by van de Wouw et al. [28], who reported TP53 overexpression by immunohistochemistry in 23 out of 48 cases (48 %). Puzzlingly, others [32] reported TP53 positivity only in 13 out of 69 specimens (19 %). Another surprising finding relates to the CUP subgroup located to head and neck lymph nodes: Although TP53 mutations are a frequent finding in other head and neck carcinomas, sequencing of exons 4–9 of TP53 in 23 specimens from head and neck lymph node CUP cases revealed no mutations at all [37]. Together, the small sample sizes and methodological differences of the above studies again make it difficult to draw firm conclusions also on the TP53 mutation frequency in CUP.

The publications cited up to now mainly relied on immunohistochemistry, and if molecular analyses were included, they were restricted to selected exons. In contrast, the advent of next-generation sequencing has enabled researchers to speed up the investigation of tumor-associated mutations by several orders of magnitude with the additional advantage that the findings are less dependent on or biased by educated guessing. Not unexpectedly, it took some years from the introduction of this methodological advance until the first results with CUP samples were published. Not until last year, Tothill et al. [16] examined tumors from 16 CUP cases by sequencing a large panel of 701 genes, which was supplemented by an array-based profiling of copy-number alterations. Twelve cases displayed mutations, deletions, or amplifications of genes for which targeted treatment approaches are available, including mutations of KRAS, PIK3CA, AKT1, and IDH1 and a homozygous deletion of BRCA1 [16]. The authors claimed that in five of these cases, there was strong clinical evidence supporting the efficacy of a drug based on the tumor genotype [16]. In addition, they argued that comparison of the mutation spectra of CUP cases with published mutation frequencies from different solid tumor entities – which they combined with clinical and immunohistochemical clues and the results of gene expression profiling – was useful for assignment of a likely site of origin [16]. With regard to pathogenetic mechanisms, it was stated that the majority of actionable mutations and copy-number alterations were identified in core mitogenic and cell growth pathways [16], but this may be biased by the fact that most of the available targeted drugs are designed to target these pathways.

A recently published larger study investigated 200 CUP specimens (125 adenocarcinomas, 75 non-adenocarcinomas) by targeted sequencing of 255 genes, thereby recording base substitutions, short insertions and deletions (indels), amplifications, homozygous deletions, and rearrangements [38]. On average, 4.2 genomic alterations were identified per case, which affected 121 genes in total. The most commonly affected gene was TP53, which was altered in 55 % of cases of both adenocarcinomas and non-adenocarcinomas. More common alterations classified as actionable by the authors involved KRAS (25 % of adenocarcinomas, 12 % of non-adenocarcinomas), CDKN2A (19 % of adenocarcinomas and non-adenocarcinomas), MCL1 (10 % of adenocarcinomas, 8 % of non-adenocarcinomas), PTEN (8 % of adenocarcinomas and non-adenocarcinomas), PIK3CA (8 % of adenocarcinomas, 9 % of non-adenocarcinomas), BRAF (6 % of adenocarcinomas, 4 % of non-adenocarcinomas), NF1 (5 % of adenocarcinomas, 3 % of non-adenocarcinomas), ERBB2/HER-2/neu (10 % of adenocarcinomas), and EGFR (8 % of adenocarcinomas) [38]. In conclusion, also these very recent data based on next-generation sequencing did not reveal genes or pathways specifically or preferentially altered in CUP. Instead, these data are compatible with the notion that there is no difference between cancers with hidden versus overt primary lesion, and hence the mutational landscape of CUP simply reflects the distribution of sites of origin.

Some more data on expression levels and mutations in additional proteins and genes can be found in the above-cited studies and references therein – and have been excellently reviewed by others [39] – but are not further discussed here. We will come back to some of these data in the next section when highlighting possible mechanisms of overwhelming metastatic spread but will otherwise not discuss these findings as they, mostly due to small sample numbers, do not contribute to our understanding of the biology of CUP.

3.7 The Pathogenesis of Overwhelming Metastatic Spread

Finally, we come back to the question why in CUP, in contrast to other solid cancers, metastases grow faster than the primary tumor (keeping in mind that there might be alternative explanations why there is no primary in a portion of cases, see Sect. 3.2 of this chapter and Fig. 3.1). Back in 1974, Yuhas and Pazmino [12] subcutaneously injected cells from a lung cancer cell line into BALB/c mice, which induced tumor formation at the injection site. When the same cell line was injected intravenously in parallel, this not only led to development of lung metastases but also slowed down the growth of tumor cells at the subcutaneous site [12]. It was therefore proposed that metastases are capable to inhibit growth of the primary tumor through elusive soluble factors. Today, it is known that tumors acquire genetic changes in a process of branched evolution, and hence metastases are genetically different from the primary lesion [40]. With regard to the genesis of CUP, the relative growth advantages of metastases might therefore be based on specific genetic alterations acquired by the metastatic subclone. Other explanations include the role of the nonmalignant microenvironment, which might inhibit the growth at the primary but not at metastatic sites, and immunological mechanisms specifically targeting the primary lesion, thereby not only slowing down its growth but sometimes possibly even completely eliminating the primary tumor. The latter hypothesis is supported by the observation that in some cases of extragonadal germ cell tumors, "burned-out" primary testicular cancers were described, which were histologically characterized by fibrous scars consistent with tumor regression at the site of origin [9]. Since other investigations have found evidence that regression of germ cell tumors is associated with interstitial inflammatory infiltration [41], it may be speculated that immune reactions against the primary are a more general phenomenon in CUP evolution.

Another study focused on head and neck squamous cell carcinomas of unknown origin [10]. In 18 cases, microsatellite analyses were performed in both cervical lymph node metastases and histologically benign mucosal biopsy specimens obtained during staging. In ten cases, mucosal specimens were found that were genetically identical to the cancer specimens, indicating that the respective mucosal regions were the likely origin of the cervical lymph node metastases [10]. It must be pointed out that these mucosal lesions of origin, although histologically benign, harbored clonal genetic alterations. This observation supports a model where, in rare instances, clonal populations may spread to metastatic sites while persisting in an otherwise nonmalignant stage. This would imply that the "classical" adenoma-carcinoma sequence where metastatic spread stands at the end of an evolutionary process involving formation of a benign clone and subsequent invasive growth may be inverted, putting metastatic spread to an earlier stage in tumor evolution and invasive growth to a later time point when clonal cells have already colonized the metastatic site, although it remains unclear how metastatic spread should occur without preceding invasion into lymphatic and blood vessels.

Up to now, we have dealt with models focused on growth inhibition of the primary lesion. Alternatively, CUP might simply be characterized by an unusually aggressive course of metastatic spread. Support for this hypothesis came from a study comparing the gene expression profiles of primary tumors and metastases [42]. This led to definition of a "metastasis signature" that was characteristic for metastatic cancers. Interestingly, a subset of primary tumors resembled metastatic tumors with respect to this gene expression signature. Analysis of a larger set of cancer cases revealed that this "metastasis signature" was associated with an increased probability for metastasis formation and a poor outcome. The authors concluded that a molecular program of metastasis that is shared by multiple solid tumor types may exist [42]. In case of CUP, this "metastasis program" may be hyperactive. Beyond that, one might speculate that somatic mutations in specific genes activate this program. Stella et al. [43] reasoned that mutations of the MET oncogene, which have been causally linked to invasive growth, might sustain premature occult dissemination of cancer cells. Sequencing of MET in 47 early metastatic cancers, which were classified as either cases where immunohistochemistry suggests a clear working hypothesis regarding the site of origin (most often the lung; 24 patients overall) or "true CUPs" lacking any working hypothesis (23 patients), revealed MET mutations in seven samples, which all belonged to the "true CUP" category, corresponding to a percentage of 30 % MET mutations within this category, whereas the usual percentage of MET mutations in cancer is about 3 % [43]. Another publication [44], however, reported MET mutations in only 6 out of

87 CUP samples (6.7 %). Hence, more data from larger numbers of cases are needed to follow up on this interesting hypothesis, which should also be tested in model systems.

A different approach considers angiogenesis, one of the hallmarks of cancer [1]: Usually, a malignant tumor is able to support the formation of blood vessels, which conversely constitute a prerequisite for the growth of a lesion beyond a certain size. Naresh [45] hypothesized that CUP reflects an angiogenic incompetence of the tumor at the primary site, with the result that its growth is not supported by sufficient blood supply. This angiogenic incompetence may be overcome at metastatic sites either because the specific environment supports growth of tumor clones without angiogenesis or because of additional genetic alterations occurring after metastatic spread [45]. Support for this hypothesis came from mouse models showing that non-angiogenic tumor cell lines produce only dormant cancers when injected into mice, while their spontaneous switch toward faster-growing cancers is associated with activation of angiogenesis, as demonstrated by gene expression profiling and examination of specific regulators both on the mRNA and protein level [46–48]. An immunohistochemical evaluation of 81 CUP specimens for expression of angiogenesis markers concluded that, based on high-level expression of VEGF in 83 % of cases and the widespread staining for CD34 as an endothelial marker in all specimens, angiogenesis is very prominent in CUP [49]. Moreover, tumor microvessel density was higher in tumors classified as unfavorable compared to more favorable subgroups [49]. In sharp contrast, a team including Naresh, who originally had formulated the hypothesis of angiogenic incompetence, published a comparison of squamous cell carcinomas of the head and neck with either known or unknown primary [50]. By assessing VEGF expression using immunohistochemistry, immunoblotting, and RT-RCR, they showed that both the protein and mRNA levels of VEGF were lower in the cases with unknown primary when compared to those with known primary, claiming that this lower activity of angiogenesis in the CUP samples experimentally confirms their hypothesis of angiogenic incompetence even at the stage of metastatic disease [50]. From a clinical perspective, however, the fact that bevacizumab, an antibody to VEGF which inhibits angiogenesis, shows promising activity in CUP [51, 52] seems to argue against widespread angiogenic incompetence in CUP tumors. It may be objected, however, that since the clinical trials involving bevacizumab were phase II trials without control group and bevacizumab was administered in combination with other drugs, conclusions on the therapeutic efficacy of bevacizumab are not warranted. Therefore, the role of angiogenesis in CUP remains largely elusive.

Tumor invasion and metastasis depend on the ability of tumor cells to degrade the surrounding extracellular matrix [53]. Important enzymes catalyzing this degradation include matrix metalloproteinases (MMPs), while in the same context, the role of tissue inhibitors of matrix metalloproteinases (TIMPs) seems to be more complex and elusive [53]. Prompted by the hypothesis that this machinery is upregulated in CUP, immunohistochemical evaluation of 75 CUP specimens revealed expression of MMP-2, MMP-9, and TIMP-1 in 69 %, 49 %, and 79 % of cases, with strong expression in 49 %, 36 %, and 44 %, respectively [53]. In addition, high-level expression of TIMP-1 significantly correlated with a shorter survival [53]. The authors conclude that the widespread expression of these proteins in CUP indicates an essential role of proteolysis in these tumors [53], although it has to be mentioned that these data are purely descriptive and do not offer any mechanistic insights.

Another process contributing to metastatic spread is epithelial-mesenchymal transition (EMT), a complex program by which cells lose their epithelial differentiation (cell-cell adhesion, polarity, and lack of motility) and acquire mesenchymal features (motility, invasiveness, and increased resistance to apoptosis) instead [54]. Stoyianni and coworkers investigated EMT in 99 CUP specimens by immunohistochemistry, defining an EMT phenotype as low-level protein expression of E-cadherin, expression of N-cadherin or vimentin, and concomitant expression of SNAIL [54]. An EMT phenotype was observed in 8 cases (8.1 %) and was significantly ($p=0.023$) associated with poor overall survival, which was 8 months when this phenotype was present versus 13 months in cases not displaying EMT [54]. Other significant correlations with EMT included high histological grade and presence of visceral metastases [54]. Furthermore, the authors noted associations between high-level expression of SNAIL and NOTCH2, and between vimentin and NOTCH3 expression [54], which may hint at a possible causal role of NOTCH2/3 activation for EMT induction. The same group, probably using the same case collection, published that NOTCH2 was expressed in 56 % and NOTCH3 in 73 % of CUP cases, respectively [55], which does not support a strict causal link between NOTCH signaling – which seems to be, in analogy with other malignancies [56], frequently activated in CUP – and the EMT phenotype, since the latter seems to be an infrequent phenomenon in CUP. Another hypothesis examined by this group is that a stem cell phenotype may contribute to rapid dissemination in CUP. These data are unpublished but mentioned in a review, where the authors state that as judged by expression of CD133 and OCT4, they failed to find any stem cell phenotype [39]. Together, it must be assumed that neither EMT nor acquisition of stem cell properties seems to play a major role in the pathogenesis of overwhelming metastatic spread in CUP.

3.8 Conclusions and Perspectives

It is time to come back to the question whether there are pathophysiological mechanisms common to all or at least a large proportion of CUPs. To us, the fact that there are many different hypotheses and no unifying theory only allows the conclusion that common biological mechanisms still remain largely elusive. Also, the diverse reasons why there might be no identifiable primary lesion and the indisputable heterogeneity of CUP in terms of histological types and sites of origin do not support the view that all CUPs share a common set of biological features. Still, some common features may exist. Accordingly, two groups of CUPs may be discriminated from each other: The first group may include cases closely related to typical organ counterparts with known primary, including some of the well-defined, prognostically favorable CUP subgroups (see Chaps. 4 and 10). The second group may be the "genuine CUP" category, comprising cases sharing more features with other "genuine" CUP cases than with typical organ cancers of the same origin. The most promising candidate for this "genuine CUP" entity seems to be CK7-positive, poorly differentiated adenocarcinomas, which, in line with data published by others [57–60], account for roughly half of our own CUP cases. Probably, most of the up-to-now fragmentary knowledge regarding the biology of CUP applies to this large group, and it might be worthwhile to restrict studies on CUP biology to this "genuine CUP" category, although it might prove difficult to find an exact definition for this group to clearly demarcate it from the rest of CUPs.

References

1. Hanahan D, Weinberg RA. The hallmarks of cancer. Cell. 2000;100(1):57–70. PubMed.
2. Pentheroudakis G, Briasoulis E, Pavlidis N. Cancer of unknown primary site: missing primary or missing biology? Oncologist. 2007;12(4):418–25. PubMed.
3. Pentheroudakis G, Golfinopoulos V, Pavlidis N. Switching benchmarks in cancer of unknown primary: from autopsy to microarray. Eur J Cancer. 2007;43(14):2026–36. PubMed.
4. Löffler H, Neben K, Krämer A. Cancer of unknown primary: epidemiology and pathogenesis. Radiologe. 2014;54(2):107–11. PubMed CUP-Syndrom : Epidemiologie und Pathogenese.
5. Sempoux C, Jibara G, Ward SC, Fan C, Qin L, Roayaie S, et al. Intrahepatic cholangiocarcinoma: new insights in pathology. Semin Liver Dis. 2011;31(1):49–60. PubMed.
6. Wick MR, Goellner JR, Wolfe 3rd JT, Su WP. Adnexal carcinomas of the skin. I. Eccrine carcinomas. Cancer. 1985;56(5):1147–62. PubMed.
7. Schmoll HJ. Extragonadal germ cell tumors. Ann Oncol. 2002;13 Suppl 4:265–72. PubMed.
8. Gatcombe HG, Assikis V, Kooby D, Johnstone PA. Primary retroperitoneal teratomas: a review of the literature. J Surg Oncol. 2004;86(2):107–13. PubMed.
9. Fabre E, Jira H, Izard V, Ferlicot S, Hammoudi Y, Theodore C, et al. 'Burned-out' primary testicular cancer. BJU Int. 2004;94(1):74–8. PubMed.
10. Califano J, Westra WH, Koch W, Meininger G, Reed A, Yip L, et al. Unknown primary head and neck squamous cell carcinoma: molecular identification of the site of origin. J Natl Cancer Inst. 1999;91(7):599–604. PubMed.
11. Motzer RJ, Rodriguez E, Reuter VE, Bosl GJ, Mazumdar M, Chaganti RS. Molecular and cytogenetic studies in the diagnosis of patients with poorly differentiated carcinomas of unknown primary site. J Clin Oncol. 1995;13(1):274–82. PubMed.
12. Yuhas JM, Pazmino NH. Inhibition of subcutaneously growing line 1 carcinomas due to metastatic spread. Cancer Res. 1974;34(8):2005–10. PubMed.
13. Pavlidis N, Briassoulis E, Bai M, Fountzilas G, Agnantis N. Overexpression of C-myc, Ras and C-erbB-2 oncoproteins in carcinoma of unknown primary origin. Anticancer Res. 1995;15(6B):2563–7. PubMed.
14. Bar-Eli M, Abbruzzese JL, Lee-Jackson D, Frost P. p53 gene mutation spectrum in human unknown primary tumors. Anticancer Res. 1993;13(5A):1619–23. PubMed.
15. Su AI, Welsh JB, Sapinoso LM, Kern SG, Dimitrov P, Lapp H, et al. Molecular classification of human carcinomas by use of gene expression signatures. Cancer Res. 2001;61(20):7388–93. PubMed.
16. Tothill RW, Li J, Mileshkin L, Doig K, Siganakis T, Cowin P, et al. Massively-parallel sequencing assists the diagnosis and guided treatment of cancers of unknown primary. J Pathol. 2013;4. PubMed.
17. Hainsworth JD, Rubin MS, Spigel DR, Boccia RV, Raby S, Quinn R, et al. Molecular gene expression profiling to predict the tissue of origin and direct site-specific therapy in patients

with carcinoma of unknown primary site: a prospective trial of the Sarah Cannon research institute. J Clin Oncol. 2013;31(2):217–23. PubMed.
18. Lengauer C, Kinzler KW, Vogelstein B. Genetic instabilities in human cancers. Nature. 1998;396(6712):643–9. PubMed.
19. Rajagopalan H, Lengauer C. Aneuploidy and cancer. Nature. 2004;432(7015):338–41. PubMed.
20. Mitelman F. Catalog of chromosome aberrations in cancer. 6th ed. New York: Wiley; 1998.
21. Hedley DW, Leary JA, Kirsten F. Metastatic adenocarcinoma of unknown primary site: abnormalities of cellular DNA content and survival. Eur J Cancer Clin Oncol. 1985;21(2):185–9. PubMed.
22. Speel EJ, van de Wouw AJ, Claessen SM, Haesevoets A, Hopman AH, van der Wurff AA, et al. Molecular evidence for a clonal relationship between multiple lesions in patients with unknown primary adenocarcinoma. Int J Cancer. 2008;123(6):1292–300. PubMed.
23. Abbruzzese JL, Lenzi R, Raber MN, Pathak S, Frost P. The biology of unknown primary tumors. Semin Oncol. 1993;20(3):238–43. PubMed.
24. Pantou D, Tsarouha H, Papadopoulou A, Mahaira L, Kyriazoglou I, Apostolikas N, et al. Cytogenetic profile of unknown primary tumors: clues for their pathogenesis and clinical management. Neoplasia. 2003;5(1):23–31. PubMed.
25. Horwich A, Shipley J, Huddart R. Testicular germ-cell cancer. Lancet. 2006;367(9512):754–65. PubMed.
26. Summersgill B, Goker H, Osin P, Huddart R, Horwich A, Fisher C, et al. Establishing germ cell origin of undifferentiated tumors by identifying gain of 12p material using comparative genomic hybridization analysis of paraffin-embedded samples. Diagn Mol Pathol. 1998;7(5):260–6. PubMed.
27. Hainsworth JD, Lennington WJ, Greco FA. Overexpression of Her-2 in patients with poorly differentiated carcinoma or poorly differentiated adenocarcinoma of unknown primary site. J Clin Oncol. 2000;18(3):632–5. PubMed.
28. van de Wouw AJ, Jansen RL, Griffioen AW, Hillen HF. Clinical and immunohistochemical analysis of patients with unknown primary tumour. A search for prognostic factors in UPT. Anticancer Res. 2004;24(1):297–301. PubMed.
29. Massard C, Voigt JJ, Laplanche A, Culine S, Lortholary A, Bugat R, et al. Carcinoma of an unknown primary: are EGF receptor, Her-2/neu, and c-Kit tyrosine kinases potential targets for therapy? Br J Cancer. 2007;97(7):857–61. PubMed.
30. Dova L, Pentheroudakis G, Georgiou I, Malamou-Mitsi V, Vartholomatos G, Fountzilas G, et al. Global profiling of EGFR gene mutation, amplification, regulation and tissue protein expression in unknown primary carcinomas: to target or not to target? Clin Exp Metastasis. 2007;24(2):79–86. PubMed.
31. Sholl LM, Xiao Y, Joshi V, Yeap BY, Cioffredi LA, Jackman DM, et al. EGFR mutation is a better predictor of response to tyrosine kinase inhibitors in non-small cell lung carcinoma than FISH, CISH, and immunohistochemistry. Am J Clin Pathol. 2010;133(6):922–34. PubMed Central PMCID: 3156055.
32. Koo JS, Kim H. Hypoxia-related protein expression and its clinicopathologic implication in carcinoma of unknown primary. Tumour Biol. 2011;32(5):893–904. PubMed.
33. Pardanani A, Tefferi A. Imatinib targets other than bcr/abl and their clinical relevance in myeloid disorders. Blood. 2004;104(7):1931–9. PubMed.
34. Dova L, Pentheroudakis G, Golfinopoulos V, Malamou-Mitsi V, Georgiou I, Vartholomatos G, et al. Targeting c-KIT, PDGFR in cancer of unknown primary: a screening study for molecular markers of benefit. J Cancer Res Clin Oncol. 2008;134(6):697–704. PubMed.
35. Leroy B, Anderson M, Soussi T. TP53 mutations in human cancer: database reassessment and prospects for the next decade. Hum Mutat. 2014;35(6):672–88. PubMed.
36. Briasoulis E, Tsokos M, Fountzilas G, Bafaloukos D, Kosmidis P, Samantas E, et al. Bcl2 and p53 protein expression in metastatic carcinoma of unknown primary origin: biological and clinical implications. A Hellenic Co-operative Oncology Group study. Anticancer Res. 1998;18(3B):1907–14. PubMed.

37. Gottschlich S, Schuhmacher O, Gorogh T, Hoffmann M, Maune S. Analysis of the p53 gene status of lymph node metastasis in the head and neck region in occult primary cancer. Laryngorhinootologie. 2000;79(7):434–7. PubMed PMID: 11005098. Analyse des p53-Gen-Status von Lymphknotenmetastasen im Kopf-Hals-Bereich bei okkultem Primärtumor.
38. Ross JS, Wang K, Gay L, Otto GA, White E, Iwanik K, et al. Comprehensive genomic profiling of carcinoma of unknown primary site: new routes to targeted therapies. JAMA Oncol. 2015 [Epub 12 Feb 2015].
39. Kamposioras K, Pentheroudakis G, Pavlidis N. Exploring the biology of cancer of unknown primary: breakthroughs and drawbacks. Eur J Clin Invest. 2013;43(5):491–500. PubMed.
40. Gerlinger M, Rowan AJ, Horswell S, Larkin J, Endesfelder D, Gronroos E, et al. Intratumor heterogeneity and branched evolution revealed by multiregion sequencing. N Engl J Med. 2012;366(10):883–92. PubMed Epub 2012/03/09. eng.
41. Schütte B, Holstein AF, Schirren C. Macrophages lysing seminoma cells in patients with carcinoma-in-situ (CIS) of the testis. Andrologia. 1988;20(4):295–303. PubMed.
42. Ramaswamy S, Ross KN, Lander ES, Golub TR. A molecular signature of metastasis in primary solid tumors. Nat Genet. 2003;33(1):49–54. PubMed.
43. Stella GM, Benvenuti S, Gramaglia D, Scarpa A, Tomezzoli A, Cassoni P, et al. MET mutations in cancers of unknown primary origin (CUPs). Hum Mutat. 2011;32(1):44–50. PubMed.
44. Pentheroudakis G, Kotteas EA, Kotoula V, Papadopoulou K, Charalambous E, Cervantes A, et al. Mutational profiling of the RAS, PI3K, MET and b-catenin pathways in cancer of unknown primary: a retrospective study of the Hellenic Cooperative Oncology Group. Clin Exp Metastasis. 2014;5. PubMed.
45. Naresh KN. Do metastatic tumours from an unknown primary reflect angiogenic incompetence of the tumour at the primary site?--a hypothesis. Med Hypotheses. 2002;59(3):357–60. PubMed.
46. Almog N, Henke V, Flores L, Hlatky L, Kung AL, Wright RD, et al. Prolonged dormancy of human liposarcoma is associated with impaired tumor angiogenesis. FASEB J. 2006;20(7):947–9. PubMed.
47. Almog N, Ma L, Raychowdhury R, Schwager C, Erber R, Short S, et al. Transcriptional switch of dormant tumors to fast-growing angiogenic phenotype. Cancer Res. 2009;69(3):836–44. PubMed.
48. Naumov GN, Bender E, Zurakowski D, Kang SY, Sampson D, Flynn E, et al. A model of human tumor dormancy: an angiogenic switch from the nonangiogenic phenotype. J Natl Cancer Inst. 2006;98(5):316–25. PubMed.
49. Karavasilis V, Malamou-Mitsi V, Briasoulis E, Tsanou E, Kitsou E, Kalofonos H, et al. Angiogenesis in cancer of unknown primary: clinicopathological study of CD34, VEGF and TSP-1. BMC Cancer. 2005;5:25. PubMed Central PMCID: 555600.
50. Agarwal B, Das P, Naresh KN, Borges AM. Angiogenic ability of metastatic squamous carcinoma in the cervical lymph nodes from unknown primary tumours. J Clin Pathol. 2011;64(9):765–70. PubMed.
51. Hainsworth JD, Spigel DR, Farley C, Thompson DS, Shipley DL, Greco FA. Phase II trial of bevacizumab and erlotinib in carcinomas of unknown primary site: the Minnie Pearl Cancer Research Network. J Clin Oncol. 2007;25(13):1747–52. PubMed.
52. Hainsworth JD, Spigel DR, Thompson DS, Murphy PB, Lane CM, Waterhouse DM, et al. Paclitaxel/carboplatin plus bevacizumab/erlotinib in the first-line treatment of patients with carcinoma of unknown primary site. Oncologist. 2009;14(12):1189–97. PubMed.
53. Karavasilis V, Malamou-Mitsi V, Briasoulis E, Tsanou E, Kitsou E, Kalofonos H, et al. Matrix metalloproteinases in carcinoma of unknown primary. Cancer. 2005;104(10):2282–7. PubMed.
54. Stoyianni A, Goussia A, Pentheroudakis G, Siozopoulou V, Ioachim E, Krikelis D, et al. Immunohistochemical study of the epithelial-mesenchymal transition phenotype in cancer of unknown primary: incidence, correlations and prognostic utility. Anticancer Res. 2012;32(4):1273–81. PubMed.
55. Krikelis D, Pentheroudakis G, Goussia A, Siozopoulou V, Bobos M, Petrakis D, et al. Profiling immunohistochemical expression of NOTCH1-3, JAGGED1, cMET, and phospho-MAPK in 100 carcinomas of unknown primary. Clin Exp Metastasis. 2012;29(6):603–14. PubMed.

56. Miele L. Notch signaling. Clin Cancer Res. 2006;12(4):1074–9. PubMed.
57. Culine S, Kramar A, Saghatchian M, Bugat R, Lesimple T, Lortholary A, et al. Development and validation of a prognostic model to predict the length of survival in patients with carcinomas of an unknown primary site. J Clin Oncol. 2002;20(24):4679–83. PubMed.
58. Hess KR, Abbruzzese MC, Lenzi R, Raber MN, Abbruzzese JL. Classification and regression tree analysis of 1000 consecutive patients with unknown primary carcinoma. Clin Cancer Res. 1999;5(11):3403–10. PubMed.
59. Petrakis D, Pentheroudakis G, Voulgaris E, Pavlidis N. Prognostication in cancer of unknown primary (CUP): development of a prognostic algorithm in 311 cases and review of the literature. Cancer Treat Rev. 2013;39(7):701–8. PubMed.
60. Seve P, Ray-Coquard I, Trillet-Lenoir V, Sawyer M, Hanson J, Broussolle C, et al. Low serum albumin levels and liver metastasis are powerful prognostic markers for survival in patients with carcinomas of unknown primary site. Cancer. 2006;107(11):2698–705. PubMed.

Chapter 4
Prognostic Factors and Their Role in the Management of CUP

Harald Löffler and Alwin Krämer

4.1 Introduction

If a category of cancers is biologically well defined, and therefore cases falling into this category are biologically closely related, prognosis is usually dictated by the stage, i.e., how disseminated the disease is and which organs are affected. CUP, in contrast, does not seem to be a biologically homogeneous category and instead seems to comprise a broad spectrum of prognostically very different cases and subcategories, some of which display a clearly better prognosis than the average CUP case.

The first difficulty is that even regarding such general information as median overall survival of unselected CUP patients, published data broadly vary between 11 weeks and 16.5 months [1, 2]. The second difficulty is that a range of different categorization systems regarding prognosis exist. As detailed in the previous chapter, we can either look at CUP as a whole, trying to find common features applicable to all or the majority of CUP cases, or follow the assumption that CUP comprises a collection of different diseases that are best described by their site of origin. Accordingly, two fundamentally different approaches to prognostication of CUP patients exist. The first approach categorizes CUP into subgroups characterized by specific working hypotheses, which should ideally be based on clear-cut criteria in order to reproducibly determine the prognosis of each respective subgroup, and to specify standardized therapeutic approaches. The other approach is to aim at establishing common prognostic factors valid for all or the majority of CUP cases by investigating cohorts of unselected CUP patients. In the following chapter sections, we will look at each of these approaches separately, but it should be noted that they are usually applied in a sequential manner: Once the diagnosis of CUP is established, the first step is to assess whether a patient should be assigned to a specified subgroup

H. Löffler (✉) • A. Krämer
Clinical Cooperation Unit Molecular Hematology/Oncology, German Cancer Research Center (DKFZ) and University of Heidelberg, Heidelberg, Germany
e-mail: h.loeffler@Dkfz-Heidelberg.de; a.kraemer@Dkfz-Heidelberg.de

A. Krämer, H. Löffler (eds.), *Cancer of Unknown Primary*,
DOI 10.1007/978-3-319-22581-4_4

requiring a specific therapeutic approach – and usually enjoying a better prognosis than the remaining CUP cases. Using classification by clinical staging, histology, and immunohistochemistry (but not gene expression profiling), 10–30 % of CUP patients can be assigned to an established subgroup, which will be discussed in the next section of this chapter. In the remaining 70–90 % of patients not belonging to such a subgroup, more general prognostic factors, which are discussed in subsequent chapter sections, will be applied.

4.2 Prognosis of Defined Subgroups

CUP subgroups may be defined on the basis of two principles, which are not mutually exclusive: First of all, any lesion that is reasonably targetable by a curative approach, i.e., a solitary tumor or lesions restricted to a single lymph node region, should be preferentially treated with curative intent. Secondly, if a constellation of clinical and histological findings is highly suggestive of a specific site of origin, this may direct the choice of therapy.

Historically, these CUP subgroups were defined in order to assign patients to therapies. In earlier times, patients who could not be reasonably assigned to such a subgroup usually did not receive any cancer-specific therapy at all, as stated in a review from 1993 [3]. Since then, several phase II studies led to the establishment of platinum-based cytostatic combination regimens as standard therapy for this "nonspecific" patient group (see Chap. 8). Although there is no randomized comparison to best supportive care and therefore no formal proof, it appears likely that these regimens have improved overall survival of this majority of patients by several months.

It does not surprise that as long as the rest of CUP patients did not receive more than supportive treatment, all these subgroups, which were assigned to entity-specific therapy, displayed a relatively favorable prognosis. Hence, they were termed "prognostically favorable." However, it should be noted that the meanwhile improved prognosis of the "nonspecific" patient group might have leveled the prognostic differences between this group and some of the "prognostically favorable" subgroups. Also, changes in the diagnostic armamentarium might influence the outcome of patients assigned to some of the subgroups. Thus, although the subgroups discussed in the following are still valid in terms of warranting specific therapeutic approaches, they may not always truly be prognostically favorable when compared to the majority of CUP cases not belonging to specific subgroups.

4.2.1 Women with Isolated Axillary Lymph Node Metastases from Adenocarcinoma

This subgroup should be treated as breast cancer. As with many of the subgroups listed here, its exact delineation may sometimes be problematic, e.g., if metastases are present not only in axillary lymph nodes but also at other sites still consistent with breast cancer, e.g., infraclavicular or parasternal nodes, or if histology is different from adenocarcinoma, e.g., poorly or undifferentiated carcinoma. In a systematic review of 24 retrospective studies with 689 patients, the mean age of patients was 52 years, and 66 % of the patients were postmenopausal [4]. The nodal status was N1 in 48 % and N2-3 in 52 %. Ductal adenocarcinoma was the most frequent histological classification (83 %). Expression of estrogen and progesterone receptors was reported in 43 % and 41 % of cases with available data, respectively, while HER-2/neu was overexpressed in 31 % of cases. A small breast primary was identified histologically in 72 % of cases where mastectomy was performed. Within these cohorts, which were heterogeneous in terms of treatment and whose recruitment spanned the long period of 1975–2006 during which therapeutic strategies changed substantially, the mean 5-year overall survival was 72 %, ranging from 59.4 to 88 %, with axillary tumor burden being the most relevant prognostic factor [4]. From these data, it may be concluded that tumor biology and prognosis of this CUP subgroup are similar to the corresponding stages of node-positive breast cancer with evident primary lesion and that there is convincing evidence that this constellation represents a prognostically favorable subset of CUP.

4.2.2 *Women with Papillary Serous Carcinoma Restricted to the Peritoneum*

This subgroup should be treated as ovarian cancer, although it should be mentioned that some authors refer to this entity as a primary peritoneal malignancy [5]. In a systematic review, Pentheroudakis and Pavlidis grouped clinical series published between 1980 and 2008 into publications before 1990, more recent studies before the taxane era, and studies in the taxane era [5]. In the first two groups, most studies reported median overall survival times in the range between 12 and 24 months, while in the taxane era, the reported median overall survival times ranged between 15 and 42 months. In this latest group of case series, the rates of both optimum surgical cytoreduction and tumor regression on chemotherapy were higher [5]. In conclusion, published data on prognosis of this CUP subset vary considerably but, compared to the data regarding survival of unselected CUP patients, ranging from 11 weeks to 16.5 months [1, 2], the peritoneal cancer subgroup seems to be associated with a favorable prognosis.

4.2.3 *Squamous Cell Carcinoma (and Other Cancers) Restricted to Cervical Lymph Nodes*

This subgroup should be treated as head and neck cancer, usually implying aggressive multimodal therapies with curative intent. Again, stricter and less strict definitions exist: While the majority of cancer cases restricted to cervical lymph nodes are indeed squamous cell carcinomas, there is a subset of roughly 25 % of cases showing different histologies including undifferentiated cancers and adenocarcinomas [6]. While some authors consider only squamous cell carcinomas, others include all cancers restricted to cervical lymph nodes in this favorable CUP subset [6–8]. It should be mentioned that this is a relatively well-investigated subgroup, but nevertheless, we face the problem that knowledge is mainly based on retrospective case series and that the reported 5-year overall survival varies between 24 and 71 % [6, 8–13]. These discrepancies are explained by several inconsistencies: First, some studies include patients selected for specific therapies, while others comprise unselected cases – of course, aggressive multimodal therapies are expected to lead to a better prognosis than less aggressive approaches. Second, restriction to histologic subsets may influence results since at least some studies have reported a better prognosis for squamous cell carcinomas [9]. Finally, a substantial proportion of the published studies include cases from many decades ago, and therapeutic approaches clearly have changed over time. Nevertheless, it seems that for this CUP subset as a whole, 5-year overall survival is about 40–60 %. A substantial proportion of patients enjoy long-term disease control, and a significant minority can be cured. Moreover, the same prognostic factors as for head and neck cancers with known primary, such as nodal stage and extracapsular nodal extension, seem to affect survival [9, 10]. We conclude that this subgroup does prognostically by far better than unselected CUP patients.

4.2.4 Squamous Cell Carcinoma Restricted to Inguinal Lymph Nodes

For this subgroup, the likelihood of an origin within the anogenital region appears high, and approaches with curative intent including radical resection, radiation, or radiochemotherapy are usually first choice. Guarischi et al. [14] identified 56 cases of CUP with inguinal node involvement, which also included non-squamous cell histologies and cases metastasized beyond the inguinal region and accounted for 0.065 % of all new cancer cases seen at a large Canadian center from 1968 to 1982. The 5-year overall survival was 27 % for the whole group and 37.5 % for 40 patients with disease restricted to inguinal with or without iliacal lymph nodes. Similarly, for the 24 cases with squamous cell carcinoma, 5-year overall survival was approximately 35 %, whereas no separate data were reported for the combination squamous cell carcinoma restricted to inguinal (and/or iliacal) nodes [14]. Interestingly, survival curves of both patient groups with squamous cell carcinoma and locally restricted disease seemed to stabilize at a plateau around 30 and 40 % long-term survival, possibly reflecting cure [14]. These data, which are in principal agreement with other smaller series [14], support the notion that the prognosis of this CUP subset is substantially better than that of unselected CUP patients.

4.2.5 Adenocarcinoma with Lower Gastrointestinal Profile

This group is usually defined by the immunohistochemical marker combination $CDX2^+/CK20^+/CK7^-$, which is typically found in colorectal adenocarcinomas but can be likewise present in small intestine cancers, the latter being much less frequent, so alternative namings include adenocarcinoma with "colon cancer" or simply "gastrointestinal" profile. A less strict definition, which is therefore less specific for lower intestinal malignancies, considers only positivity for CDX2 without paying attention to CK7 and CK20. Varadhachary et al. published a series of 74 patients, of whom 53 received a first-line colorectal cancer regimen based on FOLFOX or FOLFIRI [15]. Overall survival was separately determined for the subgroup "consistent with lower gastrointestinal profile" ($CDX2^+/CK20^+/CK7^-$; 34 cases) and patients displaying "probable lower gastrointestinal profile" ($CDX2^+$ only; 40 cases), showing median survival times of 37 and 21 months, respectively [15]. In conclusion, treatment as colorectal cancer is warranted, and prognosis of this CUP subset is favorable, especially if cases meet the stricter definition with $CDX2^+/CK20^+/CK7^-$.

4.2.6 Poorly Differentiated CUP with Midline Distribution

In the 1980s, poorly differentiated CUP was identified as a CUP subset which was prognostically favorable in comparison with other CUPs, with high response rates to cisplatin-based combination chemotherapy including complete remissions and a minority of patients enjoying long-term survival [16]. Within poorly differentiated CUP, localization of tumors to the mediastinum, retroperitoneum, or lymph nodes was associated with an even more favorable outcome, and these patients frequently showed features of germ cell tumors [16]. Consequently, this group was established as a prognostically favorable CUP subset. Later studies utilizing improved possibilities of immunohistochemistry, however, indicated that a substantial proportion of these patients actually had lymphoma or other well-treatable malignancies [17, 18], which probably accounted for many of the long-term survivors among "poorly differentiated CUP" patients. Taking into account the apparent median overall survival, which was between 1 and 2 years in the cited "poorly differentiated CUP" study [16] and is likewise in the range of 1 year in newer studies of CUP patients not selected for prognostically relevant subgroups [2, 19, 20], it is in our view far from clear that the "poorly differentiated CUP" subgroup can still be regarded as prognostically favorable. Nevertheless, it seems reasonable to treat patients with features of germ cell cancer, especially men younger than 50 years old, with germ cell cancer protocols.

4.2.7 Neuroendocrine CUP

Neuroendocrine tumors comprise a heterogeneous group of diseases, and survival largely depends on whether the histological grade is low or high, with the former usually being associated with an indolent course while the prognosis of the latter group is dismal. A systematic review of studies on neuroendocrine CUP revealed a median overall survival of 15.5 months among 294 patients with available outcome data [21]. The authors concluded that there was no evidence that in comparison with neuroendocrine tumors with known primaries, neuroendocrine CUPs behave differently in terms of biology or outcome. To us, these data seem to indicate that disseminated high-grade neuroendocrine CUPs are associated with outcomes similar to unselected CUPs while there are probably subgroups, such as low-grade tumors or localized stages, with a clearly better prognosis.

4.2.8 Metastatic Melanoma of Unknown Primary

This entity is inconsistently listed among CUP subgroups, probably because some authors consider melanoma as an entity generally not belonging to CUP. After all, its distinct histologic features, its probably distinct biology, and the distinct therapeutic options available clearly separate this entity from "standard" CUPs. Kamposioras et al. [22] published a systematic review of the literature regarding malignant melanoma of unknown primary site, comprising 4348 patients and including studies covering the long period from 1917 to 2007. Depending on disease stage, the median overall survival ranged between 24 and 127 months if metastases were restricted to lymph nodes and between 3 and 16 months in cases with visceral metastatic spread [22]. However, these data are probably outdated since several systemic therapies have been approved for metastatic melanoma in recent years, substantially improving its prognosis even in cases with visceral metastases [23–26].

4.2.9 Men with Osteoblastic Metastases and Elevated Serum PSA

This subgroup should be treated as prostate cancer [7, 27]. Based on the fact that there are several specific therapeutic options for this entity, such as androgen deprivation and radiopharmaceuticals specifically targeting bone lesions, it may be assumed that this is another prognostically favorable subset of CUP [27, 28]. However, we are not aware of any systematic study assessing survival data of this specific subgroup.

4.2.10 CUP Restricted to a Single Metastatic Site

Several CUP subgroups are characterized by localized disease stage and therefore warrant multimodal therapeutic approaches with curative intent. As detailed above, these patients usually enjoy a clearly better prognosis than the majority of CUP patients with disseminated disease. It is therefore recommended to treat patients not belonging to defined (organ specific) subgroups but nevertheless presenting with localized disease in an analogous fashion, i.e., with curative intent. This is also supported by the finding that even by autopsy, a primary cannot always be found in CUP cases [29]. Therefore, resection of a solitary CUP lesion may be truly curative in a fraction of cases (for further details, see Chap. 3). Unfortunately, systematic evidence supporting this notion by outcome data is scarce, as this category is not only rare but also heterogeneous. In our own published cohort of 223 CUP cases (restricted to adenocarcinoma or undifferentiated carcinoma), nine patients (4 %) were treated with radical resection alone and showed a median overall survival of 52.7 months, while radical resection combined with radiation was applied in seven cases (3 %), leading to a median overall survival of 27.0 months [2]. We conclude that these approaches appear sensible, but more outcome data regarding CUP restricted to a single metastatic site are needed.

4.2.11 Defined Subgroups: Conclusion

In summary, for most but not all of the traditional "prognostically favorable" subsets, there is at least some evidence that outcome is better than that of unselected CUP patients. It has to be emphasized that most of these subgroups are themselves heterogeneous, implying that it can be assumed that subsets of cases within these subgroups exist which are clearly prognostically favorable while others are not. For individual cases, it appears reasonable to apply risk predictors known from analogous entities, e.g., nodal stage in women with axillary adenocarcinoma or histological grade in neuroendocrine tumors.

4.3 Case Series of CUP Patients

In most of the subsets listed in the previous section, analogies to organ-specific cancers provide hints useful for prognostication, but one should keep in mind that these subsets account for only 10–30 % of all CUP cases. For the remaining majority of CUPs not belonging to specific subsets, it appears desirable to define generally applicable prognostic factors for outcome prediction. Such prognostic factors could be extracted from clinical drug therapy trials, but in case of CUP, we face the limitation that only small trials exist, and in addition, such trials inevitably imply patient selection, thereby further limiting the validity of prognostic factors determined in these studies. Drug therapy trials will be discussed in detail in Chap. 8. Another option to determine prognostic factors comes from series of unselected CUP cases. In fact, several such series exist, which are summarized in Table 4.1. In this table, all newer, internationally published case series that did not select patients for therapy received and did not exclusively focus on minor CUP subgroups are listed. There were some minor differences in eligibility criteria between these case series, with some studies excluding all or some of the minor subgroups listed in Sect. 4.2, while other series did not exclude these patients. As indicated in the table, some of the studies also included patients without histological confirmation.

It should be noted that these case series are the most valid evidence available regarding overall survival of unselected CUP patients. Nevertheless, reported overall survival varied between 11 weeks and 16.5 months in these publications. A closer look reveals that the worst overall survival of 11 weeks was reported by two epidemiological registries, while the best outcomes were reported by specialized oncologic centers (Table 4.1). This seems to indicate that patient selection may partly explain these discrepancies since there may be a proportion of frail or terminally ill patients that never reach a specialized oncologic center, as discussed in detail in Sect. 2.2 of this book. On the other hand, there seems to be a trend that better survival and higher rates of patients treated with cytostatics in the newer as compared to the older series reflect some improvement in therapeutic options. Prognostic factors might be useful to overcome these selection effects and predict survival of individual patients better than pooled data of heterogeneous patient cohorts.

4.4 Specific Prognostic Factors

Given the small number of publications addressing prognostic factors in CUP patients, the number of reported prognostic factors is rather high. However, when only parameters with prognostic significance confirmed by multivariate analysis in several independent investigations are considered, fewer parameters remain. Moreover, the practical utility of a given prognostic parameter is influenced by additional factors, e.g., the question whether this information is generally available for all patients or requires special tests and the related question whether this information can be determined in an unequivocal, objective, easy-to-handle fashion, which might be problematic for some parameters such as performance status or comorbidity. With the following list, we focus on the most relevant and best-established prognostic factors in CUP patients.

- *Age*: Several case series found higher age to be correlated with poorer outcome [17, 34, 37, 42, 44]. For example, Van de Wouw et al. [37] reported a median overall survival of 30 weeks in 17 patients aged less than 60 years, whereas median survival was 12 weeks in 53 patients aged 60 years or older ($p=0.016$). On the other hand, several other series including our own collection of 223 cases

Table 4.1 Case series of unselected CUP patients (in chronological order)

Citation	Study population	Survival data, selected prognostic factors, comments
Altman and Cadman (1986) [30]	1539 cases from a single center (USA), 1922–1981	Median OS 5 months. 56 % of cases received therapy, 18 % were not confirmed histologically. Histologically confirmed cases that received therapy showed a median OS of 7 months
Alberts et al. (1989) [31]	100 cases from a single center (South Africa), 1977–1984	Median OS 124 days. RF: performance status
Pavlidis et al. (1994) [32]	85 cases from three centers (Greece), 1986–1991	Aim was to study serum tumor markers. Median OS not specified, was about 5 months as indicated by figure. CA 19–9 and CA 15–3 levels correlated with number of metastases
Abbruzzese et al. (1994) [33]	657 cases from a single center (USA), 1987–1992	Median OS 11 months. An extended study of this population was published later once more [34]; see next row
Hess et al. (1999) [34]	1000 cases from a single center (USA), 1987–1994	Median OS 11 months. Two prognostic models with ten and nine groups, respectively. RF: number of metastatic sites, adenocarcinoma, liver and adrenal metastases. Protective factor: neuroendocrine carcinoma
Van de Wouw et al. (2002) [35]	1285 cases from a cancer registry (Netherlands, representing about one million inhabitants), 1984–1992	1024 cases biopsy proven, 261 only clinically diagnosed. Biopsy-proven cases: median OS 11 weeks, only supportive therapy in 67 %. Protective factors: age <50 years, lymph node metastases
Levi et al. (2002) [1]	699 cases from a cancer registry (Switzerland, representing 786.000 inhabitants), 1984–1993	543 biopsy-proven cases: median age 71 years, median OS 11 weeks. 156 only clinically diagnosed cases: median age 79 years, median OS 6 weeks. Protective factor: squamous cell carcinoma (median OS 41 weeks)
Culine et al. (2002) [36]	150 cases from a single center (France), 1989–1999	Median OS 7.5 months. RF: performance status, liver metastases, LDH
Van de Wouw et al. (2004) [37]	70 cases from a single center (Netherlands), 1990–1996	Median OS 12 weeks. RF: age ≥60 years, performance status, number of metastatic sites, liver metastases, LDH
Seve et al. (2006) [38]	317 cases from a single center (Canada), 1998–2004	Median OS 104 days. RF: liver metastases, low serum albumin, performance status
Ponce Lorenzo et al. (2007) [39]	100 cases from a single center (Spain), 2002–2006	Median OS 4.7 months. RF: performance status, number of metastatic sites, liver metastases
Trivanovic et al. (2009) [40]	145 cases from two centers (Croatia), 2002–2007	Median OS 330 days. RF: performance status, liver metastases, LDH, anemia, age, prolonged QT interval

(continued)

Table 4.1 (continued)

Citation	Study population	Survival data, selected prognostic factors, comments
Thöm et al. (2009) [41]	136 cases from a single center (Germany), 1989–1998	Median OS 7.9 months. RF: performance status, male sex
Fernandez-Cotarelo et al. (2010) [42]	265 cases from a single center (Spain),1999–2003	Median OS 2.5 months. RF: age, AP, low albumin. Protective factor: squamous cell carcinoma
Petrakis et al. (2013) [43]	311 cases from a single center (Greece), 1988–2011	Median OS 8 months. RF: performance status, leukocytosis, visceral metastases
Löffler et al. (2014) [2]	223 cases from a single center (Germany), 2006–2010	Median OS 16.5 months. RF: performance status, number of metastatic sites, liver and adrenal metastases

Abbreviations: *AP* alkaline phosphatase, *LDH* lactate dehydrogenase, *OS* overall survival, *RF* risk factor (correlated to reduced survival in comparison with reference population)

failed to find any correlation between age and prognosis [2, 33]. For example, the large series of Abbruzzese et al. [33] reported median survival times ranging from 8.7 months in patients aged 20–39 years to 6.4 months in the age group of 70 years and older, with widely overlapping confidence intervals for all age groups. Apparently, age as a prognostic factor seems to be particularly sensitive to treatment decisions since the influence of age on the decision between aggressive therapy and best supportive care might differ between institutions and might have changed over time. In conclusion, we do not think that there is evidence that age is a useful prognosis indicator.

- *Sex*: There is good evidence from several publications that male sex is associated with poorer outcome than female sex [2, 31, 33, 41]. Abbruzzese et al. [33] reported median survivals of 9.6 months in women and 6.4 months in men, and the corresponding data from our own series were 19.3 months in female versus 12.3 months in male patients [2]. It seems likely that these differences mainly reflect different distributions of sites of origin since gynecological primaries are associated with more favorable outcome, while the prognostically dismal group of smoking-related cancers is probably more frequent in men. Whether additional, more general sex-specific differences in tumor biology exist, remains an open question.
- *ECOG/WHO performance status*: The performance status according to Eastern Cooperative Oncology group [45], describing cancer-associated reduction of physical activity and also referred to as WHO, Zubrod, or ECOG score, is among the best-established prognosis predictors for CUP patients [2, 31, 36–41, 43, 46–48]. While survival seems to worsen with each step the performance status declines, patients are commonly grouped into a favorable group with a performance status of 0–1, and an unfavorable group with a performance status >1, with the latter showing survival times less than half of that of the reference group.
- *Number of metastatic sites*: To quantify metastatic dissemination, the number of involved organs sites (e.g., lymph nodes, liver, lungs) may be counted. Several publications found a correlation of this number with survival [2, 33, 34, 37, 41].

Dichotomization of prognosis groups may include patients with just one or up to two involved organ sites in the favorable group.

- *Specific sites of metastasis*: Not surprisingly, specific organ sites affected by metastases show associations with survival, and many such associations have been published. The best-established predictor of poor outcome is liver metastases, which showed significant correlations with worse survival in several independent investigations [2, 31, 33, 34, 37–40]. Adrenal metastases might be an indicator of remarkably poor prognosis, with survival being less than half of the reference group when they are present, as reported in two independent studies, although it should be mentioned that these data are based on a small number of cases [2, 34]. In our own series of 223 cases, the hazard ratio for ten patients with adrenal metastases was 2.7 (1.1–6.2), but the significance of adrenal metastases as prognostic parameter was lost after correction for confounders, especially since the overall number of metastatic organ sites was higher in this patient group [2]. Finally, some authors have reported affection of lymph nodes as being correlated with favorable outcome [33, 41], while other cohorts did not reveal this correlation, although the majority of studies showed a trend toward better survival with lymph node metastases [2, 31, 37–40], allowing the conclusion that there may be a moderate positive impact of lymph node affection on survival.
- *Specific histologic groups*: When compared to other histologic categories as reference, both squamous cell and neuroendocrine carcinomas have been reported as prognostically favorable, while adenocarcinomas – the majority of CUPs – are associated with a poorer prognosis [1, 33, 34, 42, 43]. The latter seems to result from of the fact that selecting adenocarcinomas implies a selection against most prognostically favorable subgroups. Selection of favorable subsets may also be the reason why squamous cell carcinomas are prognostically favorable since locally restricted cancers are more frequent in this histologic group. Evidence regarding the question whether squamous cell carcinomas are associated with favorable outcome also in disseminated stages is limited. For example, in the large collection of Abbruzzese et al. [33], the prognostic relevance of adenocarcinoma (conferring poor outcome) and neuroendocrine carcinoma (conferring favorable outcome) remained significant, while squamous cell histology showed no significant correlation with outcome in multivariate analysis.
- *Serum tumor markers*: Few studies exist that address the prognostic or predictive value of serum tumor markers in CUP. There is some evidence that the extent of serum tumor marker elevation in general is correlated with disease stage, and markers elevated above a threshold therefore indicate poor survival, which is expected due to the general correlation of tumor markers with tumor mass [2, 32, 43]. On the other hand, no specific tumor marker that, in comparison to other tumor markers, shows a qualitative correlation with outcome of CUP patients has been described so far. One obvious limitation of the studies published up to now is that serum tumor markers were not prospectively evaluated in all patients included, so each tumor marker was available only in a subset of the respective study population.

- *Other blood tests*: Serum lactate dehydrogenase (LDH), alkaline phosphatase (AP), and albumin levels have each been verified as prognostic parameters by several independent investigations [36–40, 42, 46, 49]. Each of these parameters, when elevated above the upper normal limit (LDH, AP) or reduced below the lower limit of normal (albumin), respectively, is associated with an overall survival less than half of that of the reference group with normal levels. Taking into account that abnormalities of these parameters affect only a minority of patients, it seems that they nonspecifically indicate an advanced disease stage. The same probably applies to other blood tests whose role in the prognostication of CUP has been less well characterized: An association with poor prognosis was also reported for leukocytosis, anemia, and lymphopenia [38, 43].
- *Other parameters*: Various prognostic factors not mentioned so far have been reported. One study found a strong association of a prolonged QT interval corrected for heart rate (QTc interval) with poor outcome [40]. An obvious disadvantage of this parameter (and probably the reason why there is only one publication addressing it) is that it is not widely assessed in routine care of CUP patients. The same probably applies to the Adult Comorbidity Evaluation 27 (ACE-27) index, a 27-item comorbidity index designed for cancer patients: Seve et al. [38] found a strong correlation of this index with outcome that remained significant in multivariate analysis, thereby being an independent prognostic parameter in addition to ECOG performance status, number of metastatic sites, and other parameters. Although application of the ACE-27 index therefore appears generally desirable and will be useful in scientific settings, we dare to predict that its establishment in routine practice will be difficult, but nevertheless oncologists should keep in mind that comorbidities are among the major factors affecting outcome of CUP patients, as it is the case for cancer in general.

Finally, it should be mentioned that some of the cited case series also analyzed the impact of therapy on prognosis. As expected, patients treated with chemotherapy or other tumor-specific therapies survived longer than patients who did not receive any tumor-specific treatment, and patients treated with surgery and/or radiotherapy survived longer than patients treated with chemotherapy, which probably reflects selection of patients suitable for these treatment modalities because of locally confined disease [2, 41, 42, 48, 49].

4.5 Prognostic Scoring Systems

Keeping in mind the above list of prognostic factors, it appears desirable to define a scoring system, ideally integrating all prognostic information into one single readout. In the following section, we will discuss, in chronological order, five different scoring systems that have been established for CUP patients. Beforehand, it should be mentioned that eligibility criteria for the respective patient cohorts varied in details between the studies discussed, some of which excluded prognostically favorable subsets by using various definitions. Nevertheless, we think that all scoring systems discussed below are generally applicable to CUP patients.

Based on regression tree analysis of 1000 consecutive CUP patients, Hess et al. [34] developed two different trees with ten and nine terminal subgroups, respectively. The regression trees incorporated different sites of involvement (liver, bones, adrenals, pleura, lymph nodes), number of metastatic sites (≤2 versus >2), histology (with neuroendocrine carcinomas as favorable group and adenocarcinomas as unfavorable group), and age (with 61.5 years as cutoff) as separate prognostic parameters. Median survival in the terminal subgroups varied between 45 and 5 months, although many groups showed overlapping confidence intervals and there was no validation cohort. We conclude that this study is a valuable resource for understanding of prognostic factors and their relative weight for the prognostication of CUP patients, but with respect to the complicated algorithms and lack of external validation, the proposed classification does not appear suitable for clinical application on a broader basis.

In contrast, Culine et al. [36] aimed to establish a simple and broadly applicable prognostic model. Considering only clinical variables in a cohort of 150 unselected CUP patients, they defined three groups (Fig. 4.1a): The favorable group, defined by a performance status of ≤1 and no liver metastases, showed a 1-year survival of 43 % and a median overall survival of 10.8 months. In the intermediate group with a performance status >1 or liver metastases, the 1-year survival was 23 % and the median survival 6.3 months. The prognostically poor group with both a performance status >1 and liver metastases displayed a 1-year survival of 0 % and a median overall survival of 2.4 months. With the addition of serum LDH levels (which were available in 81 out of the 150 patients), the independent prognostic significance of liver metastases was lost. The authors therefore defined a second prognostic model with only two groups, a favorable group with a performance status of ≤1 and normal LDH (or absent liver metastasis if LDH was unknown) and an unfavorable group comprising all other cases (Fig. 4.1b). The 1-year survivals were 45 % in the favorable versus 11 % in the unfavorable group, and the respective overall survival times were 11.7 and 3.9 months. This second model was verified in an external validation cohort generated from two prospective phase II trials, which showed 1-year survival rates of 53 % versus 23 % and median overall survivals of 12 versus 7 months ($p=0.0089$). We conclude that this prognostic model stands out due to independent validation and feasibility in routine patient care. Possible criticism may include that the presence of only two groups and the omission of several parameters known to be prognostically relevant only allows for crude classification, and that in 46 % of the study population, LDH was substituted by liver metastases as prognostic parameter, leaving open which of these parameters should be preferred in clinical practice.

Seve et al. [38] investigated 317 consecutive CUP patients, from which they deduced two prognostic groups (Fig. 4.2): The favorable group was defined by the absence of liver metastases and a normal serum albumin level, while the unfavorable group was defined by liver metastases and/or a low albumin level. The 1-year survival rates of the favorable and poor groups were 39 % and 12 %, respectively, and the corresponding median survivals were 371 and 108 days, respectively. Interestingly, a comparison of this model with the one previously published by Culine et al. revealed that using the Culine model, the relative risk of death at 1 year

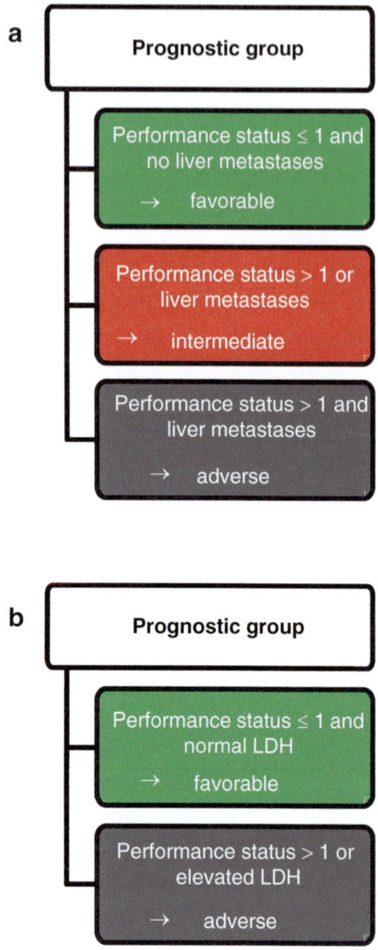

Fig. 4.1 Prognostic models for CUP published by Culine et al. [36]: (**a**) model with clinical variables only, (**b**) model with clinical and serum variables

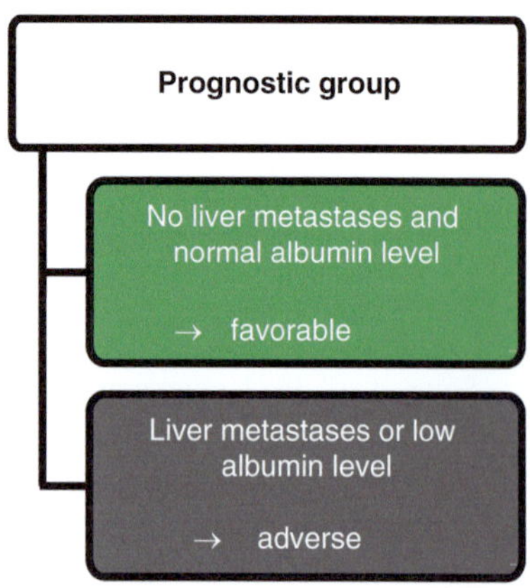

Fig. 4.2 Prognostic model for CUP published by Seve et al. [38]

in the unfavorable versus the favorable group was 2.3, whereas it was 3.4 with the Seve model [38]. Moreover, validation of the Seve model using an independent cohort of 81 patients not only approved its validity, with the relative risk of death at 1 year in the unfavorable versus the favorable group being 4.7, but also confirmed its better discriminative performance compared to the Culine model [38]. As explanation for this discordant performance, the authors put forward that 17 cases with elevated LDH that were classified as poor risk by Culine's model but as good risk according to Seve's model actually displayed a favorable median survival of 363 days [38]. Taken together, the model provided by Seve et al. is well validated, allows remarkably good discrimination between good-risk and poor-risk patients, and is feasible in routine patient care. Again, a drawback might be that several relevant prognostic factors that would possibly enable a more accurate prediction are not considered.

From prognostic data of 311 CUP cases, Petrakis et al. [43] derived a scoring system which they dubbed "Ioannina Score for CUP Outpatient Oncologic Prognostication" (I-SCOOP). Noteworthily, the authors did not exclude prognostically favorable subsets from their study. Consequently, this algorithm involved, as a first step, assignment to a clinicopathologic subgroup. It seems that the definition of these subgroups followed the classical CUP subgroup definitions as listed in Sect. 4.2, but the authors did not specify their definitions exactly. Based on this classification, the "serous peritoneal," the "axillary nodal," and the "squamous head neck" subgroups were assigned a final score of 0 (low risk). In contrast, the "nodal," "neuroendocrine," and "mucinous peritoneal" subgroups received 1 score point, while the "visceral" subgroup received 2 score points. In all subgroups with more than 0 score points, two additional parameters were considered: In case of leukocytosis of more than 10/nl, an additional score point was assigned, and in case of performance status >1, another score point was added (Fig. 4.3). Together, this led to a score ranging from 0 to 4, with the most favorable group with a score of 0 showing a median overall survival of 36 months, while cases with a score of 4 displayed a median survival of 5 months (Fig. 4.3). As evident from this description, this score is more sophisticated and demanding than the ones described above, owing to the fact that clinicopathologic subgroups are considered. In our opinion, however, it makes more sense to consider prognostically favorable subsets in a first step and only if they have been excluded, proceed to the use of a more general score. For example, thinking of a female patient with an adenocarcinoma in an axillary node, we do have clear evidence, as discussed above, to predict a 5-year overall survival of well above 50 % [4], while the I-SCOOP would predict a median overall survival of 36 months. Therefore, the more valid prediction comes from considering "axillary nodal" CUP as a separate entity first. An additional criticism regarding the I-SCOOP concerns the fact that assignment to a clinicopathologic subgroup may be frequently far from unequivocal in practice, also because the authors do not provide exact definitions of these subgroups [43]. Finally, the I-SCOOP has not yet been tested in an independent validation cohort.

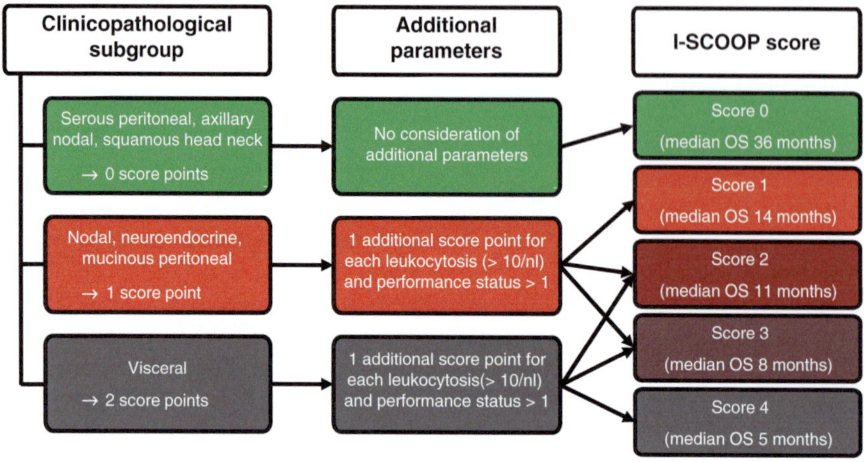

Fig. 4.3 Prognostic scoring system published by Petrakis et al. [43], termed I-SCOOP. For each final score value, the median overall survival (OS) as determined by the authors in their cohort [43] is indicated

Fig. 4.4 Prognostic model for CUP published by Löffler et al. [2]

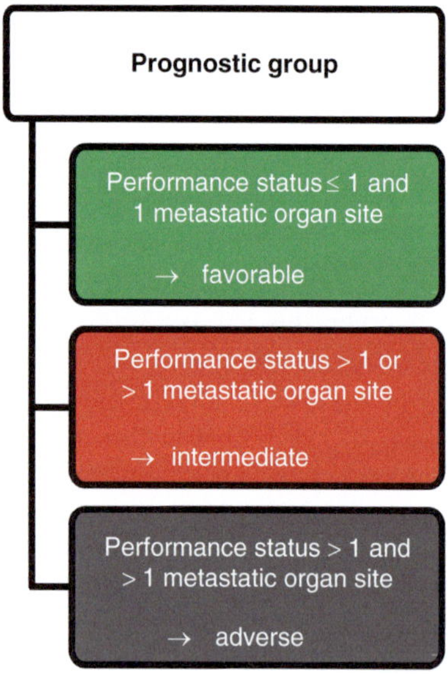

From our own cohort of 223 patients with adenocarcinomas or undifferentiated carcinomas of unknown origin [2], we derived a score solely based on clinical parameters that are available before initiation of treatment (Fig. 4.4): The favorable group with a performance status ≤1 and 1 metastatic organ site showed a median overall survival of 36.6 months, in the intermediate group with either a performance status >1 or more than 1 metastatic organ site, median survival was 12.0 months, while the unfavorable group, defined by both a performance status >1 and more than

1 metastatic organ site, displayed a median survival of 8.7 months. The significance of this scoring system remained valid when patients that were subsequently treated with resection with or without radiation – the subset including cases that might be cured – were excluded from analysis: Even then, the median overall survival of the favorable subgroup was 28.2 months [2]. Hence, we provided another easy-to-use score with good discriminative performance for unselected patients. This score has not yet been tested using an independent validation cohort. Compared to the well-validated scores published by Culine et al. [36] and Seve et al. [38], our score might have the advantage that it can be obtained without any serum blood tests.

We conclude this section with the remark that some scores have been published that incorporate a large number of prognostic parameters. This may be useful in scientific settings and these publications have surely contributed to our understanding of prognostic factors in CUP, but these tests also imply the application of sophisticated algorithms, making them less useful in routine care. In contrast, other scores have been published that are easily applicable in routine care, with the potential disadvantage that prognostic information that might be helpful in individual patients is not considered. Among these tests, the best validated ones are the scores published by Culine et al. [36] and Seve et al. [38], with the latter showing the better discriminative performance.

4.6 Conclusions

After all, CUP is still a heterogeneous disease. Hence, it is important to take prognostic information into account in every individual patient. We think that the main aim of this approach in practice will be to identify individuals with considerable better prospects than the majority of cases characterized by dismal outcomes. Accordingly, it has to be asked how the data presented in this chapter should be applied to serve this aim and also which limitations and caveats regarding the current knowledge about CUP prognostication exist.

Regarding the latter question, one difficulty when comparing different studies evaluating prognostic factors or applying such factors to individual patients is that the respective studies varied regarding their inclusion criteria. Therefore, the validity of individual prognostic factors may be confounded by whether or not specific subgroups have been included into the study. The role of specific prognostic factors may also change whenever therapeutic approaches change. This may be of special importance when different therapeutic paradigms such as nonspecific chemotherapies on one hand and gene expression profiling-guided site-specific therapies on the other hand are considered.

How do we apply prognostic information to individual patients? Here, a stepwise approach seems most appropriate, the first step being to consider whether patients belong to one of the "classical" subgroups listed in Sect. 4.2. Considering these subgroups first is not only warranted with respect to prognostication but rather an issue of general management, since subgroup assignment will first of all affect the choice of therapy. In addition, the most important prognostic information regarding these subgroups does not come from studies addressing CUP in general but from investigations dedicated to the respective subgroup, as illustrated by the example of a woman with isolated axillary nodes of an adenocarcinoma (see Sect. 4.5). In general, it seems to make little sense to consider prognostic parameters published for unselected CUP such as LDH or albumin in these specific subgroups.

Only if these "classical" subgroups have been excluded and hence we face a "classical" CUP with no clear working hypothesis, one should proceed to prognostic determinants for CUP in general, including performance status, number of metastatic sites, presence of liver or adrenal metastases, serum LDH and albumin, and so on. In practice, all prognostic information that may be of relevance to the patient should be considered. In this context, it also seems important to reflect which prognostic factors are of little importance for CUP patients, as, e.g., age, whose role as a prognosis indicator is at least controversial, or, just to give another example, brain metastases, which indicate a very poor prognosis in many other cancers, while in CUP, they do not play a prominent role in prognostication, as also underlined by our own data showing that our 18 cases with brain metastases displayed a median overall survival of 16.5 months [2].

References

1. Levi F, Te VC, Erler G, Randimbison L, La Vecchia C. Epidemiology of unknown primary tumours. Eur J Cancer. 2002;38(13):1810–2. PubMed.
2. Löffler H, Puthenparambil J, Hielscher T, Neben K, Krämer A. Patients with cancer of unknown primary: a retrospective analysis of 223 patients with adenocarcinoma or undifferentiated carcinoma. Dtsch Arztebl Int. 2014;111(27–28):481–7. PubMed.
3. Hainsworth JD, Greco FA. Treatment of patients with cancer of an unknown primary site. N Engl J Med. 1993;329(4):257–63. PubMed.
4. Pentheroudakis G, Lazaridis G, Pavlidis N. Axillary nodal metastases from carcinoma of unknown primary (CUPAx): a systematic review of published evidence. Breast Cancer Res Treat. 2010;119(1):1–11. PubMed.
5. Pentheroudakis G, Pavlidis N. Serous papillary peritoneal carcinoma: unknown primary tumour, ovarian cancer counterpart or a distinct entity? A systematic review. Crit Rev Oncol Hematol. 2010;75(1):27–42. PubMed.
6. Cerezo L, Raboso E, Ballesteros AI. Unknown primary cancer of the head and neck: a multidisciplinary approach. Clin Transl Oncol. 2011;13(2):88–97. PubMed.
7. Hainsworth JD, Fizazi K. Treatment for patients with unknown primary cancer and favorable prognostic factors. Semin Oncol. 2009;36(1):44–51. PubMed.
8. Pavlidis N, Pentheroudakis G, Plataniotis G. Cervical lymph node metastases of squamous cell carcinoma from an unknown primary site: a favourable prognosis subset of patients with CUP. Clin Transl Oncol. 2009;11(6):340–8. PubMed.
9. Beldi D, Jereczek-Fossa BA, D'Onofrio A, Gambaro G, Fiore MR, Pia F, et al. Role of radiotherapy in the treatment of cervical lymph node metastases from an unknown primary site: retrospective analysis of 113 patients. Int J Radiat Oncol Biol Phys. 2007;69(4):1051–8. PubMed.
10. Colletier PJ, Garden AS, Morrison WH, Goepfert H, Geara F, Ang KK. Postoperative radiation for squamous cell carcinoma metastatic to cervical lymph nodes from an unknown primary site: outcomes and patterns of failure. Head Neck. 1998;20(8):674–81. PubMed.

11. Issing WJ, Taleban B, Tauber S. Diagnosis and management of carcinoma of unknown primary in the head and neck. Eur Arch Otorhinolaryngol. 2003;260(8):436–43. PubMed.
12. Ligey A, Gentil J, Crehange G, Montbarbon X, Pommier P, Peignaux K, et al. Impact of target volumes and radiation technique on loco-regional control and survival for patients with unilateral cervical lymph node metastases from an unknown primary. Radiother Oncol. 2009;93(3):483–7. PubMed.
13. Shoushtari A, Saylor D, Kerr KL, Sheng K, Thomas C, Jameson M, et al. Outcomes of patients with head-and-neck cancer of unknown primary origin treated with intensity-modulated radiotherapy. Int J Radiat Oncol Biol Phys. 2011;81(3):e83–91. PubMed.
14. Guarischi A, Keane TJ, Elhakim T. Metastatic inguinal nodes from an unknown primary neoplasm. A review of 56 cases. Cancer. 1987;59(3):572–7. PubMed.
15. Varadhachary GR, Karanth S, Qiao W, Carlson HR, Raber MN, Hainsworth JD, et al. Carcinoma of unknown primary with gastrointestinal profile: immunohistochemistry and survival data for this favorable subset. Int J Clin Oncol. 2013;28. PubMed.
16. Greco FA, Vaughn WK, Hainsworth JD. Advanced poorly differentiated carcinoma of unknown primary site: recognition of a treatable syndrome. Ann Intern Med. 1986;104(4):547–53. PubMed.
17. Hainsworth JD, Johnson DH, Greco FA. Cisplatin-based combination chemotherapy in the treatment of poorly differentiated carcinoma and poorly differentiated adenocarcinoma of unknown primary site: results of a 12-year experience. J Clin Oncol. 1992;10(6):912–22. PubMed.
18. Hainsworth JD, Wright EP, Johnson DH, Davis BW, Greco FA. Poorly differentiated carcinoma of unknown primary site: clinical usefulness of immunoperoxidase staining. J Clin Oncol. 1991;9(11):1931–8. PubMed.
19. Hainsworth JD, Spigel DR, Thompson DS, Murphy PB, Lane CM, Waterhouse DM, et al. Paclitaxel/carboplatin plus bevacizumab/erlotinib in the first-line treatment of patients with carcinoma of unknown primary site. Oncologist. 2009;14(12):1189–97. PubMed.
20. Huebner G, Link H, Kohne CH, Stahl M, Kretzschmar A, Steinbach S, et al. Paclitaxel and carboplatin vs gemcitabine and vinorelbine in patients with adeno- or undifferentiated carcinoma of unknown primary: a randomised prospective phase II trial. Br J Cancer. 2009;100(1):44–9. PubMed.
21. Stoyianni A, Pentheroudakis G, Pavlidis N. Neuroendocrine carcinoma of unknown primary: a systematic review of the literature and a comparative study with other neuroendocrine tumors. Cancer Treat Rev. 2011;37(5):358–65. PubMed.
22. Kamposioras K, Pentheroudakis G, Pectasides D, Pavlidis N. Malignant melanoma of unknown primary site. To make the long story short. A systematic review of the literature. Crit Rev Oncol Hematol. 2011;78(2):112–26. PubMed.
23. Finn L, Markovic SN, Joseph RW. Therapy for metastatic melanoma: the past, present, and future. BMC Med. 2012;10:23. PubMed Central PMCID: 3308914.
24. Girotti MR, Saturno G, Lorigan P, Marais R. No longer an untreatable disease: how targeted and immunotherapies have changed the management of melanoma patients. Mol Oncol. 2014;8(6):1140–58. PubMed.
25. Robert C, Long GV, Brady B, Dutriaux C, Maio M, Mortier L, et al. Nivolumab in previously untreated melanoma without BRAF mutation. N Engl J Med. 2015;372(4):320–30. PubMed.
26. Postow MA, Chesney J, Pavlick AC, Robert C, Grossmann K, McDermott D, et al. Nivolumab and ipilimumab versus ipilimumab in untreated melanoma. New Engl J Med. 2015;372:2006–17.
27. Pavlidis N, Petrakis D, Golfinopoulos V, Pentheroudakis G. Long-term survivors among patients with cancer of unknown primary. Crit Rev Oncol Hematol. 2012;84(1):85–92. PubMed.
28. Gartrell BA, Saad F. Managing bone metastases and reducing skeletal related events in prostate cancer. Nat Rev Clin Oncol. 2014;11(6):335–45. PubMed.
29. Pentheroudakis G, Golfinopoulos V, Pavlidis N. Switching benchmarks in cancer of unknown primary: from autopsy to microarray. Eur J Cancer. 2007;43(14):2026–36. PubMed.

30. Altman E, Cadman E. An analysis of 1539 patients with cancer of unknown primary site. Cancer. 1986;57(1):120–4. PubMed.
31. Alberts AS, Falkson G, Falkson HC, van der Merwe MP. Treatment and prognosis of metastatic carcinoma of unknown primary: analysis of 100 patients. Med Pediatr Oncol. 1989;17(3):188–92. PubMed.
32. Pavlidis N, Kalef-Ezra J, Briassoulis E, Skarlos D, Kosmidis P, Saferiadis K, et al. Evaluation of six tumor markers in patients with carcinoma of unknown primary. Med Pediatr Oncol. 1994;22(3):162–7. PubMed.
33. Abbruzzese JL, Abbruzzese MC, Hess KR, Raber MN, Lenzi R, Frost P. Unknown primary carcinoma: natural history and prognostic factors in 657 consecutive patients. J Clin Oncol. 1994;12(6):1272–80. PubMed.
34. Hess KR, Abbruzzese MC, Lenzi R, Raber MN, Abbruzzese JL. Classification and regression tree analysis of 1000 consecutive patients with unknown primary carcinoma. Clin Cancer Res. 1999;5(11):3403–10. PubMed.
35. van de Wouw AJ, Janssen-Heijnen ML, Coebergh JW, Hillen HF. Epidemiology of unknown primary tumours; incidence and population-based survival of 1285 patients in Southeast Netherlands, 1984–1992. Eur J Cancer. 2002;38(3):409–13. PubMed.
36. Culine S, Kramar A, Saghatchian M, Bugat R, Lesimple T, Lortholary A, et al. Development and validation of a prognostic model to predict the length of survival in patients with carcinomas of an unknown primary site. J Clin Oncol. 2002;20(24):4679–83. PubMed.
37. van de Wouw AJ, Jansen RL, Griffioen AW, Hillen HF. Clinical and immunohistochemical analysis of patients with unknown primary tumour. A search for prognostic factors in UPT. Anticancer Res. 2004;24(1):297–301. PubMed.
38. Seve P, Ray-Coquard I, Trillet-Lenoir V, Sawyer M, Hanson J, Broussolle C, et al. Low serum albumin levels and liver metastasis are powerful prognostic markers for survival in patients with carcinomas of unknown primary site. Cancer. 2006;107(11):2698–705. PubMed.
39. Ponce Lorenzo J, Segura Huerta A, Diaz Beveridge R, Gimenez Ortiz A, Aparisi Aparisi F, Fleitas Kanonnikoff T, et al. Carcinoma of unknown primary site: development in a single institution of a prognostic model based on clinical and serum variables. Clin Transl Oncol. 2007;9(7):452–8. PubMed.
40. Trivanovic D, Petkovic M, Stimac D. New prognostic index to predict survival in patients with cancer of unknown primary site with unfavourable prognosis. Clin Oncol. 2009;21(1):43–8. PubMed.
41. Thöm I, Rogers C, Andritzky B, Witzel I, Schuch G, Hossfeld DK, et al. Single-center management of 136 patients with cancer of unknown primary site (CUP syndrome) over a period of 10 years. Onkologie. 2009;32(12):741–6. PubMed.
42. Fernandez-Cotarelo MJ, Guerra-Vales JM, Colina F, de la Cruz J. Prognostic factors in cancer of unknown primary site. Tumori. 2010;96(1):111–6. PubMed.
43. Petrakis D, Pentheroudakis G, Voulgaris E, Pavlidis N. Prognostication in cancer of unknown primary (CUP): development of a prognostic algorithm in 311 cases and review of the literature. Cancer Treat Rev. 2013;39(7):701–8. PubMed.
44. Lenzi R, Hess KR, Abbruzzese MC, Raber MN, Ordonez NG, Abbruzzese JL. Poorly differentiated carcinoma and poorly differentiated adenocarcinoma of unknown origin: favorable subsets of patients with unknown-primary carcinoma? J Clin Oncol. 1997;15(5):2056–66. PubMed.
45. Oken MM, Creech RH, Tormey DC, Horton J, Davis TE, McFadden ET, et al. Toxicity and response criteria of the Eastern Cooperative Oncology Group. Am J Clin Oncol. 1982;5(6):649–55. PubMed.
46. van der Gaast A, Verweij J, Planting AS, Hop WC, Stoter G. Simple prognostic model to predict survival in patients with undifferentiated carcinoma of unknown primary site. J Clin Oncol. 1995;13(7):1720–5. PubMed.

47. Kodaira M, Takahashi S, Yamada S, Ueda K, Mishima Y, Takeuchi K, et al. Bone metastasis and poor performance status are prognostic factors for survival of carcinoma of unknown primary site in patients treated with systematic chemotherapy. Ann Oncol. 2010;21(6):1163–7. PubMed.
48. Pasterz R, Savaraj N, Burgess M. Prognostic factors in metastatic carcinoma of unknown primary. J Clin Oncol. 1986;4(11):1652–7. PubMed.
49. Piga A, Gesuita R, Catalano V, Nortilli R, Cetto G, Cardillo F, et al. Identification of clinical prognostic factors in patients with unknown primary tumors treated with a platinum-based combination. Oncology. 2005;69(2):135–44. PubMed.

Chapter 5
Diagnostic Work-up of CUP: An Approach to Current Recommendations and Underlying Evidence

Alwin Krämer and Harald Löffler

5.1 Introduction

It is frequently claimed that there are evidence-based standard recommendations for the diagnostic work-up and subsequent management of CUP. However, the deeper one digs into the current literature, the less clear matters become. For example, many remarks that have been passed on from one review to another as established facts turn out to be based on clearly outdated original data since diagnostic and therapeutic possibilities have changed over time. Another major problem is the lack of comparability of patient selection between different studies not only because of differing definitions of CUP but also due to the advancement of diagnostic standards.

To give one example, in the 1980s, poorly differentiated carcinoma (PDC) was established as a prognostically favorable CUP subgroup, with a subset of patients enjoying long-term survival [1, 2]. A substantial fraction of this subgroup showed features of germ cell cancer. Since then, PDC compatible with germ cell cancer is listed among prognostically favorable CUP subgroups in guidelines. However, current immunohistochemical standards to distinguish lymphoma from carcinoma were not available for these early studies. Therefore, a substantial proportion of these long-term survivors might have had lymphoma, which is also supported by original data from one of the cited publications where the diagnosis of some cases originally classified as PDC was retrospectively reclassified as being lymphoma on the basis of immunostaining, which was introduced as a novel method at the time [2, 3].

These considerations prompted us to start the chapters dedicated to diagnostic work-up of CUP with some general remarks about what evidence tells us, how this

A. Krämer (✉) • H. Löffler
Clinical Cooperation Unit Molecular Hematology/Oncology, German Cancer Research Center (DKFZ) and University of Heidelberg, Heidelberg, Germany
e-mail: a.kraemer@Dkfz-Heidelberg.de; h.loeffler@Dkfz-Heidelberg.de

A. Krämer, H. Löffler (eds.), *Cancer of Unknown Primary*,
DOI 10.1007/978-3-319-22581-4_5

is translated into current guidelines, and what we conclude therefrom for practice of patient care.

5.2 Extensive Work-up or Pragmatic and Fast Decision Process?

A general rule is that every medical intervention requires appropriate diagnostics. In the case of CUP, we tend to feel some unrest because we have not been able to find or define the primary, which might drive us towards exhaustive diagnostic studies. However, we should take into account that the median life expectancy of a CUP patient is, at best, in the range of 1 year, and exhausting all up-to-date diagnostic possibilities before starting treatment might take several weeks to months, while the patient might suffer from symptoms and there usually is no cure anyway. With regard to the latter point, we should also consider whether the result of a specific diagnostic study will affect prognosis or not or whether there might be any other benefit to the patient.

Thinking about whether specific procedures should be part of routine diagnostics, it is again helpful to look at history and tradition. For example, colonoscopy was invented before the routine use of immunohistochemistry and modern cross-sectional imaging, and without the latter methodologies, it indeed made sense to routinely perform colonoscopy when searching for a primary lesion of an adenocarcinoma. Nowadays, if an adenocarcinoma expresses CK7 in the absence of CK20 and CDX2 (the majority of cases), and there is no sign of colorectal cancer in the CT scan, a colorectal primary is extremely unlikely, making colonoscopy unnecessary in this specific setting (while colonoscopy is warranted if immunohistochemistry is suggestive of colorectal carcinoma).

On the other hand, there are subgroups of CUP patients with a better prognosis, some of whom might even enjoy long-term survival if treated correctly. Hence, apart from excluding conditions other than CUP like lymphoma or mesothelioma, the main task is to exclude or confirm whether a patient belongs to one of these subgroups, which are discussed in detail in other chapters of this book.

5.3 The Implementation of Novel Methods into Routine Diagnostics – Chances and Caveats

Oncologists are constantly confronted with novel possibilities regarding both diagnostics and therapy, which provide otherwise incurable cancer patients with new hope. This hope and its biased perception by patients and physicians may induce fast-track implementation of such novel possibilities into clinical practice. On the other hand, ideally, every medical intervention should be based on a properly designed randomized controlled trial. In case of CUP, there is a substantial divergence between novel possibilities on one hand and evidence-based data on the other hand. We will briefly discuss some examples.

^{18}F-deoxyglucose (FDG)-PET/CT combines a CT scan, as standard for the workup of CUP patients, with metabolic labeling of cancer cells, which should in theory increase sensitivity and specificity for tumor detection. In fact, a meta-analysis covering 10 original publications came to the conclusion that FDG-PET (with or without CT) led to the detection of previously unrecognized metastases in 37 % and altered clinical management in 34.7 % of patients [4]. However, in only 2 out of the 10 studies included in this meta-analysis, a CT scan of the chest, abdomen, and pelvis was a regular part of the workup of CUP patients before FDG-PET was performed as additional test [4]. Therefore, in settings where high-resolution CT scans are routinely performed, the additional value of FDG-PET will probably be lower. Moreover, even if we assume that FDG-PET/CT will yield identification of hitherto undetected primaries in a fraction of cases, it still has to be proven that this will lead to a survival benefit. Finally, depending on the specific clinical setting, patient access to FDG-PET/CT might be limited, which might delay therapy. On the other hand, a timely FDG-PET/CT might save time and avoid further tests. This issue will be discussed in greater detail in the next chapter, but for now, it may be concluded that the value of FDG-PET/CT depends on the specific clinical setting.

Gene expression profiling, assessing expression levels of selected messenger or micro-RNAs, has clearly augmented the repertoire to assign a likely site of origin in CUP patients. Today, two tests are commercially available, assigning a single site of origin in 80 % of cases or more, performing well in correctly classifying cancers of known origin, and correlating well with primary sites suggested by clinical staging and immunohistochemistry [5, 6]. These tests will be discussed in Chap. 11 in greater detail. Here, we would like to point to the practical differences regarding the use of gene expression profiling in different countries: While these tests are covered by the Medicare health insurance in the USA and therefore can be widely offered to CUP patients, they are not covered by health insurances in Germany (and, as far as we know, most other countries throughout Europe and the world) and therefore cannot be offered easily to CUP patients here. In general, a site-of-origin assignment does only improve prognosis if a treatment for the identified site of origin exists that is superior to the therapy which would have been given without this information. In this regard, it is relevant that with the combined use of clinical staging and state-of-the-art immunohistochemistry, important subgroups in which a site-specific therapy leads to improved survival, such as CUP with immunohistochemical features of colorectal adenocarcinoma, can be identified with high accuracy also without gene expression profiling and that for the majority of the remaining cases, treatment schedules do not dramatically differ between CUP protocols and protocols for sites of origin typically underlying CUP, e.g., lung cancer. Moreover, as discussed in Chap. 3, there might be biological differences between a CUP originating from a given organ and the respective typical organ cancer with obvious primary. Hence, although these differences are still somewhat elusive, it cannot simply be assumed that a site-specific therapy is equally effective in a CUP assigned to the respective site of origin. All these arguments lead to the conclusion that a superiority of a therapeutic algorithm based on site-of-origin assignment by gene expression profiling, as compared to a conventional approach without gene expression profiling, should be tested in a randomized controlled trial. Up to now, only phase II data exist, showing that the gene expression-directed approach yields an overall survival of about 1 year [7], which is similar to what can be reached by nonspecific approaches [8]. Therefore, the results of randomized controlled trials such as the GEFCAPI 04 trial, a phase III trial of a French cooperative group [9], are eagerly awaited.

In addition to gene expression profiling, next-generation sequencing might become another important diagnostic tool for CUP since in principle, it might likewise be applicable to assign sites of origin, while in addition, detected molecular aberrations might be useful to predict response to molecularly targeted drugs [10]. Establishment of the clinical use of this method is far less advanced than for gene expression profiling [10]. On the other hand, mutation analysis of specific genes is already established in many clinical settings, e.g., analysis of EGF receptor mutations in lung cancer or RAS mutations in colorectal cancer, which both are important for the choice of therapy. We therefore believe that work-up of CUP patients should include mutation analysis of specific genes whenever clinical findings are suggestive for a specific entity warranting the respective analysis. This implies that in many cases of CUP, sequencing of a panel of relevant genes is justified.

All these examples suggest that there is no simple answer regarding if and when to introduce novel methods into clinical practice. The usefulness of a novel diagnostic method may depend on the specific setting, i.e., which routine methods are otherwise established in the work-up of CUP patients. This fact impedes the generalizability of study results regarding such novel methods. In practice, if an added benefit attributed to the additional use of a novel method appears plausible but has not formally been proven, it is a matter of not only medical but also political debate whether or not to use this method, which not only implies consideration of risks and benefits but also of cost-effectiveness. At this point, we will turn towards our own practical approach to the diagnostic workup of CUP patients, keeping in mind that this applies to a relatively restrictive setting regarding fast-track implementation of novel methods.

5.4 Practical Approach to the Diagnostic Work-up of CUP Patients

The starting point of the diagnostic work-up of a CUP patient is either a symptom or sign which gave reason for screening tests, e.g., ultrasound, or suspicious lesions were unexpectedly detected by a routine test or a diagnostic imaging performed for unrelated reasons (Fig. 5.1). If malignancy is suspected, the next task is to obtain a suitable biopsy for histology, preferably by means of core needle or excisional biopsy. Selection of an appropriate site for such a biopsy often already prompts

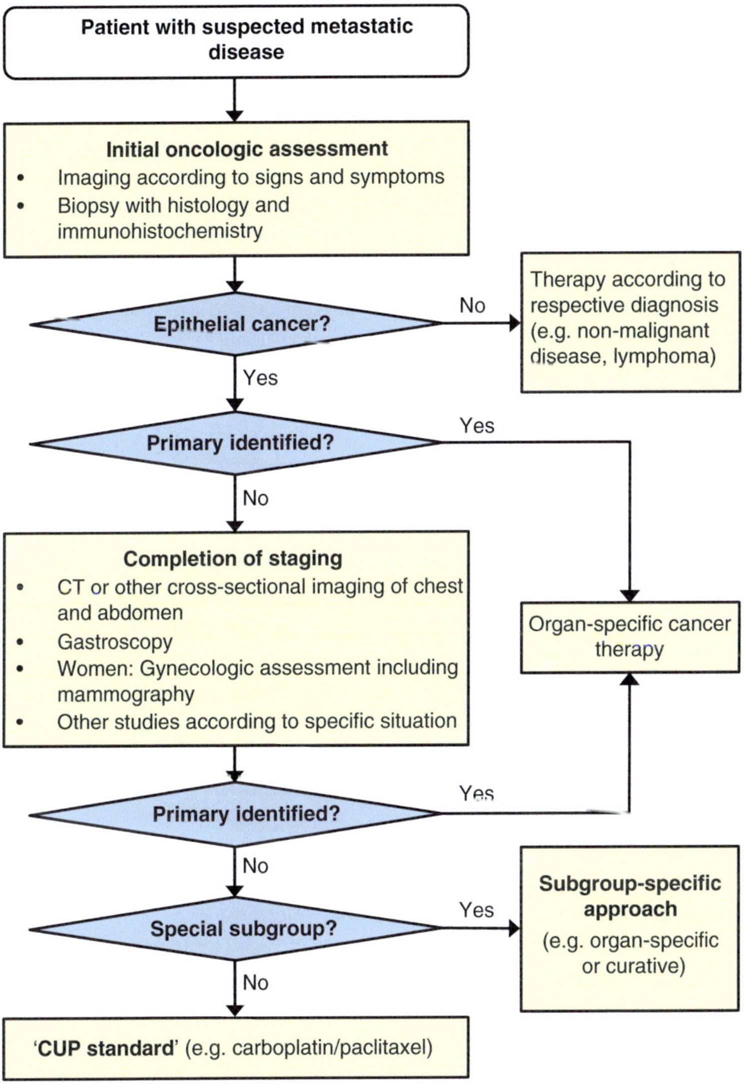

Fig. 5.1 Diagnostic workup of CUP patients. See text for discussion and further details

cross-sectional imaging. Histological diagnostics including appropriate immunohistochemistry and, where applicable, hypothesis-driven molecular diagnostics, which are covered in detail in Chap. 7, will guide the further clinical workup. Apart from a careful history and physical examination, this workup should always include cross-sectional imaging of chest and abdomen, usually by CT scan, which will also be important as baseline test for subsequent response assessment during therapy. Therefore, the interval between cross-sectional imaging and initiation of anticancer treatment should be as short as possible.

As stated before, exhaustive diagnostics regardless of expected benefit should be avoided in CUP patients. Indeed, apart from state-of-the-art histological (and possibly molecular) diagnostics and complete cross-sectional imaging, the relative contribution of additional tests to the diagnostic work-up is small. Of course, a blood test will be done, and routine parameters such as LDH will provide important information about prognosis (see previous chapter). Moreover, serum tumor markers should be evaluated, most importantly AFP, β-HCG, and, in men, PSA, which might hint at specific subgroups (see previous chapter). In addition, the most common tumor markers should be tested, e.g., in adenocarcinoma, CEA and CA 19–9, and in women, CA 125 and CA 15–3. These markers have a low diagnostic value but might be valuable for monitoring of subsequent anticancer therapy.

Gastroscopy is usually recommended since esophageal and gastric cancers often lack histologic or immunohistochemical features clearly distinguishing them from other primary sites, which implies that in the vast majority of CUP cases, they have to be considered as differential diagnoses. Taken together with its low risk of adverse events, the benefit-risk profile appears to favor the routine use of gastroscopy. Nevertheless, gastroscopy might be dispensable if histology and localization pattern clearly argue against a primary in the upper gastrointestinal tract.

As already discussed, we do not think that colonoscopy should be routinely performed in all CUP patients since immunohistochemistry typically performs well in distinguishing between colorectal cancer (positive for CK20 and CDX2 in the absence of CK7) and other primary origins [11]. There is usually no need for endoscopic confirmation that a CK7-positive, CK20-negative cancer does not originate from the colorectum. If there is any suspicion of colorectal cancer, e.g., histological clues, suspicious lesions detected by imaging, clinical symptoms or signs, then colonoscopy is warranted. Likewise, bronchoscopy should be reserved to patients with a clinical suspicion of lung cancer, also keeping in mind that CT scans are quite sensitive for detection of lung cancer. It will be unlikely to find a malignant lesion by bronchoscopy if the CT scan has been unsuspicious.

In women, screening for breast cancer, usually by palpation, ultrasound, and mammography, optionally supported by MRI, should be part of the standard workup, again with the exception of circumstances clearly arguing against breast cancer as the primary origin. We will not discuss here the different imaging modalities used for breast cancer screening in detail since they are covered in the next chapter. Routine work-up of female CUP patients should furthermore include a complete gynecological examination and transvaginal ultrasound.

Some authors recommend transrectal ultrasound of the prostate as part of the routine work-up of male CUP patients. However, metastatic prostate cancer usually shows several distinct characteristics like PSA elevation, osteoblastic lesions, and some immunohistochemical clues. In the absence of such characteristics, we do not see a clear indication for transrectal ultrasound. Hence, the serum PSA level is the only specific parameter that should be assessed with respect to prostate cancer as part of the routine work-up.

An important and well-defined specific constellation is the exclusive or predominant affection of cervical lymph nodes by squamous cell carcinoma or another cancer subtype compatible with head and neck cancer. In addition to the abovementioned studies, a panendoscopy of the upper aerodigestive tract (pharyngoscopy including nasopharynx, laryngoscopy, and esophagoscopy) should be performed, usually including directed biopsies and bilateral tonsillectomy in case of squamous cell carcinoma since the tonsils are frequent sites of hidden primaries, although there is some controversy whether tonsillectomy should be performed generally, or what the indications for tonsillectomy should be [12, 13]. It should also be noted that FDG-PET/CT is more established in this situation than for CUP in general. This will be discussed in greater detail in the next chapter.

The studies listed up to now may be amended due to individual considerations, i.e., if a clear hypothesis favoring a specified organ site exists. Again, we would like to emphasize that extensive studies in order to follow any vague possibility should be avoided since they rarely retrieve helpful results while delaying therapy.

5.5 Conclusion

In the next chapters, we will discuss specific diagnostic studies in greater detail. It should be kept in mind that the major aim of the diagnostic work-up of CUP patients is the identification of subgroups that should be treated differently and may have a better prognosis than "standard" CUP. Diagnostic studies that do not serve this aim should be avoided.

References

1. Greco FA, Vaughn WK, Hainsworth JD. Advanced poorly differentiated carcinoma of unknown primary site: recognition of a treatable syndrome. Ann Intern Med. 1986;104(4):547–53. PubMed.
2. Hainsworth JD, Johnson DH, Greco FA. Cisplatin-based combination chemotherapy in the treatment of poorly differentiated carcinoma and poorly differentiated adenocarcinoma of unknown primary site: results of a 12-year experience. J Clin Oncol. 1992;10(6):912–22. PubMed.
3. Hainsworth JD, Wright EP, Johnson DH, Davis BW, Greco FA. Poorly differentiated carcinoma of unknown primary site: clinical usefulness of immunoperoxidase staining. J Clin Oncol. 1991;9(11):1931–8. PubMed.
4. Seve P, Billotey C, Broussolle C, Dumontet C, Mackey JR. The role of 2-deoxy-2-[F-18] fluoro-D-glucose positron emission tomography in disseminated carcinoma of unknown primary site. Cancer. 2007;109(2):292–9. PubMed.
5. Meiri E, Mueller WC, Rosenwald S, Zepeniuk M, Klinke E, Edmonston TB, et al. A second-generation microRNA-based assay for diagnosing tumor tissue origin. Oncologist. 2012;17(6):801–12. PubMed Central PMCID: 3380879.
6. Erlander MG, Ma XJ, Kesty NC, Bao L, Salunga R, Schnabel CA. Performance and clinical evaluation of the 92-gene real-time PCR assay for tumor classification. J Mol Diagn. 2011;13(5):493–503. PubMed Central PMCID: 3157614.
7. Hainsworth JD, Rubin MS, Spigel DR, Boccia RV, Raby S, Quinn R, et al. Molecular gene expression profiling to predict the tissue of origin and direct site-specific therapy in patients

with carcinoma of unknown primary site: a prospective trial of the Sarah cannon research institute. J Clin Oncol. 2013;31(2):217–23. PubMed.

8. Hainsworth JD, Spigel DR, Thompson DS, Murphy PB, Lane CM, Waterhouse DM, et al. Paclitaxel/carboplatin plus bevacizumab/erlotinib in the first-line treatment of patients with carcinoma of unknown primary site. Oncologist. 2009;14(12):1189–97. PubMed.
9. Martineau G, Laplanche A, Van de Wouw AW, Gedske Daugaard G, Balana C, Penel N, et al. GEFCAPI 04: a phase III trial comparing a treatment oriented by a molecular analysis with CancerTYPE ID test to cisplatin-gemcitabine in patients with carcinoma of an unknown primary (CUP). J Clin Oncol. 2014;32, TPS11134.
10. Tothill RW, Li J, Mileshkin L, Doig K, Siganakis T, Cowin P, et al. Massively-parallel sequencing assists the diagnosis and guided treatment of cancers of unknown primary. J Pathol. 2013;4. PubMed.
11. Varadhachary GR, Karanth S, Qiao W, Carlson HR, Raber MN, Hainsworth JD, et al. Carcinoma of unknown primary with gastrointestinal profile: immunohistochemistry and survival data for this favorable subset. Int J Clin Oncol. 2013;28. PubMed.
12. Strojan P, Ferlito A, Medina JE, Woolgar JA, Rinaldo A, Robbins KT, et al. Contemporary management of lymph node metastases from an unknown primary to the neck: I. A review of diagnostic approaches. Head Neck. 2013;35(1):123–32. PubMed.
13. Cerezo L, Raboso E, Ballesteros AI. Unknown primary cancer of the head and neck: a multidisciplinary approach. Clin Transl Oncol. 2011;13(2):88–97. PubMed.

Chapter 6
The Radiologist's Approach to CUP

Philipp M. Kazmierczak, Axel Rominger, and Clemens C. Cyran

6.1 Introduction

In 2–4 % of patients with histologically proven cancer, the primary tumor cannot be localized, even by use of modern diagnostic methods. This situation is clinically described as cancer of unknown primary (CUP) [1, 2] and has a frequency similar to pancreatic cancer, renal cell carcinoma, or leukemia [3]. Even after extensive diagnostic workup using state-of-the-art methods, less than 20 % of primary tumors are localized antemortem, compared to almost 80 % of primary tumors identified in postmortem autopsy series [4].

CUP tumors are adenocarcinomas in 40–60 %, undifferentiated carcinomas in 15–20 %, squamous cell carcinomas in 5–8 %, and neuroendocrine tumors in 3–5 %; 1–3 % of all CUP belong to other entities [5]. Most frequently, primary tumors are localized in the lung (20–35 %) and the pancreas (15–20 %), followed by other gastrointestinal and gynecological malignancies. Median survival in this heterogenic group of cancer patients is only 3–11 months [6]. Imaging is essential in all four steps of the diagnostic and therapeutic management of CUP patients [7]: localization of the primary tumor, identification of all manifestations, identification of potentially treatable tumors (i.e., breast cancer, prostate carcinoma, lymphoma, etc.), and characterization of the clinicopathological entity and stratification into subsets with favorable prognosis (approximately 20 %) with differentiated and/or chemosensitive tumors for which specific treatment options are available and, on

P.M. Kazmierczak, MD • C.C. Cyran, MD (✉)
Institut für Klinische Radiologie, Klinikum der Universität München – Campus Großhadern, Marchioninistraße 15, 81377 Munich, Germany
e-mail: Clemens.Cyran@med.lmu.de

A. Rominger, MD
Klinik und Poliklinik für Nuklearmedizin, Klinikum der Universität München – Campus Großhadern, Marchioninistraße 15, 81377 Munich, Germany

A. Krämer, H. Löffler (eds.), *Cancer of Unknown Primary*,
DOI 10.1007/978-3-319-22581-4_6

the other hand, subsets with unfavorable prognosis without clear categorization (approximately 80 %) [6].

Using modern imaging methods, the detection rate for primary tumors in CUP has increased [8]. Numerable factors influence the prognosis in patients with CUP: age, sex, general condition, weight loss, histopathology, serum tumor markers, tumor burden, tumor localization, and metastatic pattern. These factors contribute to the differentiation between favorable and unfavorable subsets [9], with direct implications on the therapeutic management [10].

Imaging is of headmost importance for the reliable evaluation of tumor burden, tumor/metastatic localization, and metastatic pattern, most eminently computed tomography (CT) for whole-body staging and magnetic resonance imaging (MRI) for local tumor staging [7]. According to international guidelines (www.esmo.org, www.nccn.org), the minimum diagnostic program in patients with CUP includes clinical history and examination, lab work, as well as CT of the neck, chest, and abdomen. In women, additional mammography and transvaginal ultrasound are recommended, while male patients should undergo transrectal prostate ultrasound [11, 12]. Generally, clinical workup and the search for potential primary tumors should always follow diagnostic algorithms that balance potential benefits in survival for the patient against expenditure of time and financial aspects.

6.2 Computed Tomography (CT)

In the diagnostic algorithm of CUP, CT finds broad application for localization of the primary tumor and staging of disease, although only few studies provide detailed evidence-based data in support of its diagnostic role in CUP. CT has a high sensitivity for tumors which frequently present as metastasized disease, e.g., lung cancer, pancreatic adenocarcinoma, colon carcinoma, and renal cell carcinoma [7]. In a study with 879 patients initially presenting with metastatic disease without primary, CT was diagnostic in 86 % of patients with pancreatic carcinoma, in 36 % of patients with colon carcinoma, and in 74 % of patients with lung cancer, having an overall diagnostic accuracy of 55 % [11, 13]. CT also proved valuable for the identification of lung, liver, lymph node, and bone metastases. A meta-analysis of patient populations with metastasized head and neck squamous cell carcinoma found a detection rate for the primary tumor for CT of 22 %, for MRI of 36 %, and for combined positron-emission tomography (PET)-CT with ^{18}F-fluorodeoxyglucose (FDG) of 28–57 % [14].

In the diagnostic algorithm of CUP, particularly favorable subsets have to be identified at initial staging to allow for immediate treatment of patients with established therapy regimens and documented improved outcome [7]. At the beginning of the diagnostic algorithm, whole-body imaging is recommended to identify typical patterns of metastasis. In the case of multiple lung and liver lesions paired with paraaortic lymphadenopathy and splenomegaly, lymphoma should be mentioned as possible differential diagnosis in the report. In young men with mediastinal and/or retroperitoneal masses (midline disease) as well as extensive metastasis to the lung, liver, bone, and more rarely to the central nervous system, a possible differential diagnosis is extra-gonadal germ cell tumor [7]. However, also benign diseases mimicking malignoma have to be considered in the differential diagnosis of CUP. Multifocal osteolytic and/or osteoblastic lesions may also be consistent with Paget's disease [7]. Differential diagnosis of pulmonary nodules includes pneumonia, sarcoidosis, or hamartoma, and it is important to take all available clinical information into account.

In the diagnosis of a pulmonary primary tumor, chest CT has been shown to be superior to conventional X-ray [15]. Furthermore, chest CT allows for the additional identification of pulmonary nodules, the assessment of mediastinal lymphadenopathy, as well as the identification of lesions most suitable for biopsy. A study by Latief and coworkers investigated 32 patients with cerebral metastases and without initial primary tumor. Thirty-one patients were eventually diagnosed with lung carcinoma that were identified on conventional X-ray in 19 cases (61 %) and in chest CT in all 31 cases (100 %) [15]. Although chest CT demonstrated the highest sensitivity for the detection of the primary tumor in these cases, additional CT of the abdomen is recommended, as the primary tumor is frequently located below the diaphragm. CT exams have to be performed state-of-the-art with acquisition of an arterial phase of the abdomen, followed by a venous phase of the thorax and abdomen, as arterial phase scans of the abdomen allow for the detection of hypervascular neoplasms, such as neuroendocrine tumors [16].

6.3 Hybrid Imaging: PET/CT and PET/MRI

Smaller lesions may evade detection by CT – a particular problem in CUP [17]. The combination with ^{18}F-FDG PET has been shown to increase sensitivity [18]; however, because of cost and restricted availability, hybrid imaging with PET/CT is frequently limited to patients in good general condition and negative CT. ^{18}F-FDG is the most commonly used radiotracer in PET/CT imaging, due to the well-documented increased ^{18}F-FDG avidity of many tumor entities [19]. Accordingly, most studies investigating the value of PET/CT for CUP detection and staging have been performed using ^{18}F-FDG.

6.3.1 Cervical CUP

Around 50–70 % of cervical lymph node metastases derive from squamous cell carcinoma located in the head and neck region, especially if the lymph nodes are located in the upper two thirds of the neck [20]. Metastatic disease in the lower third of the neck is often caused by extracervical primaries, predominantly adenocarcinomas located below the level of the clavicles [20]. Cervical CUP is considered a favorable, i.e., potentially curable subset, and therefore any effort should be taken in order to assure a timely identification of the primary. ^{18}F-FDG PET/CT has been found to have a higher sensitivity for primary detection in cervical CUP as compared to contrast-enhanced CT and MRI [21]. In a prospective study, Lee and coworkers investigated patients with histologically proven cervical metastases in whom clinical and panendoscopic evaluation failed to detect the primary tumor. ^{18}F-FDG PET/CT provided a significantly higher sensitivity (69 %) than contrast-enhanced CT (16 %) and the combination contrast-enhanced CT and MRI (41 %) for identification of the primary site. However, overall sensitivity remained low, and specificities did not differ significantly [21]. It has to be noted that the CT component of the ^{18}F-FDG PET/CT was performed unenhanced in this study, a factor underlining the additional value of the PET component in this cancer subset.

6.3.2 Extracervical CUP

Primary detection in extracervical CUP benefits from ^{18}F-FDG PET/CT as well, but literature data suggest that the additional value of the ^{18}F-FDG PET component is smaller than in cervical CUP. A recent study by Møller et al. found a sensitivity of 71 % and specificity of 58 % for ^{18}F-FDG PET/CT, with a sensitivity of 61 % and a specificity of 65 % for the contrast-enhanced CT component alone, respectively [22]. In addition, ^{18}F-FDG PET/CT allows for a precise assessment of overall disease burden as an imaging biomarker for prediction of overall survival in CUP patients [23]. ^{18}F-FDG PET/CT should be considered in patients with tumor entities with documented ^{18}F-FDG avidity, such as lung tumors, lymphoma, suspected primary colorectal, transitional cell, and cholangiocellular carcinoma, as well as breast and ovarian cancer [24–27]. Limitations of diagnostic sensitivity of ^{18}F-FDG PET/CT exist for tumor entities with reportedly low or missing ^{18}F-FDG avidity, such as renal cell carcinoma, hepatocellular carcinoma, certain mucinous carcinomas, or low-grade lymphomas [28].

According to a report of the German Society of Nuclear Medicine, the most common indications for PET-based imaging (PET and PET/CT) in Germany in 2013 were lung tumors (40 %), lymphoma (8 %), gastrointestinal tumors (5 %), and neuroendocrine tumors (NET, 5 %) [29]. ^{18}F-FDG PET/CT is widely used as imaging standard of reference for bronchial carcinoma and shows a high sensitivity (around 96 %) for the detection of malignant lung nodules. Specificity remains lower (about 80 %), as false-positive results can occur in infectious or granulomatous disease of the lung [30]. Also in lymphoma, an entity with many ^{18}F-FDG-avid subtypes, ^{18}F-FDG PET/CT is now the recommended imaging standard of reference for staging and restaging [31].

6.3.3 CUP of Neuroendocrine Origin

Neuroendocrine tumors (NET) account for 3–5 % of all CUP cases [5]. High expression of somatostatin receptors (SSTR) is a distinct feature of this tumor entity, especially of low-grade variants, making NET eligible for imaging with radiolabeled somatostatin analogues, i.e., ^{68}Ga-DOTATATE [32] (Fig. 6.1). In general, the uptake of SSTR analogs in neuroendocrine tumor is primarily dependent on their degree of differentiation. While low-grade, well-differentiated tumors show high SSTR expression, undifferentiated, high-grade neuroendocrine tumors generally present with poor or without relevant SSTR expression, with a potential risk of negative PET results [33]. A retrospective study by Alonso and coworkers provided evidence for the applicability of ^{68}Ga-DOTATATE PET/CT in CUP of neuroendocrine origin [34]. In the study population, the primary tumor was successfully identified in 59 %. Furthermore, ^{68}Ga-DOTATATE PET/CT revealed additional sites of unsuspected metastatic disease, predominantly lymph nodes and mesentery, and therefore delivered staging information crucial for therapeutic management. Although it is

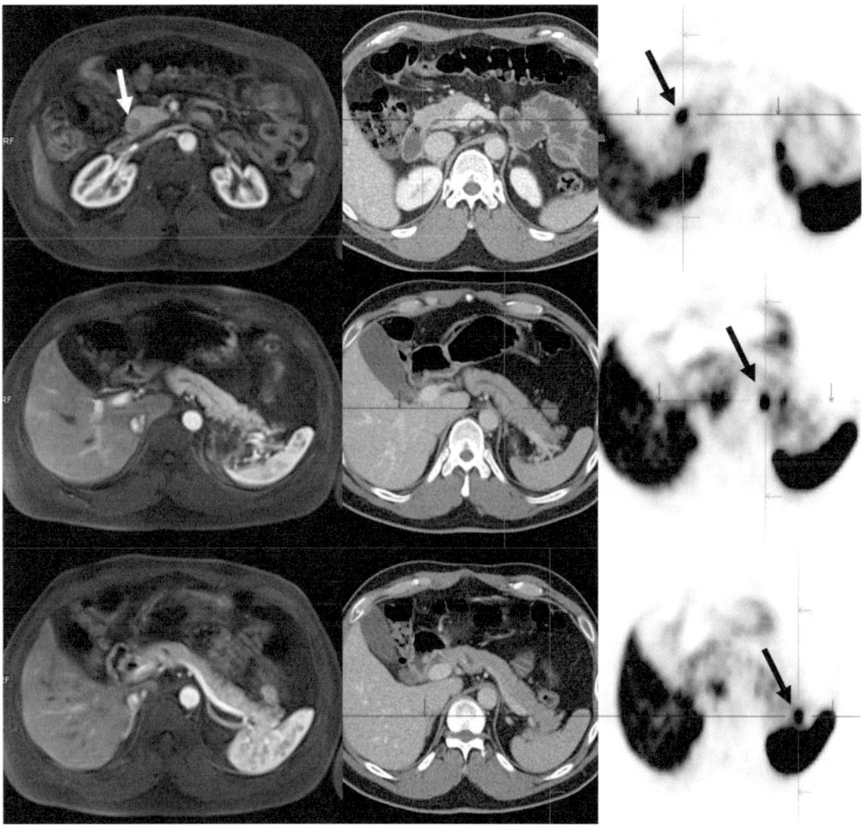

Fig. 6.1 A 43-year-old male patient with multiple endocrine neoplasia syndrome (MEN) type 1. On contrast-enhanced MRI a singular mass in the pancreatic head was observed suspicious for a neuroendocrine tumor (*top row*, *left image*, *white arrow*). ^{68}Ga-DOTATATE PET/CT demonstrated corresponding focal somatostatin receptor overexpression of the mass in the pancreatic head (*top row*, *right image*, *black arrow*) and revealed two more focal DOTATATE accumulations in the pancreatic corpus (*middle row*, *right image*, *black arrow*) and cauda (*bottom row*, *right image*, *black arrow*), consistent with multifocal NET of the pancreas. Note that the focal DOTATATE accumulations in the pancreatic corpus and cauda did not show well-defined correlates on MRI or CT

known that NET show moderate ^{18}F-FDG avidity depending on tumor grade, ^{68}Ga-DOTATATE PET/CT proved to be superior to ^{18}F-FDG PET/CT regarding the staging of well-differentiated NET, while intermediate- to high-grade NET may benefit from the combined, consecutive assessment with both ^{18}F-FDG and ^{68}Ga-DOTATATE [35]. These data suggest that histopathological findings should be taken into account when choosing the appropriate radiotracer for primary detection in CUP of neuroendocrine origin. Last but not least, ^{68}Ga-DOTATATE PET/CT is applicable for the monitoring of peptide receptor radionuclide therapy (i.e., ^{90}Y- and ^{177}Lu-DOTATATE/DOTATOC), delivering noninvasive molecular information on somatostatin receptor expression [36].

6.3.4 Hybrid Imaging for Suspected Prostate Carcinoma

Basic assessment of suspected primary prostate carcinoma in CUP includes digital rectal examination, serum prostate-specific antigen (PSA) levels, and prostate ultrasound. For local staging, the examination protocol can be extended by multiparametric pelvic MRI, which has been shown to detect 90 % of intermediate- and high-risk prostate carcinomas and additionally identifies lesions eligible for biopsy [37]. According to data from the Swedish Cancer Registry, prostate carcinoma accounts for only 2 % of all deaths in CUP, despite a high prevalence, particularly in the elderly population [38]. The reason for this finding is probably the relatively high detection rate of prostate carcinoma during the primary workup, since cases in which the primary tumor is successfully identified will not be classified as CUP. MRI accurately assesses local tumor extent and infiltration (T staging) and therefore helps to distinguish between low- and high-risk carcinomas [39] – differentiation between these subtypes has a direct impact on therapy decisions. Prostate ultrasound and multiparametric pelvic MRI are valuable tools for local tumor staging (T and N staging). However, in order to detect occult primary tumors and distant metastases (M staging), as well as an accurate assessment of the disease burden, whole-body imaging must be performed.

State-of-the-art diagnostic workup in prostate carcinoma includes hybrid whole-body imaging using the dedicated, prostate-specific radiotracer ^{68}Ga-prostate-specific membrane antigen (PSMA). ^{68}Ga-PSMA PET/CT detects a significantly higher rate of prostate carcinomas and associated metastases compared to ^{18}F-fluorocholine-PET/CT [40]. A recent trial investigated PET/MRI and PET/CT with ^{68}Ga-PSMA and found ^{68}Ga-PSMA PET/MRI to detect prostate cancer and its metastases more accurately [41]. According to the authors, this finding may be explained by the fact that MRI can be performed using organ-specific sequences and provides a higher soft tissue resolution and contrast compared to CT [41]. However, the study findings are limited as the PET/MRI examination protocol focused on the abdomen and pelvis and only included the chest if suspicious lesions were detected on the prior PET/CT scan. Furthermore, PET/MRI detected more suspicious lesions, but there was no final histopathological correlation to exclude false-positive and false-negative findings which are known to occur in hybrid imaging [42]. Advantages of PET/MRI include the lack of ionizing radiation for the MRI component, which makes it an attractive tool for repeated examinations, particularly in younger patients. On the contrary, a whole-body CT scan can be completed within several minutes, while whole-body MRI examination protocols including organ-specific sequences may last more than 60 min. In addition to that, PET/MRI is a relatively novel method, and its true diagnostic value for regional and whole-body staging remains to be investigated in prospective studies. To date, no studies exist which investigate PET/MRI for whole-body staging in CUP. An important aspect to consider is the limited availability of PET/MRI, which to date is restricted to few, mainly academic centers. To conclude, hybrid imaging with ^{68}Ga-PSMA has a significant impact on clinical decision-making and therefore plays a central role in the management of prostate carcinoma patients, especially in low PSA tumors [43]. Therefore, hybrid ^{68}Ga-PSMA whole-body imaging may be considered in all CUP patients with suspected prostate carcinoma.

6.4 CT-Guided Biopsy

In CUP, CT imaging also plays an important role for the identification of lesions eligible for biopsy. Representative tissue samples are required for histological, cytological, and immunohistochemical workup in order to diagnose malignancy and narrow down the potential origin of the primary tumor [44]. Besides lesions in the periphery, tumor manifestations may be accessible via endoscopy or bronchoscopy. CT fluoroscopy-guided biopsy (Fig. 6.2) can be applied to sample even central tumor manifestations with great precision by obtaining real-time moving images to control the positioning of the biopsy needle. This is, however, dependent on the exact anatomic localization and the local expertise and availability of interventional radiology [7]. A study by Hewitt et al. in 149 female patients with peritoneal carcinosis reported that CT- and ultrasound-guided core needle biopsies for histological and immunohistochemical workup were diagnostic in 93 % of cases. Re-biopsy was necessary in 7 % of cases in this population of mainly gynecological malignancies (81 %). Despite these limitations, the study demonstrated that CT- and

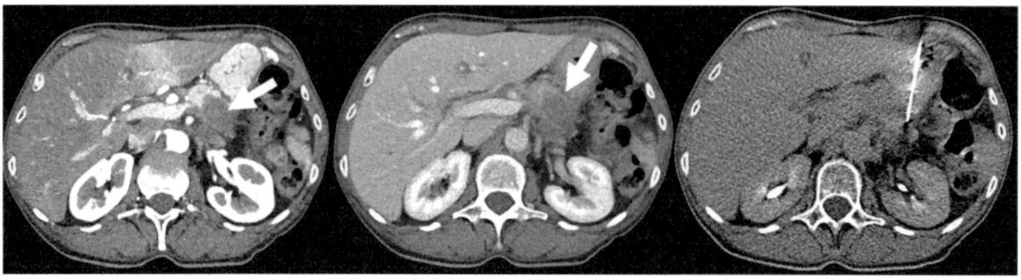

Fig. 6.2 A 57-year-old female patient with an unclear hypodense, hypovascular mass in the pancreatic corpus (*white arrows*). CT-guided transgastral biopsy (*right image*) revealed an undifferentiated ductal adenocarcinoma with CK-7 and CK-20 co-expression and weak, partial expression of CDX-2 (Images courtesy of Tobias Geith, MD)

ultrasound-guided core needle biopsies are a safe and effective diagnostic tool and, under careful consideration of contraindications, may be preferred over open or laparoscopic biopsy [45].

6.5 Magnetic Resonance Imaging (MRI)

MRI allows for staging of malignomas at high soft tissue contrast and spatial resolution [7]. In addition to the depiction of tumor morphology, functional MR imaging techniques are increasingly established for the assessment of various aspects of tumor pathophysiology, including tumor perfusion and diffusivity. Tumor microcirculation can be evaluated using contrast-enhanced or non-contrast-enhanced techniques, with dynamic contrast-enhanced (DCE) imaging as the most widely used method. Diffusion-weighted imaging (DWI) is a noninvasive method reflecting the random Brownian motion of water molecules within the tissue. Although the link between diffusivity and histology is complex, densely cellular tissues exhibit lower diffusion coefficients, and thus diffusion can be useful in tumor characterization. Evidence-based data for the detection of primary tumors using DWI is available for the female breast as well as for the identification of metastasis in whole-body staging [46–48]. Therefore, multiparametric MRI imaging protocols, including morphological and functional sequences, allow for the noninvasive characterization of different aspects of tumor pathophysiology in vivo, with the goal of increased diagnostic accuracy, sensitivity, and specificity.

6.5.1 *Whole-Body MRI*

Whole-body MRI tumor staging protocols can routinely be performed in less than 1 h examination time, depending on the kind and number of sequences acquired [7, 49, 50], as well as on the acquisition of dedicated sequences for potential characterization and local staging of the primary tumor. In some instances, however, a combination of whole-body staging and dedicated imaging of the primary tumor cannot be achieved, e.g., in breast MRI performed in prone position [7]. Whole-body MRI allows for staging of the local lymph nodes (N staging) as well as distant metastases (M staging). However, studies showed that, compared to ^{18}F-FDG PET/CT, conventional MRI sequences have lower sensitivity and specificity for nodal status assessment. For the detection of lymph node metastases, Antoch et al. observed a sensitivity of 93 % for PET/CT and 79 % for whole-body MRI [46]. This may in part be attributed to the superior spatial resolution of CT compared to MRI. Particularly lymph nodes <12 mm and lymph nodes in anatomic regions prone to pulsation and movement artifacts (hilus lymph nodes of the lung, mediastinum, diaphragm) are frequently not adequately detected in MRI [7]. Additionally, hybrid imaging with PET/CT is able to identify morphologically unsuspicious lymph node metastases by focal tracer accumulation and anatomic co-localization with CT, thereby increasing

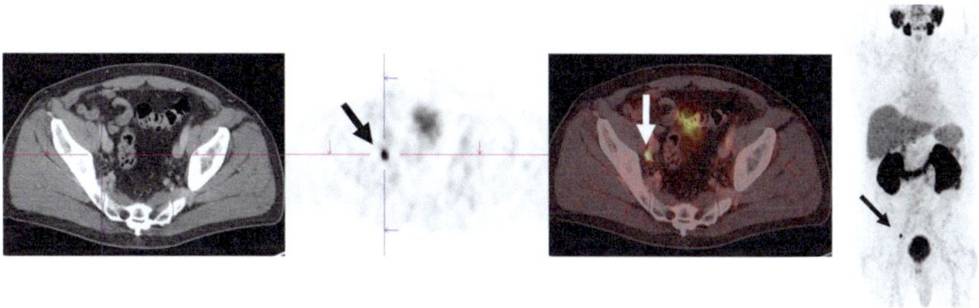

Fig. 6.3 A 67-year-old male with prostate carcinoma following radical prostatectomy 18 months ago and radiotherapy. Increase of prostate-specific antigen (PSA) levels over the last months to 1.5 ng/mL. ^{68}Ga-PSMA PET/CT was performed in search of metastasis and revealed a morphologically unsuspicious lymph node (4 mm) adjacent to the right external iliac artery with focal PSMA uptake (*arrows*). Histology confirmed a right iliac lymph node metastasis of the prostate carcinoma

diagnostic sensitivity (Fig. 6.3). To date, it has not been demonstrated that DWI MRI has the potential to augment diagnostic sensitivity compared to conventional MRI sequences in the identification of lymph node metastases [51]. Improved diagnostic sensitivity of DWI compared to ^{18}F-FDG PET/CT was reported for lung [52] but not for breast cancer [51]. Sensitivity was comparable for the detection of malignant lesions with 94 % for ^{18}F-FDG PET/CT vs. 91 % for whole-body DWI, while specificity was significantly lower for DWI (79 %) than for ^{18}F-FDG PET/CT (99 %). With regard to the identification of distant metastases (M staging), studies report similarly high sensitivity values for DWI and ^{18}F-FDG PET/CT in heterogeneous patient groups with different tumor entities (93–100 %) [46, 53].

Multiparametric MRI, applying different sequences focusing on morphological and functional parameters, is particularly applicable for the detection of metastases in the brain, soft tissue, liver, and muscle. Ultrafast spin-echo sequences, fat-saturated T2-weighted sequences, and contrast-enhanced T1 flash sequences as part of a comprehensive whole-body MRI protocol have been shown to allow for the detection of lung nodules ≤3 mm with similarly high diagnostic sensitivity as compared to multislice CT (MRI sensitivity 87–93 %) [54]. For the detection and characterization of focal liver lesions, multiphasic MRI with contrast-enhanced T1-weighted gradient-echo sequences has been shown to be superior to CT, particularly when imaging with hepatobiliary MRI contrast agents was performed [55].

6.5.2 *MRI for Organ-Specific Staging*

6.5.2.1 Prostate Carcinoma

Multiparametric MRI of the prostate, including high-resolution morphological sequences, diffusion-weighted sequences, and/or dynamic contrast-enhanced sequences and/or spectroscopy, allows for a multi-facetted characterization of gland anatomy as well as physiological processes. Depending on the imaging protocol,

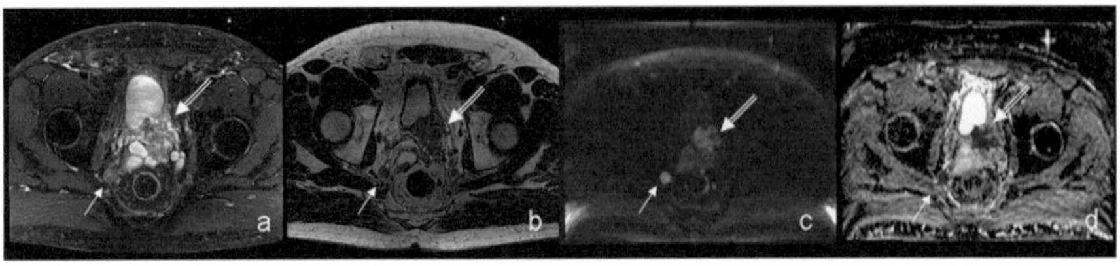

Fig. 6.4 A 68-year-old patient with increased PSA level (6.15 ng/mL). Multiparametric MRI (**a**) axial contrast-enhanced T1w, (**b**) axial T2w, (**c**) DWI b800 with corresponding Apparent Diffusion Coefficient Map, (**d**) revealed a mass (*white open arrow*) in left lobe of the prostate infiltrating the bladder and the seminal vesicles, consistent with a T4 prostate carcinoma. Note the suspicious right iliacal lymph node (*white closed arrow*). Core needle biopsy confirmed a mostly well-differentiated acinar adenocarcinoma of the prostate

prostate MRI can be performed clinically at 1.5 or 3 T with or without endorectal coil. However, several studies demonstrated that at 3 T, overall accuracy, sensitivity, and specificity for local staging in prostate cancer were not significantly different with or without endorectal coil [56]. In prostate carcinoma, conventional MRI sequences are routinely applied for the detection and precise assessment of tumor size and local extension [7, 57]. Abd-Alazeez et al. investigated the diagnostic value of multiparametric MRI in patients diagnosed with occult prostate carcinoma [58] based on negative ultrasound-guided biopsy and persisting elevated PSA levels. The authors reported a sensitivity of 76 % and a specificity of 42 % for the detection of prostate carcinomas ≥4 mm and Gleason score ≥4+3 using a multiparametric MRI protocol (T2, DWI, and dynamic contrast-enhanced MRI) at 1.5 T and 3 T with an endorectal coil. In tumors ≥6 mm and Gleason score ≥3+4, sensitivity increased to 90 % and specificity remained at 42 %. Multiparametric MRI has been shown to identify focal intraglandular lesions occult on transrectal ultrasound for consecutive biopsy planning. Multiparametric MRI with a T2-weighted sequence and at least two of three functional parameters (DWI, DCE, spectroscopy) has been shown to detect 90 % of prostate carcinomas with intermediate- to high-risk; lower diagnostic performance was demonstrated for very small tumors (<0.5 cm^3), tumors in the transitional zone and low-grade carcinomas [37]. Additionally, multiparametric MRI is a strong tool for the precise definition of tumor margins and the reliable assessment of extracapsular tumor extension and potential infiltration of adjacent anatomical structures (Fig. 6.4) [59], such as the seminal vesicles, both important parameters for the correct definition of the T-stadium [7]. Additionally, planning of therapeutic interventions such as radiation or brachytherapy is possible by high-resolution MRI data sets.

6.5.2.2 Breast Cancer

Ipsilateral axillary lymphadenopathy is the first clinical symptom in 0.3–1.0 % of all breast carcinomas [60]. Buchanan et al. investigated female patients with unilateral axillary lymphadenopathy without clinical or mammographic detection of a primary tumor in the breast and reported that contrast-enhanced MRI detected >50 % of these primarily occult breast carcinomas [47]. The authors concluded that in the diagnosis of occult breast carcinomas, MRI is superior to mammography. A study by Orel and colleagues confirmed these results and reported that 86 % of primarily occult breast carcinomas could be detected with MRI [48]. MRI also provides valuable diagnostic information for the local staging of tumors, allowing for a precise definition of tumor margins, evaluation of potential infiltration of adjacent structures such as the pectoral muscle, and the diagnosis of regional lymph node metastases. MR-guided biopsy may be applied to allow for histological sampling of otherwise occult breast carcinoma [7].

6.6 Ultrasound

Depending on the tumor entity, ultrasound can be applied for local and regional tumor staging [7]. Advantages of this fast-evolving imaging modality are low costs compared to cross-sectional imaging modalities, widespread and fast availability, as well as the absence of ionizing radiation. The main disadvantage is the high interobserver variability.

6.6.1 Ultrasound Assessment of Lymph Nodes

Ultrasound with high-frequency probes is well suited for evaluation of superficial lymph nodes. Using morphological criteria, lymph nodes can be classified as malignant, inflammatory, or normal. For the detection of cervical lymph node metastases, Ashraf et al. reported a diagnostic sensitivity of 92 % and a specificity of 97 % for Doppler ultrasound compared to a histopathological standard of reference [61]. In their study, combined ultrasound with Doppler sonography was more sensitive than CT (sensitivity 83 %, specificity 93 %). Mizrachi et al. confirmed these results in a study on cervical lymph node metastases in patients with thyroid carcinoma at a sensitivity of 95 % and a specificity of 90 % [62]. On the contrary, ultrasound showed only limited applicability for the assessment of axillary lymph node metastases in patients with breast carcinoma [63]. Negative ultrasound excludes regional lymph node metastases with high likelihood (negative predictive value 96 %). However, if suspicious lymph nodes are detected, ultrasound frequently underestimates the N status. It remains to be investigated whether contrast-enhanced ultrasound can further improve sonographic lymph node staging [64]. Initial evidence for a potential benefit of contrast-enhanced ultrasound was reported by Rubaltelli and coworkers in a population of 540 patients with malignant melanoma. Compared to fine needle aspiration as the standard of reference, the authors observed a sensitivity of 100 % and a specificity of 99.5 % for contrast-enhanced ultrasound in the detection of lymph node metastases [65].

6.7 Mammography

Women with solitary axillary lymphadenopathy are considered a particular subset of CUP patients, as 75 % will be diagnosed with breast carcinoma. Diagnosis and therapy are following the clinical guidelines for lymph node-positive breast cancer [66]. Less frequent differential diagnoses include lung cancer, amelanotic melanoma, lymphoma, and soft tissue sarcoma as primary tumors [7]. Following the clinical guidelines, diagnostic workup includes clinical history and examination, bilateral mammography in two views, as well as bilateral breast ultrasound. Suspicious lesions should undergo image-guided biopsy with histological and immunohistochemical workup including receptor status and c-erbB2 expression.

Although bilateral mammography is part of the standard workup in women with CUP syndrome, several studies suggested that mammography has only limited sensitivity for the detection of a clinically occult primary breast carcinoma in women with CUP [12, 67, 68]. Nevertheless, the diagnosis of breast carcinoma is of particular relevance, as established therapies are available for breast cancer, resulting in a significantly improved prognosis compared to other, i.e., unfavorable CUP subsets. Therefore, female patients with unremarkable clinical examination, mammography, and ultrasound should undergo contrast-enhanced MRI of the breast to identify otherwise occult carcinomas [69]. Although contrast-enhanced MRI of the breast has a high sensitivity for the diagnosis of breast carcinoma, its low specificity concurrently leads to the recommendation to biopsy suspicious lesions before surgical resection [70].

6.8 Conclusion

Imaging plays a central role in the therapeutic management of patients with CUP. Main challenges include the localization of the primary tumor, the identification of tumor entities with available dedicated therapy strategies, as well as the characterization of clinicopathological CUP subentities. Whole-body imaging stands at the beginning of the diagnostic algorithm in CUP patients, searching for potential primary tumors, identifying all manifestations, and identifying lesions for image-guided biopsy. Due to wide availability and comparably low costs, initial whole-body imaging is frequently performed by contrast-enhanced CT of the neck, chest, and abdomen, although several studies suggest improved diagnostic sensitivity of ^{18}F-FDG PET/CT for the detection of primary tumors and metastatic tumor manifestations [71]. In conclusion, the diagnostic algorithm in CUP patients should primarily aim at patient benefit with the goal to prevent overdiagnosis. Multimodality imaging helps to identify patients with favorable, i.e., treatable CUP subsets, and significantly accelerates the diagnostic workup in CUP [7].

References

1. Muir C. Cancer of unknown primary site. Cancer. 1995;75(1 Suppl):353–6.
2. van de Wouw AJ, Janssen-Heijnen ML, Coebergh JW, Hillen HF. Epidemiology of unknown primary tumours; incidence and population-based survival of 1285 patients in southeast Netherlands, 1984-1992. Eur J Cancer. 2002;38(3):409–13.
3. UK. CR: CancerStats monograph 2010. http://www.cancerresearchuk.org/cancer-info/cancer-stats/incidence/commoncancers/.
4. Pavlidis N, Briasoulis E, Hainsworth J, Greco FA. Diagnostic and therapeutic management of cancer of an unknown primary. Eur J Cancer. 2003;39(14):1990–2005.
5. Abbruzzese JL, Abbruzzese MC, Hess KR, Raber MN, Lenzi R, Frost P. Unknown primary carcinoma: natural history and prognostic factors in 657 consecutive patients. J Clin Oncol. 1994;12(6):1272–80.
6. Shaw PH, Adams R, Jordan C, Crosby TD. A clinical review of the investigation and management of carcinoma of unknown primary in a single cancer network. Clin Oncol. 2007;19(1):87–95.
7. Kazmierczak PM, Nikolaou K, Rominger A, Graser A, Reiser MF, Cyran CC. Radiological diagnostics in CUP syndrome. Radiologe. 2014;54(2):117–23.
8. Varadhachary GR, Raber MN, Matamoros A, Abbruzzese JL. Carcinoma of unknown primary with a colon-cancer profile-changing paradigm and emerging definitions. Lancet Oncol. 2008;9(6):596–9.
9. Pavlidis N, Pentheroudakis G. Cancer of unknown primary site. Lancet. 2012;379(9824):1428–35.
10. Pavlidis N, Fizazi K. Carcinoma of unknown primary (CUP). Crit Rev Oncol Hematol. 2009;69(3):271–8.
11. Abbruzzese JL, Abbruzzese MC, Lenzi R, Hess KR, Raber MN. Analysis of a diagnostic strategy for patients with suspected tumors of unknown origin. J Clin Oncol. 1995;13(8):2094–103.
12. Losa Gaspa F, Germa JR, Albareda JM, Fernandez-Ortega A, Sanjose S, Fernandez Trigo V. Metastatic cancer presentation. Validation of a diagnostic algorithm with 221 consecutive patients. Rev Clin Esp. 2002;202(6):313–9.
13. Delgado-Bolton RC, Fernandez-Perez C, Gonzalez-Mate A, Carreras JL. Meta-analysis of the performance of 18F-FDG PET in primary tumor detection in unknown primary tumors. J Nucl Med. 2003;44(8):1301–14.
14. Kwee TC, Kwee RM. Combined FDG-PET/CT for the detection of unknown primary tumors: systematic review and meta-analysis. Eur Radiol. 2009;19(3):731–44.
15. Latief KH, White CS, Protopapas Z, Attar S, Krasna MJ. Search for a primary lung neoplasm in patients with brain metastasis: is the chest radiograph sufficient? AJR Am J Roentgenol. 1997;168(5):1339–44.
16. Froeling V, Rottgen R, Collettini F, Rothe J, Hamm B, Brenner W, Schreiter N. Detection of pancreatic neuroendocrine tumors (PNET) using semi-quantitative [68Ga]DOTATOC PET in combination with multiphase contrast-enhanced CT. Q J Nucl Med Mol Imaging. 2014;58(3):310–8.
17. Pavlidis N. Forty years experience of treating cancer of unknown primary. Acta Oncol. 2007;46(5):592–601.
18. Stella GM, Senetta R, Cassenti A, Ronco M, Cassoni P. Cancers of unknown primary origin: current perspectives and future therapeutic strategies. J Transl Med. 2012;10:12.
19. Gallamini A, Zwarthoed C, Borra A. Positron emission tomography (PET) in oncology. Cancer. 2014;6(4):1821–89.
20. Strojan P, Ferlito A, Medina JE, Woolgar JA, Rinaldo A, Robbins KT, Fagan JJ, Mendenhall WM, Paleri V, Silver CE, et al. Contemporary management of lymph node metastases from an

unknown primary to the neck: I. A review of diagnostic approaches. Head Neck. 2013;35(1):123–32.
21. Lee JR, Kim JS, Roh JL, Lee JH, Baek JH, Cho KJ, Choi SH, Nam SY, Kim SY. Detection of occult primary tumors in patients with cervical metastases of unknown primary tumors: comparison of F FDG PET/CT with contrast-enhanced CT or CT/MR imaging-prospective study. Radiology. 2014;274:764–71.
22. Moller AK, Loft A, Berthelsen AK, Pedersen KD, Graff J, Christensen CB, Costa JC, Skovgaard LT, Perell K, Petersen BL, et al. A prospective comparison of 18F-FDG PET/CT and CT as diagnostic tools to identify the primary tumor site in patients with extracervical carcinoma of unknown primary site. Oncologist. 2012;17(9):1146–54.
23. Breuer N, Behrendt FF, Heinzel A, Mottaghy FM, Palmowski M, Verburg FA. Prognostic relevance of (18)F-FDG PET/CT in carcinoma of unknown primary. Clin Nucl Med. 2014;39(2):131–5.
24. Ozis SE, Soydal C, Akyol C, Can N, Kucuk ON, Yagci C, Erkek AB, Kuzu MA. The role of 18F-fluorodeoxyglucose positron emission tomography/computed tomography in the primary staging of rectal cancer. World J Surg Oncol. 2014;12:26.
25. Mertens LS, Fioole-Bruining A, Vegt E, Vogel WV, van Rhijn BW, Horenblas S. Impact of (18) F-fluorodeoxyglucose (FDG)-positron-emission tomography/computed tomography (PET/CT) on management of patients with carcinoma invading bladder muscle. BJU Int. 2013;112(6):729–34.
26. Lee JW, Lee JH, Cho A, Yun M, Lee JD, Kim YT, Kang WJ. The performance of contrast-enhanced FDG PET/CT for the differential diagnosis of unexpected ovarian mass lesions in patients with nongynecologic cancer. Clin Nucl Med. 2015;40(2):97–102.
27. Haug AR, Heinemann V, Bruns CJ, Hoffmann R, Jakobs T, Bartenstein P, Hacker M. 18F-FDG PET independently predicts survival in patients with cholangiocellular carcinoma treated with 90Y microspheres. Eur J Nucl Med Mol Imaging. 2011;38(6):1037–45.
28. Long NM, Smith CS. Causes and imaging features of false positives and false negatives on F-PET/CT in oncologic imaging. Insights Imaging. 2011;2(6):679–98.
29. Kotzerke J, Oehme L, Grosse J, Hellwig D, Arbeitsausschuss PETdDGN. Positron emission tomography 2013 in Germany. Results of the query and current status. Nuklearmedizin . 2015;54(2):53–9.
30. De Wever W, Verschakelen J, Coolen J. Role of imaging in diagnosis, staging and follow-up of lung cancer. Curr Opin Pulm Med. 2014;20(4):385–92.
31. Meignan M, Itti E, Gallamini A, Younes A. FDG PET/CT imaging as a biomarker in lymphoma. Eur J Nucl Med Mol Imaging. 2015;42:623–33.
32. Etchebehere EC, de Oliveira SA, Gumz B, Vicente A, Hoff PG, Corradi G, Ichiki WA, de Almeida Filho JG, Cantoni S, Camargo EE, et al. 68Ga-DOTATATE PET/CT, 99mTc-HYNIC-octreotide SPECT/CT, and whole-body MR imaging in detection of neuroendocrine tumors: a prospective trial. J Nucl Med. 2014;55(10):1598–604.
33. Haug AR, Cindea-Drimus R, Auernhammer CJ, Reincke M, Wangler B, Uebleis C, Schmidt GP, Goke B, Bartenstein P, Hacker M. The role of 68Ga-DOTATATE PET/CT in suspected neuroendocrine tumors. J Nucl Med. 2012;53(11):1686–92.
34. Alonso O, Rodriguez-Taroco M, Savio E, Bentancourt C, Gambini JP, Engler H. (68) Ga-DOTATATE PET/CT in the evaluation of patients with neuroendocrine metastatic carcinoma of unknown origin. Ann Nucl Med. 2014;28(7):638–45.
35. Kayani I, Bomanji JB, Groves A, Conway G, Gacinovic S, Win T, Dickson J, Caplin M, Ell PJ. Functional imaging of neuroendocrine tumors with combined PET/CT using 68Ga-DOTATATE (DOTA-DPhe1, Tyr3-octreotate) and 18F-FDG. Cancer. 2008;112(11):2447–55.
36. Oh S, Prasad V, Lee DS, Baum RP: Effect of peptide receptor radionuclide therapy on somatostatin receptor status and glucose metabolism in neuroendocrine tumors: intraindividual comparison of Ga-68 DOTANOC PET/CT and F-18 FDG PET/CT. Int J Mol Imaging. 2011;2011:524130.

37. Thompson J, Lawrentschuk N, Frydenberg M, Thompson L, Stricker P. The role of magnetic resonance imaging in the diagnosis and management of prostate cancer. BJU Int. 2013;112 Suppl 2:6–20.
38. Riihimaki M, Hemminki A, Sundquist K, Hemminki K. Causes of death in patients with extranodal cancer of unknown primary: searching for the primary site. BMC Cancer. 2014;14:439.
39. Chang AJ, Autio KA, Roach 3rd M, Scher HI. High-risk prostate cancer-classification and therapy. Nat Rev Clin Oncol. 2014;11(6):308–23.
40. Afshar-Oromieh A, Zechmann CM, Malcher A, Eder M, Eisenhut M, Linhart HG, Holland-Letz T, Hadaschik BA, Giesel FL, Debus J, et al. Comparison of PET imaging with a (68) Ga-labelled PSMA ligand and (18)F-choline-based PET/CT for the diagnosis of recurrent prostate cancer. Eur J Nucl Med Mol Imaging. 2014;41(1):11–20.
41. Afshar-Oromieh A, Haberkorn U, Schlemmer HP, Fenchel M, Eder M, Eisenhut M, Hadaschik BA, Kopp-Schneider A, Rothke M. Comparison of PET/CT and PET/MRI hybrid systems using a 68Ga-labelled PSMA ligand for the diagnosis of recurrent prostate cancer: initial experience. Eur J Nucl Med Mol Imaging. 2014;41(5).887–97.
42. Purohit BS, Ailianou A, Dulguerov N, Becker CD, Ratib O, Becker M. FDG-PET/CT pitfalls in oncological head and neck imaging. Insights Imaging. 2014;5(5):585–602.
43. Demirkol MO, Acar O, Ucar B, Ramazanoglu SR, Saglican Y, Esen T. Prostate-specific membrane antigen-based imaging in prostate cancer: impact on clinical decision making process. Prostate. 2015;75:748–57.
44. Kaufmann O, Fietze E, Dietel M. Immunohistochemical diagnosis in cancer metastasis of unknown primary tumor. Pathologe. 2002;23(3):183–97.
45. Hewitt MJ, Hall GD, Wilkinson N, Perren TJ, Lane G, Spencer JA. Image-guided biopsy in women with breast cancer presenting with peritoneal carcinomatosis. Int J Gynecol Cancer . 2006;16 Suppl 1:108–10.
46. Antoch G, Vogt FM, Freudenberg LS, Nazaradeh F, Goehde SC, Barkhausen J, Dahmen G, Bockisch A, Debatin JF, Ruehm SG. Whole-body dual-modality PET/CT and whole-body MRI for tumor staging in oncology. JAMA. 2003;290(24):3199–206.
47. Buchanan CL, Morris EA, Dorn PL, Borgen PI, Van Zee KJ. Utility of breast magnetic resonance imaging in patients with occult primary breast cancer. Ann Surg Oncol. 2005;12(12):1045–53.
48. Orel SG, Weinstein SP, Schnall MD, Reynolds CA, Schuchter LM, Fraker DL, Solin LJ. Breast MR imaging in patients with axillary node metastases and unknown primary malignancy. Radiology. 1999;212(2):543–9.
49. Schmidt GP, Haug A, Reiser MF, Rist C. Whole-body MRI and FDG-PET/CT imaging diagnostics in oncology. Radiologe. 2010;50(4):329–38.
50. Kruger DG, Riederer SJ, Grimm RC, Rossman PJ. Continuously moving table data acquisition method for long FOV contrast-enhanced MRA and whole-body MRI. Magn Reson Med. 2002;47(2):224–31.
51. Heusner TA, Kuemmel S, Koeninger A, Hamami ME, Hahn S, Quinsten A, Bockisch A, Forsting M, Lauenstein T, Antoch G, et al. Diagnostic value of diffusion-weighted magnetic resonance imaging (DWI) compared to FDG PET/CT for whole-body breast cancer staging. Eur J Nucl Med Mol Imaging. 2010;37(6):1077–86.
52. Usuda K, Sagawa M, Motono N, Ueno M, Tanaka M, Machida Y, Matoba M, Kuginuki Y, Taniguchi M, Ueda Y, et al. Advantages of diffusion-weighted imaging over positron emission tomography-computed tomography in assessment of hilar and mediastinal lymph node in lung cancer. Ann Surg Oncol. 2013;20(5):1676–83.
53. Schmidt GP, Baur-Melnyk A, Herzog P, Schmid R, Tiling R, Schmidt M, Reiser MF, Schoenberg SO. High-resolution whole-body magnetic resonance image tumor staging with the use of parallel imaging versus dual-modality positron emission tomography-computed tomography: experience on a 32-channel system. Invest Radiol. 2005;40(12):743–53.
54. Frericks BB, Meyer BC, Martus P, Wendt M, Wolf KJ, Wacker F. MRI of the thorax during whole-body MRI: evaluation of different MR sequences and comparison to thoracic multidetector computed tomography (MDCT). J Magn Reson Imaging . 2008;27(3):538–45.

55. Bottcher J, Hansch A, Pfeil A, Schmidt P, Malich A, Schneeweiss A, Maurer MH, Streitparth F, Teichgraber UK, Renz DM. Detection and classification of different liver lesions: comparison of Gd-EOB-DTPA-enhanced MRI versus multiphasic spiral CT in a clinical single centre investigation. Eur J Radiol. 2013;82(11):1860–9.
56. Kim BS, Kim TH, Kwon TG, Yoo ES. Comparison of pelvic phased-array versus endorectal coil magnetic resonance imaging at 3 Tesla for local staging of prostate cancer. Yonsei Med J. 2012;53(3):550–6.
57. Mazaheri Y, Shukla-Dave A, Muellner A, Hricak H. MRI of the prostate: clinical relevance and emerging applications. J Magn Reson Imaging . 2011;33(2):258–74.
58. Abd-Alazeez M, Ahmed HU, Arya M, Charman SC, Anastasiadis E, Freeman A, Emberton M, Kirkham A. The accuracy of multiparametric MRI in men with negative biopsy and elevated PSA level-can it rule out clinically significant prostate cancer? Urol Oncol. 2013;32:17–22.
59. Counago F, Recio M, Del Cerro E, Cerezo L, Diaz Gavela A, Marcos FJ, Murillo R, Rodriguez Luna JM, Thuissard IJ, Martin JL. Role of 3.0 T multiparametric MRI in local staging in prostate cancer and clinical implications for radiation oncology. Clin Transl Oncol. 2014;16(11):993–9.
60. de Bresser J, de Vos B, van der Ent F, Hulsewe K. Breast MRI in clinically and mammographically occult breast cancer presenting with an axillary metastasis: a systematic review. Euro J Surg Oncol. 2010;36(2):114–9.
61. Ashraf M, Biswas J, Jha J, Nayak S, Singh V, Majumdar S, Bhowmick A, Dam A. Clinical utility and prospective comparison of ultrasonography and computed tomography imaging in staging of neck metastases in head and neck squamous cell cancer in an Indian setup. Int J Clin Oncol. 2011;16(6):686–93.
62. Mizrachi A, Feinmesser R, Bachar G, Hilly O, Cohen M. Value of ultrasound in detecting central compartment lymph node metastases in differentiated thyroid carcinoma. Eur Arch Otorhinolaryngol. 2014;271:1215–8.
63. Schipper RJ, van Roozendaal LM, de Vries B, Pijnappel RM, Beets-Tan RG, Lobbes MB, Smidt ML. Axillary ultrasound for preoperative nodal staging in breast cancer patients: is it of added value? Breast. 2013;22(6):1108–13.
64. Delorme S. Ultrasound in oncology: screening and staging. Internist. 2012;53(3):271–81.
65. Rubaltelli L, Beltrame V, Scagliori E, Bezzon E, Frigo AC, Rastrelli M, Stramare R. Potential Use of contrast-enhanced ultrasound (CEUS) in the detection of metastatic superficial lymph nodes in melanoma patients. Ultraschall Med. 2013;35:67–71.
66. Senkus E, Kyriakides S, Penault-Llorca F, Poortmans P, Thompson A, Zackrisson S, Cardoso F, Group EGW. Primary breast cancer: ESMO clinical practice guidelines for diagnosis, treatment and follow-up. Ann Oncol. 2013;24 Suppl 6:vi 7–23.
67. Kirsten F, Chi CH, Leary JA, Ng AB, Hedley DW, Tattersall MH. Metastatic adeno or undifferentiated carcinoma from an unknown primary site--natural history and guidelines for identification of treatable subsets. Q J Med. 1987;62(238):143–61.
68. Stevens KJ, Smith SL, Denley H, Pinder SE, Evans AJ, Chan SY. Is mammography of value in women with disseminated cancer of unknown origin? Clin Oncol. 1999;11(2):90–2.
69. Destounis S. Breast magnetic resonance imaging indications. Top Magn Reson Imaging. 2014;23(6):329–36.
70. Taylor MB, Bromham NR, Arnold SE. Carcinoma of unknown primary: key radiological issues from the recent national institute for health and clinical excellence guidelines. Br J Radiol. 2012;85(1014):661–71.
71. Schramm N, Rominger A, Schmidt C, Morelli JN, Schmid-Tannwald C, Meinel FG, Reiser MF, Rist C. Detection of underlying malignancy in patients with paraneoplastic neurological syndromes: comparison of 18F-FDG PET/CT and CT. Eur J Nucl Med Mol Imaging. 2013;40(7):1014–24.

Chapter 7
Cancer of Unknown Primary: The Pathologist's Approach

Albrecht Stenzinger and Wilko Weichert

7.1 Introduction

About 15 % of all malignant tumors present as metastatic disease at diagnosis. According to the literature, in about 70 % of these cases, the primary tumor can be identified, while this is not successful in the remaining cases. Therefore, cancer of unknown primary (CUP) is not a rare disease but comprises 2–5 % of all diagnosed malignancies [1]. Worldwide, CUP syndrome presumably represents the seventh- and eight-most frequent malignant tumor "entity" in men and women, respectively [2]. In Germany, the estimated age-standardized incidence is about 3.9–9.1/100,000 population (2000–2010), and the rate of new cases in 2010 (for men and women combined) was about 12,300 cases, or, about 2.5 % of all malignant new cases (see Fig. 7.1) [2]. These data are comparable with observations from the United States as well as other European countries [1].

7.2 Definition

CUP is defined as a histologically confirmed metastatic neoplasm for which the localization of the primary cannot be identified using standardized diagnostic procedures [4]. Currently, there is no conclusive consensus on the minimum diagnostic requirements that ultimately define a CUP. For many experts, in addition to the detailed past and present medical history of the patient and physical examination, a

A. Stenzinger • W. Weichert (✉)
Institute of Pathology, University Hospital Heidelberg,
Im Neuenheimer Feld 224, 69120 Heidelberg, Germany

National Center for Tumor Diseases (NCT), Heidelberg, Germany
e-mail: albrecht.stenzinger@med.uni-heidelberg.de; wilko.weichert@med.uni-heidelberg.de

A. Krämer, H. Löffler (eds.), *Cancer of Unknown Primary*,
DOI 10.1007/978-3-319-22581-4_7

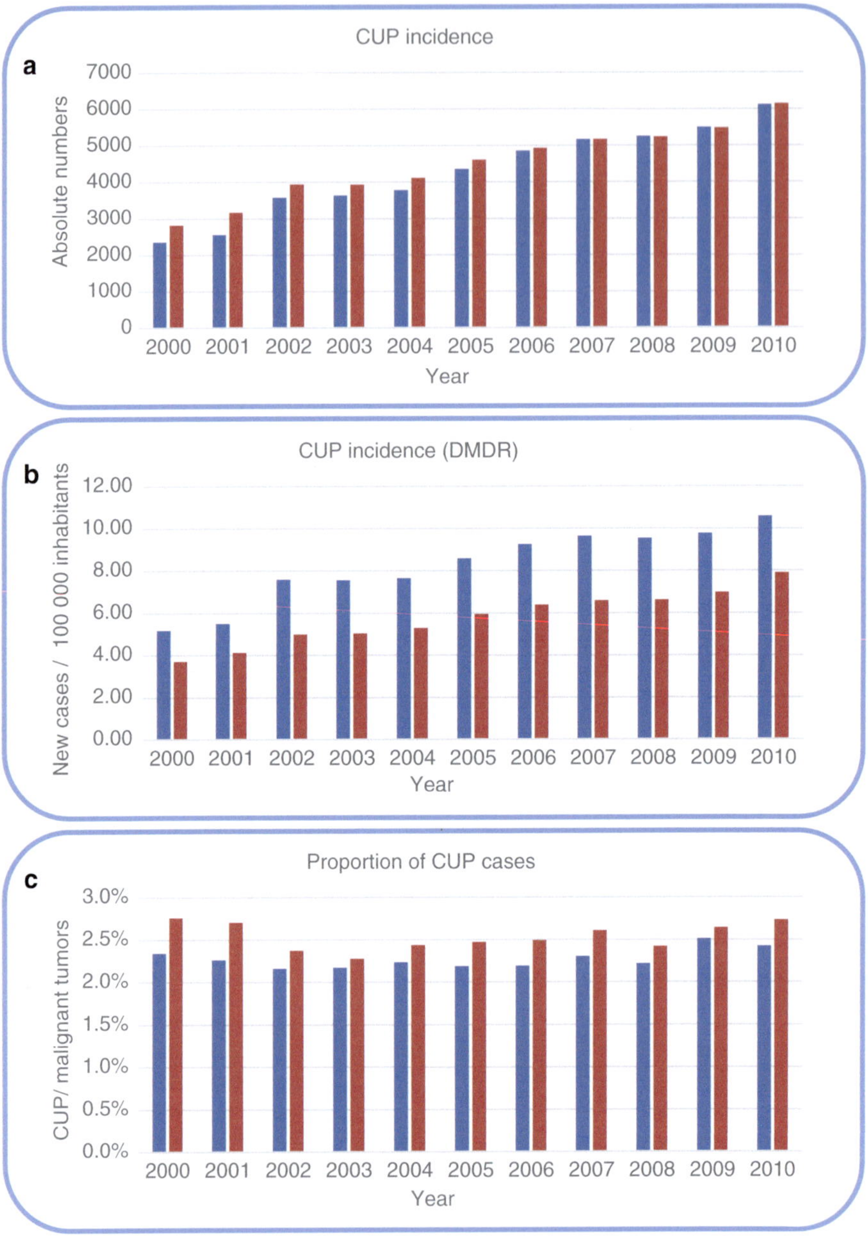

Fig. 7.1 Frequencies of the CUP syndrome in Germany (The data was made available from the Robert Koch Institute (see [3]) and adapted from [2]). (**a**) Absolute CUP numbers for men (*blue color*) and women (*red color*) in Germany from 2000 to 2010. Note the significant rise from 2400 and 2800 (2000) to approximately 6100 (2010). (**b**) Age-standardized CUP incidence rates (DMDR) for men and women in Germany from 2000 to 2010. Note the significant increase (105 and 140 %) from 5.19 and 3.70 (2000) to 10.6 and 7.9 (2010) per 100,000 inhabitants. (**c**) Percentage of CUP syndromes of all new malignant diagnoses in Germany (2000–2010). Note the relative stability of the respective numbers. The proportion is on average 0.2 % lower among men than among women

full blood count, chemical laboratory data, and a computerized tomography (CT) of the thorax, abdomen, and pelvis are essentially required. Further diagnostic investigations (gastroscopy, colonoscopy, panendoscopy, others) may be required depending on the clinical picture. Other image-generating methods (PET-CT, others) are also being discussed as mandatory [5].

7.3 Clinical Picture and Biology

In contrast to the typical clinical presentation of a malignant tumor, CUP shows a different temporal as well as spatial behavior, which impedes detection of the primary tumor by currently available diagnostic methods [4]. Metastases occur at an early stage and/or the pattern of metastasis is unusual or non-typical. At the time of diagnosis, more than 50 % of CUP patients have metastases in multiple locations, most frequently in the liver; lungs; brain; cervical, axillary, or inguinal lymph nodes; and in the pleural and abdominal cavity.

Following these clinical observations, basically two theories on the pathogenesis of CUP have emerged [6], which partially overlap. The first theory postulates a specific and independent biology for all CUP tumors, which allows for very early and aggressive metastatic spreading, while the primary tumor is either growing slowly or not at all (dormancy) or regresses and "disappears." In this context, it has also been postulated that a prototypical CUP tumor does not develop gradually through premalignant intermediates, but that tumor cell clones evolve very rapidly with the capability to metastasize and possibly regress locally after metastatic colonization of distant organs. This biological process leads to a clinical picture where the tumor is already and only obvious as systemic disease at the time of diagnosis. The second theory postulates organ-specific, functionally heterogeneous mechanisms for the occurrence of a CUP. According to this theory, there is no common "one size fits all" CUP biology, but several organ-specific CUP-defining molecular makeups. However, also according to this theory, entity-specific regression phenomena and the development of a very early metastatic potency appear to play a central role [7].

7.4 Autopsy Data

Large autopsy studies have shown that the most common primary tumors of a CUP syndrome are found in the lung and pancreas (each about 20–25 %), followed by the liver and bile ducts, colorectum, renal and adrenal glands, genitals, and stomach (each about 5–10 %) [8]. However, in these studies, a putative primary tumor could only be detected in about 60–80 % of the cases, leaving a significant percentage of CUP cases without evidence of a primary tumor even after meticulous autopsy diagnostics.

7.5 Tumor Subtypes and Prognosis

Histologically, about 90 % of the CUP cases are carcinomas; the remaining 10 % comprise mainly melanomas and sarcomas. Within the group of carcinomas, well-to-moderately differentiated adenocarcinomas (60 %) dominate over poorly differentiated adenocarcinomas (30 %). Squamous cell carcinomas and undifferentiated carcinomas are relatively rare (each about 5 %).

In general, median survival times of patients diagnosed with CUP are short and range between approx. 10 weeks and 17 months [1, 2, 4–9]. Only 25 % of the CUP patients survive the first year after diagnosis. The median age of patients at diagnosis is 65–70 years; CUP syndromes in children are extremely rare. From a clinical-pathological point of view, patients with CUP can be divided into a smaller subgroup with a relatively good prognosis (20 % of the patients) and in a second, larger subgroup with relatively poor prognosis [10]. The first group, which responds comparably well to chemotherapy, is quite heterogeneous and comprises patients with papillary adenocarcinoma in the peritoneal cavity, adenocarcinoma exclusively located in the axillary lymph nodes, isolated involvement of cervical or inguinal lymph nodes by squamous cell carcinoma, poorly differentiated carcinomas of the midline (midline tumor), male patients with osteoblastic metastases of adenocarcinoma and elevated PSA levels, patients with adenocarcinomas with a morphology and immunophenotype highly suggestive of colon cancer, as well as patients with a small and potentially resectable metastatic tumor.

Apart from the latter group, from a pathological point of view, the link between the tumors in this heterogeneous mixture of neoplasms is fairly obvious: although these tumors are formally and correctly classified as CUP (if a primary cannot be identified), the particular pattern of metastasis and/or tumor differentiation points toward a specific organ of origin (e.g., in the same order as above: ovarian cancer, breast cancer, squamous cell carcinoma of the head and neck, testicular germ cell tumor, prostate carcinoma, etc.). Hence, if these patients are treated according to the clinically undetectable but putative primary tumor, this group of patients will likely benefit from those chemotherapy regimens that have been established for the corresponding primaries [10].

The majority of CUP patients (80 %), however, follow an unfavorable clinical course. This applies to patients with non-intestinal-type metastases of adenocarcinomas located in the liver and other organs, multiple cerebral or multiple pulmonary/pleural metastases, evidence of non-papillary adenocarcinoma in ascites, squamous cell carcinoma in the abdomen or in the lesser pelvis, and patients with multiple osteolytic bone metastases as well as too many other very heterogeneous clinical constellations.

7.6 Aim of the Pathological Diagnosis

The primary aim of every pathological diagnosis is the most accurate and precise characterization of a tumor using histomorphology and immunohistochemical methods [10] as well as adjunct molecular approaches (see below) to guide and support optimal clinical management. In addition to a precise classification of a given tumor, the identification of clinically actionable molecular alterations by genotyping and other molecular profiling methods (e.g., transcriptomics, proteomics) will become increasingly important in the near future.

7.7 Current Principles of Conventional Pathological Diagnosis: Tissue Preparation

Whenever possible, a clinically accessible lesion of a CUP patient should be biopsied with the goal to retrieve at least a proper tissue core cylinder. Cytology specimens and cellular smears do not show the association of the tumor to its surrounding microenvironment; therefore, only cytological (cellular atypia) but not histological criteria (growth pattern, architecture) can be evaluated. The latter, however, do play a crucial role and contribute strongly to the pathological diagnosis, particularly in CUP tumors where diagnosis is challenging. Even in the tissue core biopsy setting, however, the amount of material obtained is usually small, so that on average only about 15–25 histological slides with sufficient tumor cellularity can be prepared from the standard paraffin-embedded biopsy tissue material. Since a considerable number of these tissue slides have to be used for the mandatory conventional morphological assessment and immunohistochemical staining, and subsequent slightly thicker slice preparations are necessary for morphology-controlled extraction of nucleic acids (for further molecular analysis on the mRNA, miRNA, or DNA level), the effective and efficient use of the tissue is of paramount importance. Hence, technical optimization of methodologies as well as consideration of all available and clinically relevant information (medical history of the patient, imaging, laboratorial chemical parameters) plays a crucial role in the diagnostic process. Optimized processing of tissue includes: (1) the use of immunohistochemical double stainings (see below), (2) a precisely planned initial workup procedure comprising sufficient numbers of blank slides at the first incision of the paraffin block to avoid loss of tissue by recutting, and (3) the use of well-established molecular assays for which the minimum amount of nucleic acids and the minimum tumor cell content that still yields valid data have been thoroughly determined. In addition, the use of multiplex molecular assays is clearly preferred over the use of sequential single marker molecular testing (see below).

7.8 The Diagnostic Gold Standard: Combination of Histomorphology, Immunohistochemistry, and Targeted Molecular Analysis

For the standard diagnostic workup of CUP, a gradual, synthetic diagnostic approach (Fig. 7.2) is recommended. In daily pathological routine, deviations from the gold standard approach may be necessary and meaningful in single cases. However, a stringent constructive approach must be maintained in order to get results, which are *reliable*, *clinically useful*, and *fast* while *protecting tissue resources*. An overview of the standard diagnostic steps is presented in Box 7.1.

Box 7.1: Multistep Algorithm of Morphological CUP Diagnostics

Step 1. Histomorphological confirmation that the lesion which is clinically observed is contained in the tissue material

Step 2. Histomorphological *confirmation* that the lesion which is clinically observed is in fact a *malignant tumor*

Step 3. Differential diagnostic *exclusion of a local primary tumor*

Step 4. Identification of the *tumor type/lineage* (carcinoma, sarcoma, melanoma, lymphoma)

Step 5. Identification of the *tumor subtype* (e.g., adenocarcinoma, squamous cell carcinoma)

Step 6. Identification of a putative *tissue of origin (organ)*

Step 7. Further *molecular tests* for prognostication and/or prediction of therapy response

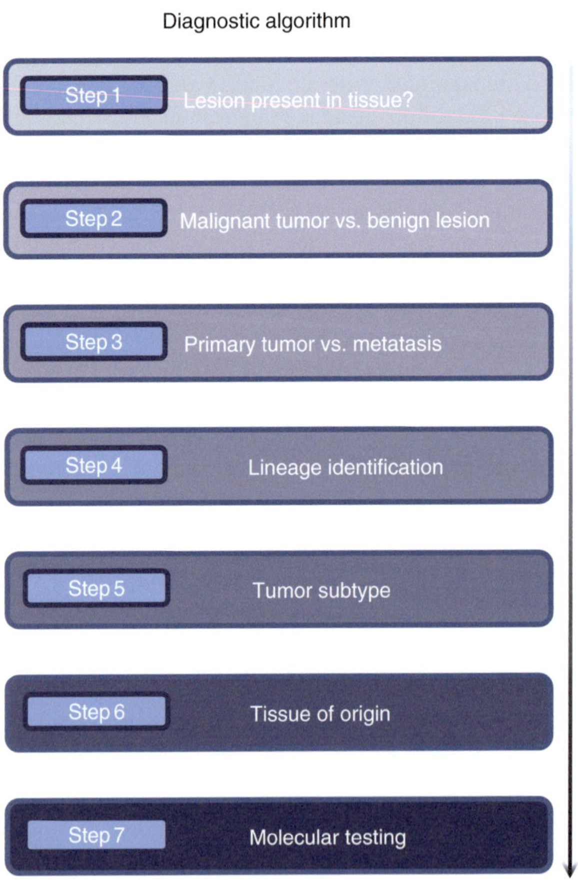

Fig. 7.2 Flowchart to visualize the initial step-by-step CUP diagnostic procedure (The figure is adapted from [2])

The first step of diagnosis is always based on the histomorphological evaluation of the tissue, usually stained with hematoxylin and eosin (HE) and periodic acid-Schiff (PAS). First, it is important to determine whether the clinically observed lesion is included in the biopsy. In this context, it may be necessary to level the tissue block to obtain deeper, potentially more significant tissue sections. It has been shown that in approximately 15 % of the cases, after conventional histology workup, the available tissue material is insufficient (quantitatively and/or qualitatively) for further diagnostic procedures [10]. In such cases, the clinical colleagues must be informed by the pathologist, and an additional biopsy should be obtained whenever possible. Classification of a tumor as CUP on the basis of insufficient tissue material is inadequate and may compromise the prognosis of the CUP patient.

If a lesion is identified, it has to be checked whether the lesion is a malignant tumor. This is achieved by the evaluation of conventional cytological (e.g., nuclear atypia, increased (atypical) mitoses) and histological (e.g., patterns of growth, invasion of the surrounding tissue, blood vessels, or nerves) criteria of malignancy. To determine whether the tumor is a local primary or a metastasis, histomorphology is crucial in addition to mandatory clinical information (a single lesion or multiple lesions of similar nature in the same/different location(s)). In this context, the histological findings have to be carefully integrated to obtain a precise and meaningful picture (e.g., direct association with the tissue of origin, presence of precursor lesions, spatial relationship to the organ system). For example, an adenocarcinoma in the muscular wall of the colon with direct contact to the surface epithelium and dysplastic adenoma at the borders of the tumor is almost certainly a primary, while an adenocarcinoma in deep wall layers of the colon without contact to the mucosa and without accompanying precursor lesion may be rather a metastasis. The initial meticulous morphological evaluation of the tissue is absolutely indispensable and is the basis for all types of additional typing approaches, either by immunohistochemical or molecular means.

If morphology is not definite, immunohistochemistry (IHC) is used to determine the major lineage/origin of the tumor (epithelial = carcinoma, lymphoid = lymphoma, mesenchymal = sarcoma, melanocytes = melanoma) [11] (for examples see: Fig. 7.3, graph Fig. 7.4). The primary immunohistochemical approach for CUP diagnosis is based on the combined morphological features of the tumor. If morphology is entirely unclear, the primary IHC approach comprises: (1) pancytokeratin antibodies for the detection of epithelial differentiation and (2) antibodies for detecting of melanocytic and (3) lymphoid cells. The differential diagnosis of a mesenchymal neoplasm is primarily based on the negativity for epithelial, melanocytic, and lymphoid markers, respectively, and simultaneous detection of (4) expression of the "first-line marker" vimentin. The latter, however, should be interpreted with caution as vimentin is frequently expressed in a variety of tumors including poorly differentiated carcinomas undergoing EMT [12]. Hence, integrated evaluation of the other IHC staining results is mandatory. The final diagnosis of a carcinoma, sarcoma, melanoma, or leukemia/lymphoma requires the appropriate morphology of the tumor as well as appropriate immunohistochemical results and additional genetic investigations where necessary.

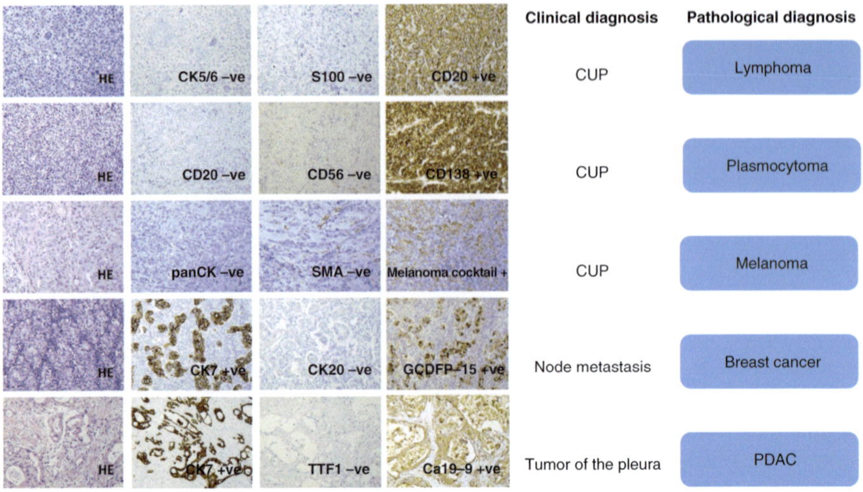

Fig. 7.3 Prototypical diagnostic examples. In these cases of essentially undifferentiated tumor, further subtyping is achieved by immunohistochemistry. *CD* cluster of differentiation, *CK* cytokeratin, *GCDFP* gross cystic disease fluid protein, *HE* hematoxylin and eosin, *SMA* smooth muscle actin, *TTF* thyroidal transcription factor, *PDAC* pancreatic ductal adenocarcinoma (The figure is adapted from [2].)

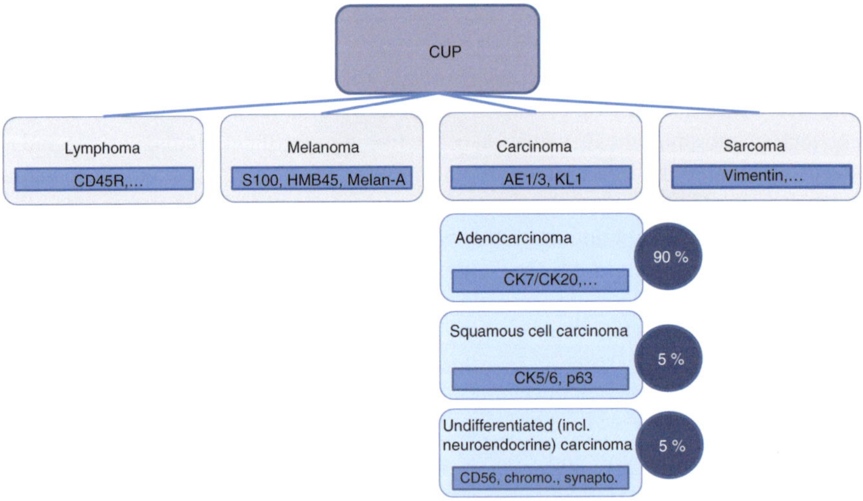

Fig. 7.4 Percentage of different histologies in CUP syndrome and first steps for class typing in cases with noncharacteristic morphology (The figure is adapted from [2])

In this context, some general principles apply for the definition of the tumor lineage.

- In addition to conventional morphology, immunohistochemically detectable expression of keratins and organ-specific marker profiles is indicative of carcinomas.

- Besides morphological criteria, subtyping of sarcomas can be achieved by a variety of markers (e.g., vimentin, actin, desmin, MyoD1, S100, CD34, CD99, c-KIT, many others) as well as genetic approaches (particularly translocation analysis; see also below) [12].
- For the diagnosis of malignant melanoma, immunohistochemical detection of S100 and melan-A as well as the use of the antibody clone HMB45, which recognizes the cytoplasmic glycoprotein gp100, may be helpful. Mutation analyses (see below) may be informative [13].
- For differential diagnosis of lymphatic or hematopoietic neoplasms, numerous immunohistochemically detectable cluster of differentiation (CD) antigens and other marker proteins can be used. In addition, molecular analysis (particularly cytogenetics) may help to establish the correct diagnosis [14].

7.9 Algorithms for Carcinoma Subtyping

For the differential diagnosis and subtyping of carcinomas, which comprise the largest group of CUP, morphology in conjunction with immunohistochemical marker panels plays an important role (step 5, Box 7.1). In an ideal setting, these markers are used in diagnostically meaningful double staining combinations to spare tissue slides (Fig. 7.5). In some cases, this method allows to determine the tissue of origin (step 6, Box 7.1). To identify squamoid neoplasms, particularly squamous differentiation markers such as high molecular weight cytokeratins

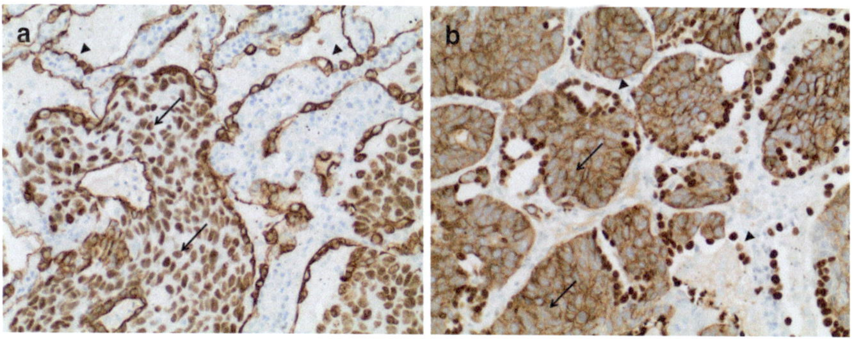

Fig. 7.5 Tissue-sparing combinations of antibodies used in simultaneous double staining procedures. (**a**) Squamous cell carcinoma of the lung. Staining for p63 (nuclear) is combined with staining for CK7 (cytoplasmic). Note p63 positivity and CK7 negativity within the tumor (*arrows*), while the epithelial lining of alveolar walls shows CK7 positivity (*arrowheads*). (**b**) The same squamous cell carcinoma of the lung stained with a different antibody cocktail comprising CK5/6 (cytoplasmic) as well as TTF1 (nuclear) antibodies. Note that the tumor stains for CK 5/6 (*arrows*) but not TTF1, while the alveolar lining is positive for TTF1 (*arrowheads*). In both cases, an antibody against a cytoplasmic protein is combined with an antibody directed against a nuclear protein. In most cases, only one of the two proteins is expressed due to intelligent combination of antibodies (The figure is adapted from [15])

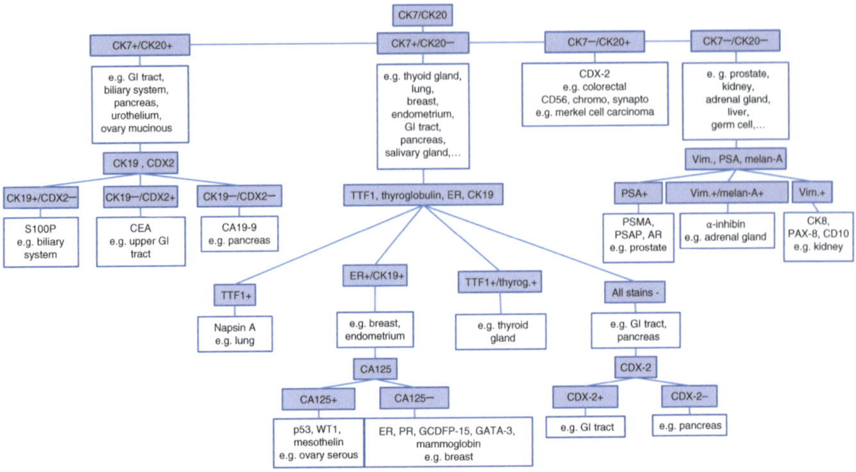

Fig. 7.6 Decision tree for immunohistochemical subtyping of adenocarcinomas (Adapted from [2, 4–7]). The presented entity and marker combinations are only examples and not exhaustive; the marker combinations are also not completely specific for these tumor entities; for further details, please refer to the main text

(e.g., CK5/6) are used. While the expression of cytokeratins 5 and 6 is very sensitive, but not specific for squamous cell carcinoma, additional detection of nuclear p40 and/or p63 staining yields a specificity of about 90 % and sensitivity of about 70 % [16]. Squamous cell carcinomas are usually negative for cytokeratins 7 and 20 – two cytokeratins that are often expressed by adenocarcinomas. Among others, determination of neuroendocrine lineage is achieved by the detection of the very specific antigens chromogranin A and synaptophysin as well as CD56 (neural cell adhesion molecule, N-CAM), which is very sensitive but less specific than the two aforementioned markers [17]. A fourth antigen indicating neuroendocrine differentiation, NSE (neuron-specific enolase), is a very sensitive but even less specific marker, so that its diagnostic utility and significance are rather limited. Adenocarcinomas (and some other epithelial neoplasms), which form the largest group of CUPs, can initially be classified into four broad diagnostic categories on the basis of the expression of the two cytokeratins CK7 and CK20 (Fig. 7.6) [1, 2, 4–14, 16–18].

1. CK20+/CK7+: e.g., gastrointestinal adenocarcinoma, transitional cell carcinoma andmucinous ovarian tumors
2. CK20+/CK7–: e.g., colorectal adenocarcinoma and neuroendocrine tumors of Merkel cell type
3. CK20–/CK7–: e.g., prostate carcinoma, hepatocellular carcinoma (HCC), clear cell renal cell carcinomas (RCC), small cell carcinoma
4. CK20–/CK7+: e.g., pancreatic cancer, bile duct carcinoma, breast carcinoma, pulmonary adenocarcinoma, salivary gland carcinoma, and endometrial carcinoma

It should be noted, however, that this list is by no means exhaustive and that aberrant immunophenotypes that significantly hamper diagnostic accuracy are not rare in CUP disease.

After initial classification, markers which facilitate determination of the organ of origin are used for further classification of adenocarcinomas. For prostate carcinomas, this includes immunohistochemical detection of the androgen receptor, PSMA and PSA [19], for pulmonary adenocarcinoma the markers napsin A and TTF1 [20], and for colorectal/gastrointestinal adenocarcinomas CDX2 (caudal-type homeobox transcription factor-2) [19]. The typing of breast cancer can be achieved through detection of the antigens GCDFP-15, mammaglobin, and GATA3 as well as through the detection of estrogen receptor (ER) and progesterone receptor (PR) expression. Many adenocarcinomas of the ovary are positive for CA-125, mesothelin, PAX8, and WT1 (nuclear) as well as ER [21]. For diagnosis of renal cell carcinoma, the coexpression of vimentin, CD10, PAX8, and cytokeratins is corroborative. In addition, in some cases, the expression of the brush-border proteins of the proximal renal tubule can be demonstrated by the RCC antibody [22]. Thyroid carcinomas show a positive immune reaction for TTF1 and thyroglobulin [22], while alpha-inhibin and melan-A are considered as established markers for adrenal carcinoma [23]. Hepatocellular carcinomas are identified by the presence of OCH1E5 as well as arginase-1 expression [24, 25]. However, although many efforts have been made to identify organ-specific markers (i.e., proteins/antigens), it is important to note that for a variety of common neoplasms, specific markers are still missing (e.g., cholangiocarcinoma, pancreatic ductal carcinoma, gastric carcinoma), and aberrant expression patterns may occur.

For squamous cell carcinoma, site-specific markers are entirely lacking. Metastatic squamous cell carcinoma of the head and neck region cannot be distinguished from squamous tumors originating from the esophagus, urinary system, uterine cervix, anus, skin, and other rare primary locations by conventional histology and immunohistochemistry. Currently, the only exception is the detection of HPV genome, which strongly points toward a primary from either the oropharyngeal region or the uterine cervix. For example, HPV analysis has been successfully used to delineate primary pulmonary squamous cell carcinomas from lung metastasis of squamous cell carcinomas of the head and neck region [26]. This is a prototypical example where a single molecular analysis may contribute valuable information to CUP diagnostics. HPV detection in this context can either be done by in situ as well as PCR-based methods (Fig. 7.7).

Common immunohistochemical markers for organ typing are exemplarily shown in Table 7.1. However, the authors would like to emphasize that these markers achieve diagnostic significance exclusively and only in conjunction with the histomorphological findings. Moreover, the immunohistochemical characterization of a tumor reaches sufficient specificity only by the interpretation of positive and negative staining results of the entire antibody panel (i.e., the *entire staining pattern*), *not* by isolated consideration of single proteins.

The latter two points are of paramount importance for diagnosis, because on the one hand, the proteins listed in Table 7.1 are also expressed in normal, nonmalignant

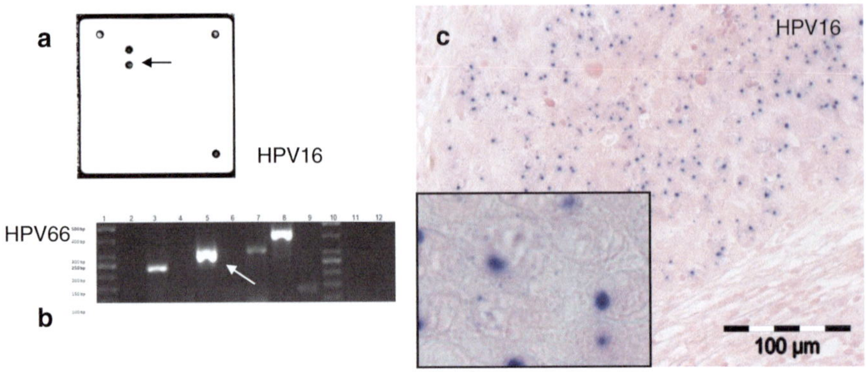

Fig. 7.7 Different methods of detecting HPV in tumor tissue (in this case in an oropharyngeal squamous cell carcinoma). (**a**) Detection of HPV and further subtyping with specific hybridization probes in a small-scale array format. This diagnostic procedure is performed with nucleic acid extracts from tumor tissue. (**b**) HPV detection and subtyping by multiplex PCR and gel electrophoresis from nucleic acid extracts. (**c**) In situ detection of HPV genomic material by chromogene in situ hybridization (CISH) (The figure is adapted from [26])

Table 7.1 Markers for immunohistochemical typing of CUP

Identification of the tumor lineage	
Carcinoma	*AE1/3*, KL1, other cytokeratin-antibody 'cocktails'
Melanoma	*S100*, HMB45, melan-A, MITF
Lymphoma/leukemia	*CD45R* (common leukocyte antigen), CD34
Sarcoma	Vimentin(with limitations; please refer to main text for further information)
Identification of the tumor subtype	
General	
Adenocarcinoma	CK7, CK20, other LMW cytokeratins
Squamous cell carcinoma	CK5/6, other HMW cytokeratins, p40, p63
Specific	
Neuroendocrine carcinoma	Chromogranin A, synaptophysin, CD56, NSE
Transitional cell carcinoma	CK7, CK20, uroplakin III, GATA3
Renal cell carcinoma	CD10, PAX8, vimentin
Thyroid carcinoma	TTF1, thyreoglobulin, PAX8
Adrenal carcinoma	Melan-A, α-inhibin
Hepatocellular carcinoma	OCH1E5, glypican-3, arginase-1
Germ cell tumor	PLAP, OCT4, CD30, SALL4, AFP, ßHCG
Mesothelioma	Calretinin, D2-40, WT1
Identification of the tissue of origin (organ)	
Lung	TTF1, napsin, surfactant protein A
Pancreatobiliary	CA19-9
Colon	CDX2, villin
Breast	GCDFP-15, mammaglobin, ER, PR, GATA3
Ovary	CA-125, WT1, mesothelin, ER, PAX8
Prostate	PSA, AR, PSMA

CAVE The list is not exhaustive and the mentioned markers are only of limited specificity; for further details, please refer to the main text.

tissue as well as in benign neoplasms, and on the other hand, each tumor represents a unique biological entity, and therefore single marker or marker profiles are never 100 % specific for a certain tumor entity. Thus, aberrant expression of a protein in a primary tumor (e.g., TTF1 expression in gynecological malignancies, urogenital tumors [27–29] and colon cancer [30]) is not unusual, also for so-called organ-specific markers. Furthermore, "organ-specific" as well as broader immunohistochemical markers usually select groups of organs rather than individual organs/sites of origin (e.g., androgen receptor is expressed in prostate carcinomas, some salivary gland tumors, and many other rare tumor entities).

Once a differential diagnosis has been narrowed down or a firm diagnosis has already been established by morphology and immunohistochemistry, screening for molecular alterations can be performed. This may be necessary (1) to further support the classification of a specific tumor (i.e., increasing diagnostic accuracy) and (2) to detect putative therapeutic targets (see below).

The first point may be important if morphology- and immunohistochemistry-based findings are not entirely conclusive. In this context, typical molecular characteristics of a tumor entity can be helpful to establish a definite diagnosis. This might apply to the detection of simple somatic mutations (e.g., detection of a BRAF mutation in a putative thyroid cancer) but is particularly true for the detection of entity-defining genetic translocations. Although more common in sarcomas and lymphomas, specific translocations are increasingly identified in carcinomas, e.g. TMPRSS-ERG in prostate cancer, MECT1-MAML2 in salivary mucoepidermoid carcinoma (Fig. 7.8), and others [32–35]. Some examples for characteristic molecular alterations in carcinomas are presented in Table 7.2.

It should be noted that single molecular tests are increasingly replaced by comprehensive multiplex molecular analyses. Such combinatorial tests (e.g., multigene ultradeep next-generation sequencing) will certainly contribute to a more precise CUP subtyping in the near future (see also below).

As for immunohistochemistry, the same limitations and restrictions also apply for genetic analyses: the detection of, e.g., genetic aberrations alone is not diagnostic (e.g., *BRAF* mutations can occur in a variety of tumors other than papillary thyroid carcinoma, such as lung cancer and colorectal cancer among many others), so that molecular results must always be interpreted with caution and integrated with all available pathological and clinical data.

7.10 The CUP Concept and Sarcomas, Melanomas, and Lymphomas

The constellation for sarcomas with "unknown" primary is different from the situation in epithelial CUP described above. This is for several reasons. First, many soft tissue tumors cannot be attributed to a single "organ system" but may occur as primary tumor at many different sites of the body. This is not surprising since the tissue of origin of sarcomas (the mesenchyme/soft tissue) can be found in almost every body part. Therefore, a liposarcoma may occur as a primary originating from fat tissue of

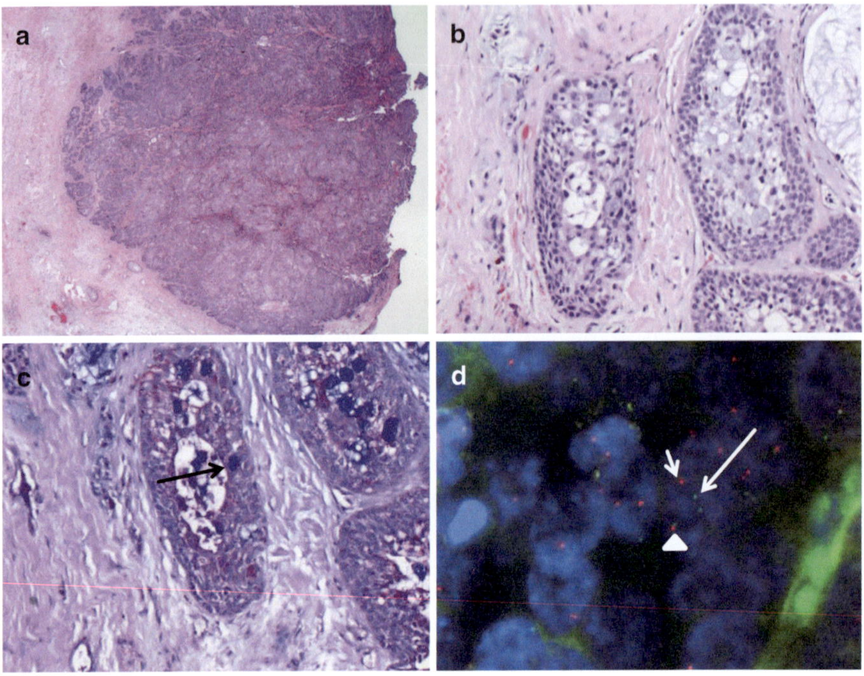

Fig. 7.8 Mucoepidermoid carcinoma of the parotid gland as an example for translocation-associated carcinomas. (**a**, **b**) HE stainings of the carcinoma highlight the presence of squamoid differentiation features typical for this tumor entity. (**c**) Alcian-PAS special stains reveal the presence of goblet cells (*arrows*), another typical feature of mucoepidermoid carcinoma. (**d**) *MAML2-FISH* break apart assay. Note the distance between the *red* (*short arrow*) and *green* (*long arrow*) signal, both representing *MAML2* hybridization probes, in a cell with a translocation involving the *MAML2* gene. In the direct vicinity, a cell with a non-translocated *MAML2* gene can be seen (*arrowhead*); here, both signals are adjacent to each other (The figure is adapted from [31])

such diverse sites as the breast, deep soft tissue of the leg, the retroperitoneum, subcutaneously, or even in/close to parenchymatous organs such as the pancreas. The second major point which must be taken into account is that current clinical strategies for treating metastasized sarcomas are rarely site specific. For example, a metastasized angiosarcoma of the breast is treated with the same chemotherapy regimen as a metastasized angiosarcoma of the skin. Therefore, particularly entity typing but not so much determination of the initial localization is paramount in metastasized sarcoma. The latter is only of importance in cases without widespread metastatic disease which can be treated with curative intent by surgery and radiation. Hence, for the determination whether a given sarcoma at a specific location is a primary or a metastasis (step 3 in Box 7.1), the definition of the entity type is usually of minor importance, as the respective delineation strongly relies on clinical data (general prevalence of this tumor type at a specific age at the given location, radiographic findings, metastasis pattern).

As already mentioned above, defining the entity (e.g., angiosarcoma) is mandatory for clinical management and therapeutic approaches and can help to predict

Table 7.2 Molecular alterations including simple somatic mutations and translocations as well as viral DNA useful as adjunct diagnostics aiding tumor typing. Some of these alterations can also be detected by mutation-specific antibodies (e.g., BRAF)

Cancer type	Genetic aberration
Prostatic adenocarcinoma	*TMPRSS-ERG* (t)
Papillary thyroid carcinoma	*BRAF*
Pancreatic ductal adenocarcinoma	*KRAS*
Mucoepidermoid carcinoma	*MECT1-MAML2* (t)
Adenoid cystic carcinoma	*MYB-NFIB* (t)
Melanoma	*BRAF*, *NRAS*
Oropharyngeal SQCC	HPV
Uterine cervival SQCC	HPV
Nasopharyngeal carcinoma	EBV

t translocation, *SQCC* squamous cell carcinoma. *CAVEAT:* This list is non-exhaustive and none of the listed SNVs is specific and thus diagnostic for a certain tumor but may support tumor typing in conjunction with other parameters including morphology and expression data. In the case of simple somatic mutations, it may be helpful to refer to specific databases, such as COSMIC (catalogue of somatic mutations in cancer), to check for specific mutations within a certain gene that have been described as recurrent for this entity (e.g., specific somatic *KIT* mutations in exon 11 of GIST (gastrointestinal stroma tumor)).

response to therapy. In general, the diagnostic workup in sarcomas follows the same steps as described for carcinomas. After careful evaluation of histology, immunophenotyping is used to clarify the broad lineage (muscle, neuronal, bone, fat, others) and specific subentity. In addition, in sarcomas, molecular methods are frequently used to ultimately confirm the suspected tumor entity. This specifically applies to those tumor entities for which disease-defining molecular events are known. For sarcomas, this is far more frequently the case than for carcinomas. Usually, these alterations are translocations or specific amplifications, which can be detected by fluorescence in situ hybridization (FISH), simple PCR-based methods, or next-generation sequencing. For further details including the use of new technologies in this context, the reader is referred to the respective literature (e.g., [36]). A comprehensive list of diagnostically useful specific molecular alterations in sarcomas can be found in the current literature as well [37].

In principle, all issues raised above for sarcomas also apply for melanoma. Melanomas can occur as primaries at every region of the skin but also in the mucosal lining of the gastrointestinal, respiratory, and urogenital tract and at the choroidea (as uveal melanoma). The occurrence at other sites is comparably rare. However, if entity typing confirms a metastatic CUP to be a melanoma, the clinical management will be the same as for metastatic melanoma with a known primary site. Treatment of melanoma today heavily relies on the prior establishment of the presence/absence of specific molecular alterations such as *BRAF*, *NRAS*, or *KIT* mutations as well as on antibody-based immunotherapy with so-called checkpoint inhibitors (e.g. PDL-1 inhibition). For a comprehensive summary, the reader is referred to the current literature [38]. As the prevalence of these mutated genes that can be comprehensively interrogated by next-generation sequencing methods differs with respect to the primary site of a melanoma, specific mutated genes may help to infer the primary. As discussed above, however, in a metastatic setting, the clinical significance of detecting the primary is only of limited value. Identification of the primary is only of consequence for locally confined tumors which can be treated by surgery. In this scenario, mainly clinical information is being used (route of spread in lymph nodes) to localize the primary.

With lymphomas [39] the situation is even more difficult. Lymphocytes are per se able to invade tissue and "metastasize," and consequently, an identifiable primary source of tumor "seeding" is usually not present. Therefore, the concept of CUP should probably not be used in the context of lymphomas. However, certain lymphomas (e.g., Hodgkin's lymphoma) also tend to grow locally and spread to more distant sites only late and stepwise in the course of disease. Again, as for melanoma and sarcoma, tumor typing but not tumor localization primarily governs clinical management of these patients.

7.11 Predictive Biomarkers in CUP

With respect to the detection of clinically actionable genetic targets in CUP [40], it should be noted that the prognostic or predictive power of a particular genetic alteration determined in clinical trials and studies for a specific primary tumor cannot be simply transferred to CUP. The significance of molecular alterations arises from the biology of the respective tumor and is certainly not the same for each tumor entity. For example, a mutated oncogene, such as *EGFR*, driving subtypes of lung cancer, may play a different role in the carcinogenesis in an unknown primary tumor, so that the clinical benefit of a specific anti-EGFR therapy remains uncertain. This being said, however, it is important to note that genetic screening of potentially druggable targets may be therapeutically helpful in individual cases and especially in patients with CUP syndrome, who quickly develop resistance against conventional chemotherapy [41, 42]. Such approaches have also been suggested for trials stratifying CUP patients for treatment with multiple different targeted therapies by comprehensively determining the molecular makeup of these tumors [43]. For further details, the reader is referred to the respective chapters of this book.

7.12 Limitations of the Approach

The methods described above have limitations and are not always satisfactory from a clinical as well as pathological point of view. One of these limitations concerns the fact that the worldwide established (TNM) tumor staging system, which is the basis for all study and treatment concepts of a tumor entity, relies on the identification of a definite primary tumor. To achieve this, organ-specific pathological tumor typing always considers clinical information about the origin of the tumor (e.g., biopsy taken from a lesion in the stomach that is suspicious of gastric cancer) or the primary tumor is macroscopically located in the resected organ/organ part subjected for pathological workup. Hence, precise tumor diagnosis is generally achieved by the synopsis of the clinical *and* macroscopic *and* histological *and* immunohistochemical findings. The accuracy of diagnosis increases with the synthesis of the available data. This *diagnostic synthesis* is naturally not possible for CUP syndromes, and the significance and validity of predictions that rely on morphological, immunohistochemical, and molecular studies alone (without knowledge of the location of the primary tumor) are limited in many cases. Another problem concerns the fact that CUPs are often tumors with poor or even absent lineage differentiation, which additionally hampers diagnosis by morphology and immunohistochemistry alone. Aggravating this situation further, pathological diagnosis of CUP is often established on small biopsies with little tumor cell content, large necrotic tumor areas, and tissue artifacts, which interfere with morphology, antigen detection, and other molecular readouts.

7.13 New Horizons in CUP Diagnostics: Molecular Multimarker Profiling

With the advent of quantitative high-throughput technologies for the determination of gene expression profiles (GEP) of a tumor, assays have been developed which are able to identify the tissue/organ of origin of a CUP on the basis of such profiles. This approach is interesting as the classical, gradual single diagnostic marker is replaced by parallel interrogation of multiple markers. Currently, two GEP-based methods for CUP diagnosis are commercially available and at least partially validated.

The Cancer Type ID (CTID) assay [44] is based on mRNA expression profiles of tumor tissue and can be conducted on formalin-fixed, paraffin-embedded tissue (FFPE) biopsies and even cytology material. The test detects the expression level of 92 mRNAs by RT-PCR [44]. The second commercially available test, miRview mets 2 [45], determines the expression of 64 miRNAs by means of an array technology and can also be performed on FFPE material. The applicability of these assays on FFPE material is mandatory, because tissue used for pathological – primarily morphology based – routine diagnostics is always paraffin embedded, to ensure optimal conservation and histological assessment.

Both assays rely on databases in which prototypical expression profiles of a certain number of tumor types and subtypes are deposited. The expression profile of a given CUP, as determined by RT-PCR or transcription arrays, is compared with the profiles stored in the database, and on the basis of these data, subsequently, a score is calculated that indicates the degree of similarity between the expression profile of the CUP case and the expression profiles deposited in the databases. On the basis of these results, a putative tissue of origin for the respective CUP is predicted. This approach has an apparent limitation: molecular profiles of tumor types and subtypes not stored in the database can obviously not be classified. The tests have been reported to have a very high specificity (≥99 %) and show a variable sensitivity (approximately 70–95 %) [45, 46]. It should be noted, however, that these data are estimates that rely on ex post classifications of known primaries and do not reflect the true specificity and sensitivity of the test to trace back CUPs.

Several studies [45–47] compared the classical morphology- and IHC-based approach with the accuracy of commercially available GEP assays. The results showed that GEP approaches need less tissue (average of three tissue sections vs. average of eight tissue sections for the classical approach). Interestingly, two of the studies also reported that with the classical combined diagnostic approach, the accuracy and confidence of the diagnosis decreased with increasing numbers of immunohistochemical stainings required to establish a diagnosis in comparison to the GEP-based diagnosis [10]. This is in line with our observations and emphasizes that the classical combined diagnostic approach will be of high accuracy, if the pathologist has a clear idea of the differential diagnoses obtained by thorough evaluation of histomorphology and supported by a first immunohistochemical panel. In these cases, GEP-based tests do not appear to be diagnostically superior. In CUP cases that are morphologically and immunohistochemically difficult to grasp, however, GEP-based diagnostic procedures seem to add important information.

Larger prospective studies that aim at validating the usability in a real-life setting and investigating cost-effectiveness of GEPs are still missing so that GEP-based diagnostics are currently considered as a useful adjunct but do not replace the conventional pathological approaches discussed above. Hence, GEPs for CUP diagnosis are not widely established in daily clinical practice yet.

7.14 Next-Generation Sequencing

In recent years, massive parallel sequencing techniques (NGS, next-generation sequencing) have revolutionized our understanding of genomic alterations in human tumors. These efforts have revealed typical sets of recurrent mutations for those entities which have been profiled. It has also been shown that genomic profiles may be used for entity subtyping in specific cases. In analogy to GEPs, this is specifically true for morphologically and immunohistochemically nondescript dedifferentiated neoplasms. For example, large cell carcinomas of the lung can be classified by exome sequencing data as being either of squamous cell carcinoma or of adenocarcinoma origin [48]. This, in principle, can also be applied to CUP diagnostics [40, 42–48]. Since it is currently neither cost-effective nor efficient to apply high-throughput exome sequencing in clinical routine diagnostics of CUP, the use of deep massive parallel sequencing of a defined set of informative genes (10–500) is favored by the authors. Since mutational profiles are usually not entity specific but show a broad overlap between different even biologically extremely divergent tumor families, their overall diagnostic impact appears to be of limited value and may aid tumor typing only in certain diagnostic settings (e.g., simultaneous interrogation of a large number of entity-specific genetic translocations in a morphologically and immunohistochemically nondescript sarcoma) [49]. In addition to its putative role in tumor diagnostics, genotyping may help to identify druggable targets (see also above).

7.15 Other High-Throughput Techniques

Multiplexing protein expression analytics by mass spectrometry on minimal tissue amounts can possibly be used for the classification of a CUP in the future [50]. Tissue-based techniques such as MALDI-TOF but also extraction-based quantitative mass spectrometry oligomarker approaches may become more important in the near future. However, currently, these methods are not ready for routine diagnostics yet. High-throughput epigenetic profiling by 450 K chips has been applied for tumor typing, e.g., in brain tumors with some success [51], and it may well be that this method will also be applied as adjunct tool for CUP diagnostics over the next couple of years.

7.16 Integration of Diagnostic Procedures

Approaches that rely on the integration of all available tissue-based diagnostic tools to classify a CUP (histomorphology, expression profiles on an individual marker level by immunohistochemistry, mRNA and miRNA expression profiles, and possibly mutation profiles of gene panels) provide the most reliable way to classify ambiguous tumors with some precision [52]. However, histomorphology is still the basis of tumor diagnosis: it supplies by far the fastest and cheapest means to answer the very basic question as to whether a tumor is present in the biopsy specimen. In addition, in combination with immunohistochemistry, it almost always allows to narrow in on a cancer superfamily and in many cases further subtyping of the tumor [11]. In ambiguous neoplasms, mRNA/miRNA expression profiles may be diagnostically supportive. The results of these tests, however, should be assessed exclusively in synthesis with the morphological and immunohistochemical findings (*congruence of results*). The role of the mutational profile of a tumor for the diagnosis and possibly therapy of a CUP has not been assessed systematically, but is likely to become increasingly important in the future.

7.17 Integration of All Findings

Despite all opportunities, tissue-based tumor mapping is often insufficient and remains incomplete. A clinically meaningful diagnosis can only be established by carefully evaluating all available pathology data in conjunction with clinical and radiological findings (see also other chapters of this book). Hence, continuous interdisciplinary communication (e.g., in specific tumor boards) is the key to clinical success and requires close interaction between all disciplines involved in the treatment of a CUP patient.

In conclusion, the authors dare to say that interdisciplinary communication is probably the most powerful and important "diagnostic approach" in the workup of a patient with CUP.

Acknowledgments We acknowledge excellent editorial assistance of Sandra Schork. Current data on the epidemiology of CUP in Germany were kindly provided by Dr. Klaus Kraywinkel, Robert Koch-Institut (RKI), Berlin, Germany (as presented in [2]). We thank Dr. Mark Kriegsmann for support with figures.

References

1. Pavlidis N, Pentheroudakis G. Cancer of unknown primary site. Lancet. 2012;379:1428–35.
2. Stenzinger A, Kriegsmann M, Weichert W. The role of pathology in the diagnostics of CUP syndrome. Radiologe. 2014;54:124–33.
3. Berlin: Center for Cancer Registry Data, Robert Koch-Institute (RKI), Berlin, Germany.
4. Varadhachary GR, Raber MN. Cancer of unknown primary site. N Engl J Med. 2014;371:757–65.
5. Pavlidis N, Briasoulis E, Pentheroudakis G, et al. Cancers of unknown primary site: ESMO Clinical Practice Guidelines for diagnosis, treatment and follow-up. Ann Oncol. 2010;21:228–31.
6. Pentheroudakis G, Briasoulis E, Pavlidis N. Cancer of unknown primary site: missing primary or missing biology? Oncologist. 2007;12:418–25.
7. Stella GM, Senetta R, Cassenti A, et al. Cancers of unknown primary origin: current perspectives and future therapeutic strategies. J Transl Med. 2012;10:12.
8. Pentheroudakis G, Golfinopoulos V, Pavlidis N. Switching benchmarks in cancer of unknown primary: from autopsy to microarray. Eur J Cancer. 2007;43:2026–36.
9. Greco FA, Pavlidis N. Treatment for patients with unknown primary carcinoma and unfavorable prognostic factors. Semin Oncol. 2009;36:65–74.
10. Hainsworth JD, Rubin MS, Spigel DR, et al. Molecular gene expression profiling to predict the tissue of origin and direct site-specific therapy in patients with carcinoma of unknown primary site: a prospective trial of the Sarah Cannon research institute. J Clin Oncol. 2013;31:217–23.
11. DeYoung BR, Wick MR. Immunohistologic evaluation of metastatic carcinomas of unknown origin: an algorithmic approach. Semin Diagn Pathol. 2000;17:184–93.
12. Heim-Hall J, Yohe SL. Application of immunohistochemistry to soft tissue neoplasms. Arch Pathol Lab Med. 2008;132:476–89.
13. Ivan D, Prieto VG. Use of immunohistochemistry in the diagnosis of melanocytic lesions: applications and pitfalls. Future Oncol. 2010;6:1163–75.
14. Garcia CF, Swerdlow SH. Best practices in contemporary diagnostic immunohistochemistry: panel approach to hematolymphoid proliferations. Arch Pathol Lab Med. 2009;133:756–65.
15. Warth A, Stenzinger A, Weichert W. Novel morphological and molecular aspects of lung cancer. Pathologe. 2013;34:419–28.
16. Kim MJ, Shin HC, Shin KC, et al. Best immunohistochemical panel in distinguishing adenocarcinoma from squamous cell carcinoma of lung: tissue microarray assay in resected lung cancer specimens. Ann Diagn Pathol. 2013;17:85–90.
17. Spigel DR, Hainsworth JD, Greco FA. Neuroendocrine carcinoma of unknown primary site. Semin Oncol. 2009;36:52–9.
18. Taliano RJ, LeGolvan M, Resnick MB. Immunohistochemistry of colorectal carcinoma: current practice and evolving applications. Hum Pathol. 2013;44:151–63.

19. Downes MR, Torlakovic EE, Aldaoud N, et al. Diagnostic utility of androgen receptor expression in discriminating poorly differentiated urothelial and prostate carcinoma. J Clin Pathol. 2013;66:779–86.
20. Mani H, Zander DS. Immunohistochemistry: applications to the evaluation of lung and pleural neoplasms: part 1. Chest. 2012;142:1316–23.
21. Shen SS, Truong LD, Scarpelli M, et al. Role of immunohistochemistry in diagnosing renal neoplasms: when is it really useful? Arch Pathol Lab Med. 2012;136:410–7.
22. Lloyd RV, Buehler D, Khanafshar E. Papillary thyroid carcinoma variants. Head Neck Pathol. 2011;5:51–6.
23. Sangoi AR, Fujiwara M, West RB, et al. Immunohistochemical distinction of primary adrenal cortical lesions from metastatic clear cell renal cell carcinoma: a study of 248 cases. Am J Surg Pathol. 2011;35:678–86.
24. Radwan NA, Ahmed NS. The diagnostic value of arginase-1 immunostaining in differentiating hepatocellular carcinoma from metastatic carcinoma and cholangiocarcinoma as compared to HepPar-1. Diagn Pathol. 2012;7:149.
25. Fan Z, van de Rijn M, Montgomery K, Rouse RV. Hep par 1 antibody stain for the differential diagnosis of hepatocellular carcinoma: 676 tumors tested using tissue microarrays and conventional tissue sections. Mod Pathol. 2003;16:137–44.
26. Weichert W, Schewe C, Denkert C, Morawietz L, Dietel M, Petersen I. Molecular HPV typing as a diagnostic tool to discriminate primary from metastatic squamous cell carcinoma of the lung. Am J Surg Pathol. 2009;33:513–20.
27. Matoso A, Singh K, Jacob R, Greaves WO, Tavares R, Noble L, Resnick MB, Delellis RA, Wang LJ. Comparison of thyroid transcription factor-1 expression by 2 monoclonal antibodies in pulmonary and nonpulmonary primary tumors. Appl Immunohistochem Mol Morphol. 2010;18:142–9.
28. Kubba LA, McCluggage WG, Liu J, Malpica A, Euscher ED, Silva EG, Deavers MT. Thyroid transcription factor-1 expression in ovarian epithelial neoplasms. Mod Pathol. 2008;21:485–90.
29. Bejarano PA, Baughman RP, Biddinger PW, Miller MA, Fenoglio-Preiser C, al-Kafaji B, Di Lauro R, Whitsett JA. Surfactant proteins and thyroid transcription factor-1 in pulmonary and breast carcinomas. Mod Pathol. 1996;9:445–52.
30. Reis HG, Metz CH, Baba HA, et al. TTF-1 (8G7G3/1) positive colon adenocarcinoma: diagnostic implications. Pathologe. 2011;32:349–51.
31. Stenzinger A, Kriegsmann M, Weichert W. Pathology of head and neck cancer– epidemiology and histological subtypes. Onkologe. 2014;20:116–29.
32. Salagierski M, Schalken JA. Molecular diagnosis of prostate cancer: PCA3 and TMPRSS2:ERG gene fusion. J Urol. 2012;187:795–801.
33. Tomlins SA, Rhodes DR, Perner S, Dhanasekaran SM, Mehra R, Sun XW, Varambally S, Cao X, Tchinda J, Kuefer R, Lee C, Montie JE, Shah RB, Pienta KJ, Rubin MA, Chinnaiyan AM. Recurrent fusion of TMPRSS2 and ETS transcription factor genes in prostate cancer. Science. 2005;310:644–8.
34. Tonon G, Modi S, Wu L, Kubo A, Coxon AB, Komiya T, O'Neil K, Stover K, El-Naggar A, Griffin JD, Kirsch IR, Kaye FJ. t(11;19)(q21;p13) translocation in mucoepidermoid carcinoma creates a novel fusion product that disrupts a Notch signaling pathway. Nat Genet. 2003;33:208–13.
35. Hunt JL. An update on molecular diagnostics of squamous and salivary gland tumors of the head and neck. Arch Pathol Lab Med. 2011;135:602–9.
36. van de Rijn M, Guo X, Sweeney RT, Beck AH, West RB. Molecular pathological analysis of sarcomas using paraffin-embedded tissue: current limitations and future possibilities. Histopathology. 2014;64:163–70.
37. Ordóñez JL, Osuna D, García-Domínguez DJ, Amaral AT, Otero-Motta AP, Mackintosh C, Sevillano MV, Barbado MV, Hernández T, de Alava E. The clinical relevance of molecular genetics in soft tissue sarcomas. Adv Anat Pathol. 2010;17:162–81.
38. Bastian BC. The molecular pathology of melanoma: an integrated taxonomy of melanocytic neoplasia. Annu Rev Pathol. 2014;9:239–71.

39. Bradish JR, Cheng L. Molecular pathology of malignant melanoma: changing the clinical practice paradigm toward a personalized approach. Hum Pathol. 2014;45:1315–26.
40. Gatalica Z, Millis SZ, Vranic S, Bender R, Basu GD, Voss A, Von Hoff DD. Comprehensive tumor profiling identifies numerous biomarkers of drug response in cancers of unknown primary site: analysis of 1806 cases. Oncotarget. 2014;15:12440–7.
41. Tan DS, Montoya J, Ng QS, et al. Molecular profiling for druggable genetic abnormalities in carcinoma of unknown primary. J Clin Oncol. 2013;31:237–9.
42. Tothill RW, Li J, Mileshkin L, Doig K, Siganakis T, Cowin P, Fellowes A, Semple T, Fox S, Byron K, Kowalczyk A, Thomas D, Schofield P, Bowtell DD. Massively-parallel sequencing assists the diagnosis and guided treatment of cancers of unknown primary. J Pathol. 2013;231:413–23.
43. Pentheroudakis G, Pavlidis N. Perspectives for targeted therapies in cancer of unknown primary site. Cancer Treat Rev. 2006;32(8):637–44.
44. Weiss LM, Chu P, Schroeder BE, et al. Blinded comparator study of immunohistochemical analysis versus a 92-gene cancer classifier in the diagnosis of the primary site in metastatic tumors. J Mol Diagn. 2013;15:263–9.
45. Varadhachary GR, Abbruzzese JL, Lenzi R. Diagnostic strategies for unknown primary cancer. Cancer. 2004;100:1776–85.
46. Kulkarni A, Pillai R, Ezekiel AM, et al. Comparison of histopathology to gene expression profiling for the diagnosis of metastatic cancer. Diagn Pathol. 2012;7:110.
47. Handorf CR, Kulkarni A, Grenert JP, et al. A multicenter study directly comparing the diagnostic accuracy of gene expression profiling and immunohistochemistry for primary site identification in metastatic tumors. Am J Surg Pathol. 2013;37:1067–75.
48. Clinical Lung Cancer Genome Project (CLCGP), Network Genomic Medicine (NGM). A genomics-based classification of human lung tumors. Sci Transl Med. 2013;30:209.
49. Qadir MA, Zhan SH, Kwok B, Bruestle J, Drees B, Popescu OE, Sorensen PH. ChildSeq-RNA: a next-generation sequencing-based diagnostic assay to identify known fusion transcripts in childhood sarcomas. J Mol Diagn. 2014;16:361–70.
50. Meding S, Nitsche U, Balluff B, et al. Tumor classification of six common cancer types based on proteomic profiling by MALDI imaging. J Proteome Res. 2012;11:1996–2003.
51. Koelsche C, Hovestadt V, Jones DT, Capper D, Sturm D, Sahm F, Schrimpf D, Adeberg S, Böhmer K, Hagenlocher C, Mechtersheimer G, Kohlhof P, Mühleisen H, Beschorner R, Hartmann C, Braczynski AK, Mittelbronn M, Buslei R, Becker A, Grote A, Urbach H, Staszewski O, Prinz M, Hewer E, Pfister SM, von Deimling A, Reuss DE. Melanotic tumors of the nervous system are characterized by distinct mutational, chromosomal and epigenomic profiles. Brain Pathol. 2015;25:202–8.
52. Centeno BA, Bloom G, Chen DT, et al. Hybrid model integrating immunohistochemistry and expression profiling for the classification of carcinomas of unknown primary site. J Mol Diagn. 2010;12:476–86.

Chapter 8
Treatment of Disseminated CUP

Gerdt Hübner

8.1 Background

CUP as a distinct tumor entity was identified in the 1940s, initially as lymph node metastases in the neck [1, 2]. CUP in visceral organs was described 20 years later [3, 4]. The treatment of CUP has developed over several decades. In an era of therapeutic nihilism in metastatic cancer, the first generation of studies of CUP were mainly retrospective large single institution surveys and series of autopsies [5–10]. The search for the primary and the account of certain diagnostic procedures were the focus of many studies; for instance, radiographic procedures of the intestine proved to be of little value [11] in contrast to CT scans [12]. Most of the favorable subsets were recognized and descriptive data on the biology, presentation, and prognosis of CUP were established.

8.2 Treatment Overview

Treatment of patients with CUP falls in two major categories:

1. Subsets of patients requiring specific treatment

   These are often named "favorable" because the prognosis of patients falling into these well-defined subsets differs favorably from the remainder of CUP patients.

G. Hübner, MD
Department of Hematology and Medical Oncology, Sana Kliniken Ostholstein GmbH, Eutin/Oldenburg/Holstein, Germany
e-mail: gerdt.huebner@sana.de
http://www.sana-oh.de; http://www.ostholstein-onkologie.de; http://www.krebsgesellschaft.de

A. Krämer, H. Löffler (eds.), *Cancer of Unknown Primary*,
DOI 10.1007/978-3-319-22581-4_8

2. Treatment of patients with disseminated disease not fitting to any of these subsets

These are often named "unfavorable" in spite of the heterogeneous course of disease with survival ranging from only a few days to years.

While CUP is a very heterogeneous disorder, only 15–25 % of patients fall into well-defined subgroups requiring specific therapy [13] – treatment of these patients is covered in Chap. 10. This chapter will focus on the majority of patients with CUP: 75–85 % of patients are suffering from a cancer without known primary tumor, spread to several metastatic sites, and histologically adenocarcinoma or poorly differentiated (adeno)carcinoma in the vast majority with a few cases of squamous cell carcinoma or anaplastic carcinoma, not otherwise specified. Unfortunately, the therapist's guess of the probable primary tumor is often not evidence based but related primarily to personal experience or a pathologist's comment and can be misleading, thus resulting in suboptimal treatment.

Prognosis is dismal in the majority of patients. Median survival is 3–11 months; the 1-year survival rate is 25–40 % [14–18]. Long-term survival is rare but possible with 5-year survival rates between 3 and 15 %. The primary is identified in less than 10 % during lifetime [19]. Patients frequently present with multiple metastases in lymph nodes, liver, bones, and lung [15] (see Chaps. 3 and 4).

Therapy in disseminated CUP is guided by several factors:

- Presenting site and pattern of metastases
- Performance status
- Age
- Histology and immunohistochemistry
- Genetic tumor profile
- Patient's requests and preferences

8.3 Specific Subsets

It is of upmost importance not to miss the subgroups with favorable prognosis (see Table 8.1 and Chap. 10).

8.4 Unfavorable Disseminated CUP

8.4.1 Single-Armed Phase II Trials

The first generation of treatment studies on CUP from 1964 to 1989 were mostly one armed and small and dealt with substances proven effective in other tumors including doxorubicin, 5-fluorouracil, mitomycin, methotrexate, vinca alkaloids, cisplatin, and cyclophosphamide [20–24]. Median survival ranged from a few

Table 8.1 Favorable subgroups requiring specific therapy

Resectable disease("oligometastatic")	Involvement of one lymph node area only (e.g., inguinal nodes), solitary lesions, resectable liver metastases
Cervical node metastases with squamous or undifferentiated histology	Strong resemblance to head and neck cancer
Axillary node metastases in women	To be regarded as node-positive breast cancer if not proven otherwise
Peritoneal carcinomatosis in women, especially papillary or serous adenocarcinoma	To be regarded as ovarian cancer or primary peritoneal carcinoma if not proven otherwise
Extragonadal germ cell tumors	Men, <50 years, undifferentiated carcinoma, retroperitoneal/mediastinal/pulmonary involvement, rapidly progressive, isochromosome i12p
Neuroendocrine tumors and carcinomas	NET I-II°, somatostatin receptor positive NET III-IV°: resembling small cell lung cancer (SCLC)
Adenocarcinoma with colon-type histology	Immunohistochemistry positive for cytokeratin 20 and CDX2, negative for cytokeratin 7 (CK7−, CK20+, CDX2+)
Hormone-sensitive cancers	Expression of estrogen or progesterone receptor (ER+, PR+) mainly in women or androgen receptor or PSA in men
Non-carcinomatous-specific histology	For example, melanoma, sarcoma, lymphoma, etc.

weeks to 8 months. Therapeutic nihilism dominated the view of many treating physicians.

The second generation of treatment trials from about 1990 to 2003 were prospective, mono- or oligocentric phase II studies, most of which investigated only a single-treatment option. Obviously, one-armed trials in CUP are subject to considerable selection bias – the investigators simply will include patients whom they believe to benefit from this type of therapy while others are not included. Furthermore, favorable subsets (see Table 8.1) were not systematically excluded. These studies established a role for platinum compounds (mainly carboplatin), taxanes, and gemcitabine in the treatment of disseminated CUP with overall survival ranging from 7 to 13 months in selected patients [16, 25–28].

8.4.2 Randomized Clinical Trials (RCT)

Only RCT can minimize the major confounder in CUP treatment studies: selection bias. Unfortunately, randomized trials are scarce with less than 1000 patients included in all published trials to date (986 as of February 2015). Nevertheless, the first study was published as early as 1980 in the *New England Journal of Medicine* [29]. Several further first-generation studies followed (Table 8.2).

Relevant results regarding modern chemotherapy treatment were added by the next generation of CUP trials (Table 8.3). These studies systematically excluded favorable subsets and were randomized, thus minimizing selection bias. One phase

Table 8.2 First-generation randomized clinical trials

Author	*N*	Regimen	ORR (%)	PFS months	OS months
Woods et al.(1980) [29]	47	C/M/FU MMC/Doxo	4 36		1.7 4.5
Eagan et al.(1987) [30]	55	MMC/Doxo MMC/Doxo/Cis	14 27		5.5 4.6
Milliken et al.(1987) [31]	95	MMC/Doxo Cis/Vbl/Bleo	42 32		4.5 6.2
Falkson andCohen (1998) [32]	84	MMC/Epi/Cis MMC	50 17		9.4 5.4
Dowell et al.(2001) [33]	34	Carbo/Eto Pac/FA/FU	19 19		8.4 6.5
Assersohn et al.(2003) [34]	88	FU cont FU cont/MMC	12 20	3.6 4.1	4.7 6.7

N number, *ORR* overall remission rate, *PFS* progression-free survival, *OS* overall survival, *C* cyclophosphamide, *M* methotrexate, *FU* 5-fluorouracil, *MMC* mitomycin C, *Doxo* doxorubicin, *Cis* cisplatin, *Vbl* vinblastine, *Bleo* bleomycin, *Epi* epirubicin, *Pac* paclitaxel, *FA* folinic acid, *cont* continuous infusion

Table 8.3 Second-generation randomized clinical trials

Author	*N*	Regimen	ORR (%)	PFSmonths	OSmonths	Survivalrate
Culine et al.(2003) [17]	80	Cis/Gem Cis/Iri	55 38		8 6	
Palmeri et al.(2006) [35]	66	Cis/Gem/Pac Cis/Gem/Vino	49 42		9.6 13.6	
Hübner et al. (2009) [14]	92	Carbo/Pac Gem/Vino	24 20	6.1 3.2	11.0 7.0	38 % @1y 29 % @1y
Hainsworthet al. (2010) [36]	198	Carbo/Pac/Eto Gem/Iri	18 18	3.3 5.3	7.4 8.5	28 % @1y 35 % @1y
Gross-Goupil et al. (2012) [37]	52	Cis/Gem Cis	19 16	5 3	11 8	46 % @1y 35 % @1y
Hainsworth et al. (2015) [38]	89	Carbo/Pac/ Belino Carbo/Pac	45 21	5.4 5.3	12.4 9.1	

N number, *ORR* overall remission rate, *PFS* progression-free survival, *OS* overall survival, *y* year, *Carbo* carboplatin, *Eto* etoposide, *Pac* paclitaxel, *Cis* cisplatin, *Gem* gemcitabine, *Iri* irinotecan, *Vino* vinorelbine, *Belino* belinostat

III trial – the biggest trial ever published – had to stop short of its aim and recruited 198 patients [36]. The remainder were randomized phase II studies with 80–100 patients included [14, 17, 37, 38]. Taken together, these trials built the basis of current first-line treatment of disseminated CUP with adenocarcinoma or poorly differentiated carcinoma. Platinum compounds, taxanes, gemcitabine, and irinotecan evolved as active compounds in CUP treatment. Tandem combinations outrivaled triple combinations because of comparable efficacy and less toxicity.

Table 8.4 Meta-analysis [18]

	N	OS	@1 year (%)	@2 year (%)	Significance
32 trials	1830	9.0	36	19	
Carbo-/cisplatin	1450	9.4	37	20	N.S.
No platinum	425	7.2	30	12	
Pacli-/docetaxel	808	9.6	41	21	$P=0.03$
No taxane	1067	8.3	31	16	
Platinum + taxane	755	9.6	42	22	$P=0.06$
No platinum + no taxane	358	6.6	28	14	

N number, *OS* overall survival, *N.S.* not significant

A recent meta-analysis of 1830 "unfavorable" CUP patients in 32 trials including 7 randomized trials showed a significant advantage of taxanes versus no taxanes and a nonsignificant trend of platinum vs. no platinum (Table 8.4, Ref. [18]). This meta-analysis on one hand suffers from the scarcity of robust data; on the other hand, its findings underline the efficacy of taxane and platinum compounds in the empirical treatment of unfavorable CUP.

8.4.3 *Squamous Cell Carcinoma*

Squamous cell carcinoma is common in cervical lymph node metastasis with unknown primary but rare in unfavorable disseminated CUP, making up about 5–7 % of cases. Meaningful treatment trials do not exist – in contrast to squamous cell carcinoma affecting cervical nodes. Some groups simply include these patients into their adenocarcinoma and poorly differentiated carcinoma trials, but the numbers are too small to reach meaningful conclusions.

In effect, treatment recommendations extrapolate experiences of squamous cell carcinoma of known primary to situations with unknown primary. Cisplatin combined with fluorouracil is a common and quite effective combination, especially in regional disease combined with concurrent irradiation. Carboplatin/taxane combinations are a reasonable alternative, especially in patients with renal failure or reduced performance status. Based on results in non-small cell lung cancer, nab-paclitaxel may also be effective. Considering the efficacy of EGFR antibodies in the head and neck and non-small cell lung cancer as well as some adenocarcinomas, they may be an option in individual patients as well.

8.4.4 *Colon Cancer-Like Treatment*

Two trials report treatment that is effective in colon cancer as first-line therapy of disseminated CUP, applying capecitabine, oxaliplatin, and irinotecan [39, 40]. In these single-armed phase II trials, the study populations were dominated by patients

Table 8.5 Second-line therapy

Author	*N*	Regimen	ORR (%)	PFS	OS	
Culine et al. (2001) [41]	25	FA/FU	0		3	After cisplatin
Hainsworth et al. (2001) [42]	39	Gem	8	4		After platinum and taxane
Pouessel et al. (2003) [43]	15	Gem/Doce	29		8	After cisplatin
Hainsworth et al. (2005) [44]	40	Gem/Iri	10		4.5	
Hainsworth et al. (2007) [45]	51	Erlotinib/Beva	10		7.4	14 pts 1st line, 24 pts2nd line, 14 pts 3rd line
Moller et al. (2010) [46]	25	Cape/Ox	13	2.3	3.9	After cisplatin, paclitaxel,and gemcitabine
Hainsworth et al. (2010) [47]	48	Cape/Ox	19	3.7	9.7	

N number, *ORR* overall remission rate, *PFS* progression-free survival, *OS* overall survival, *FA* folinic acid, *FU* 5-fluorouracil, *Gem* gemcitabine, *Doce* docetaxel, *Iri* irinotecan, *Beva* bevacizumab, *Cape* capecitabine, *Ox* oxaliplatin, *pts* patients

with features hinting to a gastrointestinal primary though typical colon cancer-like histology (favorable subset) was excluded. The results were uniformly poor with progression-free survival of 2.5–3.5 months and overall survival well below 10 months. In second-line treatment, the combination of oxaliplatin and capecitabine performed as well as in the first-line setting (see Table 8.6). Taken together, colon cancer-like regimens are not indicated as first-line therapy in disseminated CUP. They may be an option in second-line treatment.

8.4.5 Second-Line Treatment

Only few small one-armed trials investigated the role of second-line chemotherapy in unfavorable CUP. These trials hint at a potential role of gemcitabine, irinotecan, oxaliplatin, and capecitabine as moderately active drugs after platinum-based first-line chemotherapy (Table 8.5).

8.4.6 Supportive and Palliative Care

Because of the dismal prognosis in the majority of patients, supportive and palliative care is of utmost importance from the beginning. Treatment with bisphosphonates or denusomab is indicated in the presence of bone metastases or hypercalcemia. Painful local (skeletal and other) metastases should be irradiated. Adequate treatment of pain and other symptoms should be a matter of course.

Table 8.6 First-line treatment options

Drug	Dose	Application	Time
Carboplatin/paclitaxel [14]			
Paclitaxel	175 mg/m²	180 min. i.v.	Day 1
Carboplatin	AUC 5	30–60 min. i.v.	Day 1
Every 3 weeks			
Cisplatin/gemcitabine("French regimen") [37]			
Gemcitabine	1250 mg/m²	30 min. i.v.	Day 1+8
Cisplatin	100 mg/m²	30–60 min. i.v.	Day 1
Every 3 weeks			
Gemcitabine/irinotecan [36]			
Gemcitabine	1000 mg/m²	30 min. i.v.	Day 1+8
Irinotecan	100 mg/m²	30 min. i.v.	Day 1+8
Every 3 weeks			

8.4.7 Actual Standard of Care and National Guidelines

The goal of treatment is to prolong life and/or improve or maintain quality of life. The empirical treatment in disseminated CUP consists of chemotherapy in the majority of cases. Whether to choose a combination or a monotherapy depends on age, performance status, comorbidity, and functional status according to the criteria of geriatric assessment.

Based on randomized clinical trials, several combination treatment options are available for patients with disseminated CUP (Table 8.6). Taxane/platinum combinations are supported by the biggest body of evidence. They can be considered a kind of "standard of care" despite all limitations, yielding a median survival of 8–11 months, a 1-year survival rate of 37–45 % and a 2-year survival rate of 18–26 % [18].

This is reflected in available national guidelines (ESMO Clinical Practice Guidelines from 2011 [48], German Onkopedia Guidelines from 2014 [49] and the NCCN Guidelines, version 1.2015 [50]).

In patients with reduced performance status or relevant comorbidity, single-agent therapies are feasible in spite of lack of studies to prove their efficacy. The renouncement of chemotherapy may be the best choice in frail patients with reduced performance status or severe comorbidity.

Second-line therapy is not well established and its benefit is unknown. Some options for suitable patients are given in Table 8.7.

8.5 Changing Paradigms and Future Perspectives

Gene expression profiling and the identification of druggable targets as well as new developments in immunotherapy are currently changing the world of cancer therapy. Treatment decisions in CUP should particularly be facilitated by these developments:

Table 8.7 Second-line treatment options

Drug	Dose	Application	Time
Erlotinib/bevacizumab [45]			
Erlotinib	150 mg	p.o.	qd
Bevacizumab	15 mg/kg KG	30–90 min. i.v.	Day 1
Every 3 weeks			
Gemcitabine/irinotecan [44]			
Gemcitabine	1000 mg/m^2	30 min. i.v.	Day 1+8
Irinotecan	100 mg/m^2	30 min. i.v.	Day 1+8
Every 3 weeks			
Capecitabine/oxaliplatin [46, 47]			
Capecitabine	1000 mg/m^2	p.o.	Bid day 1–14
Oxaliplatin	130 mg/m^2	120 min. i.v.	Day 1
Every 3 weeks			
Gemcitabine [42]			
Gemcitabine	1000 mg/m^2	30 min. i.v.	Day 1+8+15
Every 4 weeks			

while the primary site of a cancer may still be unknown, molecular pathways, driver mutations, and immune checkpoint ligands will not. Hopefully, this will enable individual and more precise treatment recommendations in patients with disseminated CUP in the foreseeable future. Chapters 11 and 12 will focus on these developments. Nonetheless, it should be kept in mind that up to date, there is no robust evidence of these advances to build the basis for treatment recommendations in CUP.

Potential Conflicts of Interests Within the last 15 years, the corresponding author has received grants for the conduction of clinical and experimental studies in CUP syndrome by Lilly Oncology, Bristol-Myers-Squibb, Sanofi-Aventis, Roche Oncology, and Agendia BV. He is or has been member of advisory boards of Roche Oncology, Boehringer Ingelheim, and Teva Pharmaceutical.

He confirms that he has no financial relationships to any firm relevant to the treatment of CUP syndrome. The presentation of the topic is independent, and the contents of the chapter are free of any influences from third parties including pharmaceutical firms.

References

1. Deuel H. Primäre Halsgeschwülste und deren Differentialdiagnose gegenüber Lymphknotenmetastasen. Radiol Clin. 1942;11:297–316.
2. Martin H, Morfit HM. Cervical lymph node metastasis as the first symptom of cancer. Surg Gynecol Obstet. 1944;78:133–59.
3. Fenster LF, Klatskin G. Manifestations of metastatic tumors of the liver. Am J Med. 1961;31:238–48.
4. Johnson RO, Castro R, Ansfield FJ. Response of primary unknown cancers to treatment with 5-fluorouracil. Cancer Chemother Rep. 1964;38:63–4.
5. Didolkar MS, Fanous N, Elias EG, Moore RH. Metastatic carcinomas from occult primary tumors. A study of 254 patients. Ann Surg. 1977;186:625–30.

6. Hübner G, Tamme C, Wildfang I, Schöber C, Schmoll H-J. Management of patients with carcinoma of unknown primary (CUP-Syndrome). J Cancer Res Clin Oncol. 1990;116(Suppl Part I):190.
7. Altman E, Cadman E. An analysis of 1539 patients with cancer of unknown primary site. Cancer. 1986;57:120–4.
8. Muir C. Cancer of unknown primary site. Cancer. 1995;75(1 Suppl):353–6.
9. Snee MP, Vyramuthu N. Metastatic carcinoma from unknown primary site: the experience of a large oncology centre. Br J Radiol. 1985;58:1091–5.
10. Le Chevalier T, Cvitkovic E, Caille P, Harvey J, Contesso G, Spielmann M, et al. Early metastatic cancer of unknown primary origin at presentation. A clinical study of 302 consecutive autopsied patients. Arch Intern Med. 1988;148:2035–9.
11. Nystrom JS, Weiner JM, Wolf RM, Bateman JR, Viola MV. Identifying the primary site in metastatic cancer of unknown origin Inadequacy of roentgenographic procedures. JAMA. 1979;241:381–3.
12. McMillan JH, Levine E, Stephens RH. Computed tomography in the evaluation of metastatic adenocarcinoma from an unknown primary site. A retrospective study. Radiology. 1982;143:143–6.
13. Yi JH, La CY, Lee SJ, Ahn HK, Baek KK, Lim T, et al. Clinical presentation of carcinoma of unknown primary: 14 years of experience. Tumour Biol. 2011;32(1):45–51.
14. Hübner G, Link H, Kohne CH, Stahl M, Kretzschmar A, Steinbach S, et al. Paclitaxel and carboplatin vs gemcitabine and vinorelbine in patients with adeno- or undifferentiated carcinoma of unknown primary: a randomised prospective phase II trial. Br J Cancer. 2009;100:44–9.
15. Hess KR, Abbruzzese MC, Lenzi R, Raber MN, Abbruzzese JL. Classification and regression tree analysis of 1000 consecutive patients with unknown primary carcinoma. Clin Cancer Res. 1999;5(11):3403–10.
16. Greco FA, Burris III HA, Litchy S, Barton JH, Bradof JE, Richards P, et al. Gemcitabine, Carboplatin, and Paclitaxel for patients with carcinoma of unknown primary site: a minnie pearl cancer research network study. J Clin Oncol. 2002;20(6):1651–6.
17. Culine S, Lortholary A, Voigt JJ, Bugat R, Theodore C, Priou F, et al. Cisplatin in combination with either gemcitabine or irinotecan in carcinomas of unknown primary site: results of a randomized phase II study–trial for the French Study Group on Carcinomas of Unknown Primary (GEFCAPI 01). J Clin Oncol. 2003;21(18):3479–82.
18. Lee J, Hahn S, Kim DW, Kim J, Kang SN, Rha SY, et al. Evaluation of survival benefits by platinums and taxanes for an unfavourable subset of carcinoma of unknown primary: a systematic review and meta-analysis. Br J Cancer. 2013;108(1):39–48.
19. Greco FA, Spigel DR, Yardley DA, Erlander MG, Ma XJ, Hainsworth JD. Molecular profiling in unknown primary cancer: accuracy of tissue of origin prediction. Oncologist. 2010;15(5):500–6.
20. Moertel CG, Reitemeier RJ, Schutt AJ, Hahn RG. Treatment of the patient with adenocarcinoma of unknown origin. Cancer. 1972;30:1469–72.
21. Bedikian AY, Bodey GP, Valdivieso M, Burgess MA. Sequential chemotherapy for adenocarcinoma of unknown primary. Am J Clin Oncol. 1983;6:219–24.
22. Fiore JJ, Kelsen DP, Gralla RJ, Casper ES, Magill G, Cheng E, et al. Adenocarcinoma of unknown primary origin: treatment with vindesine and doxorubicin. Cancer Treat Rep. 1985;69:591–4.
23. Kelsen D, Coit D, Houston C, Martin D, Sawyer R, Colofiore J. Phase II trial of pala, methotrexate (Mtx), fluorouracil (FU), and leucovorin (L) in adenocarcinoma of unknown primary site (ACUP). Proc ASCO. 1989;8:A1141.
24. Bécouarn Y, Brunet R, Barbe-Gaston C. Fluorouracil, doxorubicin, cisplatin and altretamine in the treatment of metastatic carcinoma of unknown primary. Eur J Cancer Clin Oncol. 1989;25:861–5.
25. Hainsworth JD, Erland JB, Kalman LA, Schreeder MT, Greco FA. Carcinoma of unknown primary site: treatment with 1-hour paclitaxel, carboplatin, and extended-schedule etoposide. J Clin Oncol. 1997;15(6):2385–93.

26. Briasoulis E, Kalofonos H, Bafaloukos D, Samantas E, Fountzilas G, Xiros N, et al. Carboplatin plus paclitaxel in unknown primary carcinoma: a phase II hellenic cooperative oncology group study. J Clin Oncol. 2000;18(17):3101–7.
27. Munoz A, Barcelo JR, Lopez-Vivanco G. Gemcitabine and docetaxel as front-line chemotherapy in patients with carcinoma of an unknown primary site. Cancer. 2004;101(3):653–4.
28. Park YH, Ryoo BY, Choi SJ, Yang SH, Kim HT. A phase II study of paclitaxel plus cisplatin chemotherapy in an unfavourable group of patients with cancer of unknown primary site. Jpn J Clin Oncol. 2004;34(11):681–5.
29. Woods RL, Fox RM, Tattersall MH, Levi JA, Brodie GN. Metastatic adenocarcinomas of unknown primary site: a randomized study of two combination-chemotherapy regimens. N Engl J Med. 1980;303:87–9.
30. Eagan RT, Therneau TM, Rubin J, Long HJ, Schutt AJ. Lack of value for cisplatin added to mitomycin-doxorubicin combination chemotherapy for carcinoma of unknown primary site. A randomized trial. Am J Clin Oncol. 1987;10:82–5.
31. Milliken ST, Tattersall MH, Woods RL, Coates AS, Levi JA, Fox RM, et al. Metastatic adenocarcinoma of unknown primary site. A randomized study of two combination chemotherapy regimens. Eur J Cancer Clin Oncol. 1987;23:1645–8.
32. Falkson CI, Cohen GL. Mitomycin C, epirubicin and cisplatin versus mitomycin C alone as therapy for carcinoma of unknown primary origin. Oncology. 1998;55:116–21.
33. Dowell JE, Garrett AM, Shyr Y, Johnson DH, Hande KR. A randomized phase II trial in patients with carcinoma of an unknown primary site. Cancer. 2001;91(3):592–7.
34. Assersohn L, Norman AR, Cunningham D, Iveson T, Seymour M, Hickish T, et al. A randomised study of protracted venous infusion of 5-fluorouracil (5-FU) with or without bolus mitomycin C (MMC) in patients with carcinoma of unknown primary. Eur J Cancer. 2003;39(8):1121–8.
35. Palmeri S, Lorusso V, Palmeri L, Vaglica M, Porta C, Nortilli R, et al. Cisplatin and gemcitabine with either vinorelbine or paclitaxel in the treatment of carcinomas of unknown primary site: results of an Italian multicenter, randomized, phase II study. Cancer. 2006;107(12):2898–905.
36. Hainsworth JD, Spigel DR, Clark BL, Shipley D, Thompson DS, Farley C, et al. Paclitaxel/carboplatin/etoposide versus gemcitabine/irinotecan in the first-line treatment of patients with carcinoma of unknown primary site: a randomized, phase III Sarah Cannon Oncology Research Consortium Trial. Cancer J. 2010;16(1):70–5.
37. Gross-Goupil M, Fourcade A, Blot E, Penel N, Negrier S, Culine S, et al. Cisplatin alone or combined with gemcitabine in carcinomas of unknown primary: results of the randomised GEFCAPI 02 trial. Eur J Cancer. 2012;48(5):721–7.
38. Hainsworth JD, Daugaard G, Lesimple T, Hübner G, Greco FA, Stahl MJ, et al. Paclitaxel/carboplatin with or without belinostat as empiric first-line treatment for patients with carcinoma of unknown primary site: a randomized, phase 2 trial. Cancer. 2015;121:1654–61.
39. Briasoulis E, Fountzilas G, Bamias A, Dimopoulos MA, Xiros N, Aravantinos G, et al. Multicenter phase-II trial of irinotecan plus oxaliplatin [IROX regimen] in patients with poor-prognosis cancer of unknown primary: a hellenic cooperative oncology group study. Cancer Chemother Pharmacol. 2008;62(2):277–84.
40. Schuette K, Folprecht G, Kretzschmar A, Link H, Koehne CH, Gruenwald V, et al. Phase II trial of capecitabine and oxaliplatin in patients with adeno- and undifferentiated carcinoma of unknown primary. Onkologie. 2009;32(4):162–6.
41. Culine S, Ychou M, Fabbro M, Romieu G, Cupissol D. 5-fluorouracil and leucovorin as second-line chemotherapy in carcinomas of unknown primary site. Anticancer Res. 2001;21(2B):1455–7.
42. Hainsworth JD, Burris III HA, Calvert SW, Willcutt NT, Scullin Jr DC, Bramham J, et al. Gemcitabine in the second-line therapy of patients with carcinoma of unknown primary site: a phase II trial of the Minnie Pearl Cancer Research Network. Cancer Invest. 2001;19(4):335–9.
43. Pouessel D, Culine S, Becht C, Romieu G, Fabbro M, Ychou M, et al. Gemcitabine and docetaxel after failure of cisplatin-based chemotherapy in patients with carcinoma of unknown primary site. Anticancer Res. 2003;23(3C):2801–4.

44. Hainsworth JD, Spigel DR, Raefsky EL, Kuzur ME, Yost K, Kommor M, et al. Combination chemotherapy with gemcitabine and irinotecan in patients with previously treated carcinoma of an unknown primary site: a Minnie Pearl Cancer Research Network Phase II trial. Cancer. 2005;104(9):1992–7.
45. Hainsworth JD, Spigel DR, Farley C, Thompson DS, Shipley DL, Greco FA. Phase II trial of bevacizumab and erlotinib in carcinomas of unknown primary site: the Minnie Pearl Cancer Research Network. J Clin Oncol. 2007;25(13):1747–52.
46. Moller AK, Pedersen KD, Abildgaard J, Petersen BL, Daugaard G. Capecitabine and oxaliplatin as second-line treatment in patients with carcinoma of unknown primary site. Acta Oncol. 2010;49(4):431–5.
47. Hainsworth JD, Spigel DR, Burris III HA, Shipley D, Farley C, Dias-Perez IM, et al. Oxaliplatin and capecitabine in the treatment of patients with recurrent or refractory carcinoma of unknown primary site: a phase 2 trial of the Sarah Cannon Oncology Research Consortium. Cancer. 2010;116(10):2448–54.
48. Fizazi K, Greco FA, Pavlidis N, Pentheroudakis G. Cancers of unknown primary site: ESMO Clinical Practice Guidelines for diagnosis, treatment and follow-up. Ann Oncol. 2011;22 Suppl 6:vi64–8.
49. Hübner G, Borner M, Neben K, Stöger H (2014) Onkopedia Leitlinien: CUP-Syndrom – Krebserkrankungen mit unbekanntem Primärtumor. https://www.dgho-onkopediade/de/onkopedia/leitlinien/cup-syndrom-krebserkrankungen-mit-unbekanntem
50. NCCN Guidelines (2015) Occult primary. https://www.nccnorg/store/login/loginaspx?ReturnURL=http://www.nccnorg/professionals/physician_gls/pdf/occultpdf; 1.205

Chapter 9
Concepts of Radiotherapy in Cancer of Unknown Primary

David Krug and Florian Sterzing

9.1 Curative Treatment Concepts

9.1.1 Axillary Cancer of Unknown Primary

9.1.1.1 Introduction

Axillary cancer of unknown primary (CUP) is defined as the infiltration of axillary lymph nodes by (adeno) carcinoma without the detection of a primary tumor on standard imaging. The first three cases of axillary CUP were published by William S. Halsted. The incidence of axillary CUP ranges between 0.12 and 0.67 % of all malignant neoplasms [2]. Due to this fact, practically all publications are based on retrospective case series, mostly from single institutions, and many treatment approaches have been deduced from the treatment of breast cancer patients.

Diagnostic imaging plays a key role in the establishment of a diagnosis of CUP. In a meta-analysis by Pentheroudakis et al., the lack of sensitivity of historic imaging modalities is reflected by the fact that in patients with suspected axillary CUP who had mastectomy, a clinically occult primary tumor could be identified in 72 % of the specimens [2]. Recently, the introduction of MRI has changed the diagnostic management of axillary CUP substantially. Pooled sensitivity and specificity were 90 and 31 % in a systematic review of breast MRI [3].

D. Krug • F. Sterzing (✉)
RadioOnkologie und Strahlentherapie, UniversitätsKlinikum Heidelberg,
Im Neuenheimer Feld 400, Heidelberg 69120, Germany
e-mail: david.krug@med.uni-heidelberg.de

A. Krämer, H. Löffler (eds.), *Cancer of Unknown Primary*,
DOI 10.1007/978-3-319-22581-4_9

9.1.1.2 General Management

Although some older studies have used axillary lymph node sampling followed by axillary radiotherapy, axillary lymph node dissection (ALND) has been considered a standard procedure due to an improved locoregional control rate and the prognostic relevance of accurate axillary staging [2].

The optimal treatment of the ipsilateral breast is controversial. Available options are observation, mastectomy, and whole breast radiotherapy. In a survey of the American Society of Breast Surgeons, 43 % voted for mastectomy, 37 % preferred whole breast radiotherapy, and 6 % recommended observation [4].

Observation after axillary surgery is associated with unacceptably high rates of locoregional relapse. In a meta-analysis by Pentheroudakis et al., 42 % of patients developed a recurrence in the ipsilateral breast after a median latency period of 4–64 months. Other retrospective series have shown locoregional recurrence rates of up to 70–80 % after observation only [5–9].

Local treatment of the breast by mastectomy can improve locoregional control and also disease-free and overall survival. In a retrospective study on 51 patients, Wang et al. could show that mastectomy compared to observation reduced the risk of any recurrence from 77 to 26 % while improving median overall survival from 23 to 76 months [10]. Similarly, Blanchard and Farley showed significantly better disease-free and overall survival in patients undergoing ipsilateral mastectomy compared to observation [11].

9.1.1.3 Breast-Conserving Treatment

In the 1980s, first reports of breast-conserving treatment in axillary CUP were published [12]. In analogy to breast-conserving therapy in breast cancer, where adjuvant radiotherapy reduces the risk of any recurrence by approximately 50 % leading to an absolute survival benefit of 4 % after 15 years [13], whole breast radiotherapy was added after axillary dissection to eradicate clinically occult disease in the ipsilateral breast. In the first reports, 10-year survival rates of 72 % were achieved while breast preservation was feasible in 75 % of patients [12]. Since then, numerous studies on breast-conserving treatment in patients with axillary CUP have been published (for a summary, see Table 9.1).

In a nationwide retrospective study from Korea, 142 patients could be identified that received treatment between 1990 and 2009 [14]. About two thirds of the population had N1 disease. Overall, 23 % underwent ALND and 40 % received additional whole breast radiotherapy or mastectomy, respectively. There was a trend toward improved 10-year overall survival with whole breast radiotherapy (98 %) and mastectomy (93 %) compared to ALND alone (81 %, $p=0.061$), but patients with N3 disease were overrepresented in the ALND-only subgroup and advanced nodal status emerged as the only significant prognostic factor. Interestingly, a matched cohort analysis is presented in the publication which suggests that for patients with N1 disease, survival is significantly better for axillary CUP than for breast cancer, while there was no significant difference for N2/N3 status.

Table 9.1 Studies comparing observation, radiotherapy, and mastectomy after axillary lymph node dissection for patients with axillary CUP

Author	Study period	*N*	Follow-up	LRC (Obs/RT/M)			OS (Obs/RT/M)		
Barton [5]	1975–2009	48	68 m	34 %	87 %	–	83 %	92 %	–
Ellerbroek [7]	1944–1987	42	131 m	43 %	83 %	–	–	–	–
Foroudi [6]	1979–1996	20	73 m	17 %	75 %	–	–	–	–
Masinghe [8]	1974–2003	53	9 y	46.3 %	71.7 %	–	58.3 %	72.8 %	–
Rueth [15]	2000–2011	36	64 m		100 %	100 %		100 %	100 %
Shannon [9]	1975–2001	29	44 m	31 %	87.5 %	–	–	–	–
Sohn [14]	1990–2009	142	78 m				81 %	98 %	93 %
Vlastos [18]	1951–1998	45	7 y	–	85 %	83 %	–	75 %	79 %
Walker [16]	1983–2006	750	SEER	–	–	–	63.5 %	67.1 %	

Adapted from Krug et al. [1]
LRC locoregional control, *OS* overall survival, *Obs* observation, *RT* radiotherapy, *M* mastectomy, *m* months, *y* years, *SEER* surveillance, epidemiology, endpoints and results

The most recent publication is a retrospective study of 36 patients treated at MD Anderson Cancer Center between 2000 and 2011 [15]. Most of the patients had N1 disease, and more than 90 % had a breast MRI to rule out an occult breast tumor. Breast conservation was performed in 75 % of the patients, and 92 % had radiotherapy to the breast/chest wall and 77 % to the supra-/infraclavicular lymph node area. Almost all patients received systemic therapy, mostly in the neoadjuvant setting. The overall survival with a median follow-up of 64 months was 97.2 % with only one distant recurrence, ultimately resulting in the death of the patient. There were no local or regional recurrences.

The largest study is an epidemiological report from the Surveillance, Epidemiology, and End Results (SEER) database including 750 patients [16]. During the timeframe of the study, there was a significant decline in the use of mastectomy from 50 % before 1998 to 42 % during 1998 and afterward. Walker et al. showed that both mastectomy and whole breast radiotherapy conferred a significant overall survival benefit over ALND or selective lymph node excision alone, while there was no significant difference in 10-year cancer-specific survival between patients receiving mastectomy or whole breast radiotherapy. In a multivariate analysis, negative estrogen receptor status, 10 or more involved lymph nodes and resection of 10 or less lymph nodes emerged as negative prognostic factors.

9.1.1.4 National and International Guidelines

The NCCN guidelines for CUP and breast cancer offer recommendations on diagnostic and therapeutic management of patients with axillary CUP. Mastectomy and whole breast radiotherapy with or without nodal irradiation are being presented as equal alternatives. The use of breast MRI is recommended due to its higher sensitivity compared to mammography and ultrasound.

The German working group for Gynecologic Oncology (AGO) also recommends the use of breast MRI in patients with axillary CUP in their yearly updated guidelines. In contrast to the NCCN guidelines, mastectomy is not advised, especially not in patients with a negative breast MRI [17]. There is no clear recommendation for or against whole breast radiotherapy, although the guidelines state that there should be a discussion with the patient about its possible benefits in terms of local control and survival. This is also inconsistent with the NCCN recommendations.

9.1.1.5 Radiotherapy Treatment

Due to the limited evidence available for axillary CUP, most treatment recommendations are derived from publications on breast cancer. Radiotherapy dose, fractionation, and target volume were not consistently reported in the abovementioned studies. In the studies giving at least some treatment information concerning radiotherapy [5–7, 18], treatment was performed in analogy to breast cancer. The most common dose and fractionation regimen to the whole breast was 50–50.4 Gy in 25–28 fractions, although hypofractionation (40 Gy in 15 fractions) was used in a minority of patients in two publications [5, 6]. Barton et al. provided a subgroup analysis and were unable to show a benefit of a dose escalation beyond 50 Gy (or 40 Gy in hypofractionation) regarding locoregional recurrence and recurrence-free survival, but this analysis was limited to a total of 31 CUP patients [5]. Since the publication of the 10-year follow-up results of the major hypofractionation trials, hypofractionation has been acknowledged as a treatment standard in most national and international guidelines for the treatment of breast cancer [19, 20].

In breast-conserving treatment of breast cancer, the application of a boost dose of 10–16 Gy in 5–8 fractions to the tumor bed is commonly used and reduces the local recurrence risk by about 50 % without an effect on survival [21]. In the treatment of axillary CUP, there usually is no indication for the application of a boost, albeit there is residual tumor and a reexcision is not possible.

In the case of a complete axillary dissection, the axillary lymphatic levels I–III are typically not included in the clinical target volume in breast cancer although especially level I receives an incidental dose due to the close proximity to the breast. Indications to include the axilla in the clinical target volume are an incomplete axillary dissection, residual tumor with no possibility of reexcision, and advanced nodal disease, typically N3 with a ratio of involved to uninvolved lymph nodes over 0.75. In patients with 4 or more involved lymph nodes, the periclavicular lymphatic drainage should be included in the clinical target volume. Two large randomized trials have recently suggested that there might be a benefit of locoregional radiotherapy treatment (including the periclavicular and the parasternal lymphatic drainage) on locoregional recurrence and also distant recurrence in patients with breast cancer and N1 disease as well as selected patients with negative nodes and high-risk features, but these results have still not been fully published. Thus, a definitive conclusion on the role of locoregional radiotherapy in N0/N1 disease cannot be made [22].

Postmastectomy radiotherapy (PMRT) has mostly been recommended in breast cancer patients with at least 4 involved lymph nodes, but recently, an update of the EBCTCG meta-analysis showed that the benefit of PMRT is similar in patients with 1–3 involved lymph nodes with an absolute improvement in breast cancer-specific survival of about 8 % after 20 years [23].

Treatment of the chest wall and the regional lymphatic drainage in breast cancer patients is typically delivered using normofractionation although some patients after mastectomy and locoregional radiotherapy were included in the hypofractionation trials [19].

Axillary CUP with adjuvant breast irradiation with or without inclusion of the supraclavicular fossa can be adequately treated with 3D conformal radiotherapy in most cases. Intensity-modulated radiotherapy (IMRT) can be useful in the case of special anatomic situations, especially pectus excavatum [24]. Figure 9.1 shows a

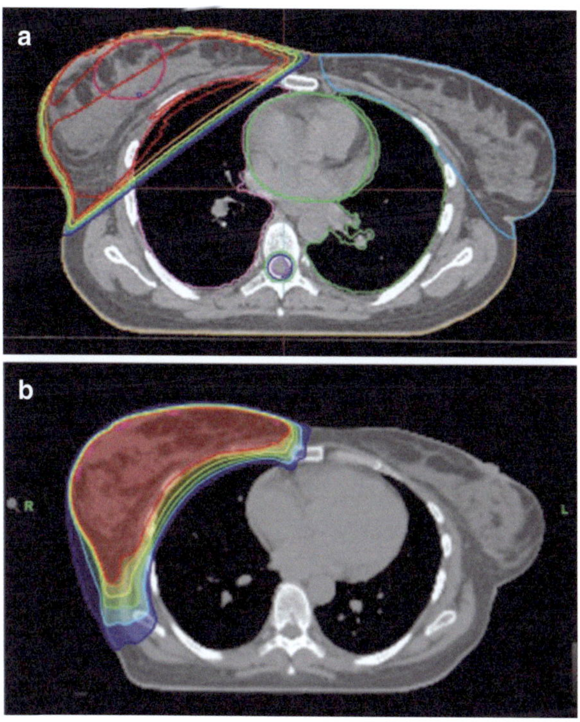

Fig. 9.1 Comparison of 3D conformal radiotherapy (**a**) and IMRT performed as a helical tomotherapy (**b**) in a patient with special anatomy. IMRT offers improved sparing of the right lung

comparison of 3D conformal radiotherapy and IMRT in a sample case with an accentuated curvature of the thoracic wall.

IMRT might also be advantageous if the internal mammary chain is included in the target volume [25].

9.1.1.6 Conclusions

The evidence on the use of radiotherapy in axillary CUP is limited. Many retrospective studies show that whole breast radiotherapy is a safe alternative to mastectomy and that there is a significant benefit on local control and in some studies on survival compared to axillary dissection alone. However, this benefit might be related to the low quality of imaging and the suboptimal systemic treatment used in these studies. Nevertheless, there are no data that support the omission of the local treatment of the breast (whole breast radiotherapy or mastectomy) in the context of a negative breast MRI as suggested by the AGO guidelines. In breast cancer, prospective studies have shown that breast MRI does not result in a lower rate of reexcisions and does increase the likelihood of performing a mastectomy.

Keeping in mind the negative impact of mastectomy on quality of life, especially body image and sexual functioning in breast cancer patients [26], the low rates of severe late toxicity with modern radiotherapy techniques, and the comparable survival rates, whole breast radiotherapy offers a reasonable alternative to mastectomy in patients with axillary CUP. In the absence of clinical data on the role of PMRT and locoregional radiotherapy in patients with axillary CUP, these indications should be based on the available recommendations for breast cancer patients with involvement of the axillary lymph nodes.

9.1.2 Cervical CUP

Cervical CUP is an uncommon entity and accounts for only about 5 % of the malignancies in the head and neck region. Histologically, most cases reveal lymph node metastasis of a squamous cell carcinoma, although in a minority a diagnosis of undifferentiated carcinoma, adenocarcinoma, or malignant melanoma is made [27].

Concerning risk factors, a German retrospective analysis showed that 80 % of patients were current or former smokers [28]. HPV status was also assessed, and about half of the patients had evidence of HPV-DNA and/or were positive on p16-INK4A immunohistochemistry. Several publications could show that p16 and/or HPV positivity predicts oropharyngeal location of previously undetected primaries [29, 30]. Similarly, positivity for EBV or evidence of lymphoepithelial carcinoma can indicate a tumor location in the nasopharynx.

Before diagnosing a cervical CUP, patients should receive a systematic staging consisting of panendoscopy, CT, and/or MRI of the head and neck region and CT or x-ray of the chest. FDG-PET can further increase the sensitivity of diagnostic imaging, but its additional value decreases if panendoscopy and other imaging modalities have already been utilized [31].

9.1.2.1 General Management

Main approaches to cervical CUP are primary surgery with neck dissection followed by adjuvant radiotherapy compared to lymph node biopsy followed by definitive radio(chemo)therapy. Important prognostic factors are the extent of nodal disease [32–35], extracapsular extension of nodal metastases [32, 35–38], and the performance status at first diagnosis [33, 39].

Several articles have addressed the role of the extent of surgery in patients with cervical CUP. For example, Christansen et al. [40], Hauswald et al. [38], and Issing et al. [41] found a significantly lower rate of nodal relapses in the neck after more extensive surgery, i.e., neck dissection and in the latter two publications tonsillectomy versus biopsy before radiotherapy. Nonetheless, a systematic review including 18 retrospective studies with a total of 1726 patients showed no significant influence of the extent of surgery on survival, although the 5-year overall survival was numerically higher in patients with more extensive surgery [42]. Possible reasons for the positive results of the previously mentioned trials include a selection bias due to comorbidities or technical irresectability precluding a surgical approach and underestimation of the clinical tumor stage in patients undergoing definitive radiotherapy.

In patients with residual disease after definitive radio(chemo)therapy, a salvage neck dissection can be discussed [43].

9.1.2.2 Radiotherapy Target Definition

In cervical CUP, radiotherapy targets not only the areas of nodal involvement but also potential sites of occult mucosal disease. Historical series using surgery alone have shown that metachronous emergence of a primary tumor in the mucosa is a relevant endpoint in cervical CUP. In a publication by the Danish DAHANCA group, mucosal failure after 5 years occurred in 54 % of patients treated with surgery alone compared to 23 and 13 % of patients receiving radiotherapy to the neck alone or to the neck and the mucosa, respectively [33]. The most common location of an emerging primary tumor was the oropharynx in about half of the patients followed by the lung and the esophagus.

A subgroup that might be managed without adjuvant radiotherapy are patients with N1 disease without extracapsular extension after neck dissection since relapse rates are low, and the long-term outcome is favorable for these patients [36, 44].

An important area of debate is if the contralateral neck should be irradiated in patients with unilateral disease since bilateral radiotherapy increases both acute and late toxicities [37, 45]. Several publications reported that nodal or mucosal relapses are not significantly more common after unilateral radiotherapy (see Table 9.2). It is

Table 9.2 Studies comparing unilateral (UL) and bilateral radiotherapy (BL) in cervical CUP

Author	Study period	*n*	Follow-up	LC UL/BL	DFS UL/BL	OS UL/BL	Details
Fakhrian [37]	1988–2009	65	64 m	n.a.	58 %/62 %	44 %/49 %	79 % ND 87 % N1–N2b
Grau [33]	1975–1995	277	137 m	27 %/51 % ($p=0.05$)	n.a.	28 %/45 % (DSS)	2 % ND 62 % N1–N2b
Ligey [39]	1990–2007	95	3.3 y	66 %/75 %		22 %/23 %	83 % ND 67 % N1–N2b 45 % Chemo
Perkins [46]	1989–2008	46	4.6 y	n.a.	n.s.	77 % overall	80 % ND 76 % N1–N2b
Reddy [45]	1974–1989	52	n.a.	66 %/73 %	53 %/47 %	n.a.	60 % ND 51 % N1–N2b

Adapted from Krug et al. [1]
LC local control, *DFS* disease-free survival, *DSS* disease-specific survival, *OS* overall survival, *ND* neck dissection, *m* months, *y* years, *n.a* not analyzed, *n.s* not stated

important to state that most of the patients in these series received adjuvant radiotherapy after neck dissection. About 40 % had N1 or N2a disease, whereas definitive radiotherapy and negative prognostic factors like N3 disease were usually more common in the bilateral treatment groups, representing a possible selection bias [39, 46]. Grau et al. provided results for 277 patients mostly treated by definitive bilateral radiotherapy including potential mucosal tumor sites after lymph node biopsy [33]. After adjustment for clinical covariates, unilateral radiotherapy was associated with a relative risk of 1.9 for locoregional failure, while the difference in disease-specific survival was not statistically significant. A study by Reddy and Marks provides treatment outcomes by nodal stage. While there was no significant difference between unilateral and bilateral radiotherapy for N1 patients, bilateral radiotherapy significantly increased nodal and mucosal control rates in patients with N2/N3 stage [45]. Survival was similar in both groups. Thus, unilateral adjuvant radiotherapy represents a treatment option mainly for patients with limited nodal disease after initial neck dissection [44].

There have been some publications addressing the question of elective mucosal coverage in cervical CUP. In patients without involvement of lymph node level III, exclusion of the hypopharynx and larynx still resulted in a 5-year mucosal control rate of 100 % [34]. Based on their data from 87 patients, Glynne-Jones et al. suggested to exclude the nasopharynx from the elective irradiation target volume. However, the nasopharynx was the second most common site of mucosal relapse in 4 out of 19 patients with omission of radiotherapy to this area [47]. Mourad et al. treated 68 patients with limited field radiotherapy including the oropharynx, the retropharyngeal nodes, and the bilateral neck. The locoregional control rate was 95.5 % after 3.5 years with one mucosal and two nodal recurrences.

It is crucial to remember that most of the abovementioned results were achieved with outdated imaging and radiotherapy techniques. With the combination of modern imaging modalities, parameters allowing for a prediction of the location of an occult primary tumor such as p16-INK4A, and more advanced radiotherapy techniques, individualization of the postoperative treatment volume will be an important issue in the near future.

9.1.2.3 Combined Chemoradiotherapy

In definitive radiotherapy of locally advanced head and neck squamous cell carcinomas (laHNSCC), a clear benefit of concurrent chemotherapy has been shown in terms of local control and overall survival [48]. In the setting of adjuvant radiotherapy for laHNSCC, concomitant chemotherapy is typically recommended in patients with adverse factors such as residual tumor and extracapsular extension of lymph node metastases [49].

In cervical CUP, the indication for combined chemoradiotherapy is usually based on the same factors, but specific evidence is limited.

Argiris et al. analyzed outcomes of 25 patients treated on different prospective protocols with combined chemoradiotherapy for cervical CUP [50]. The treatment consisted of split-course radiotherapy with a 5-FU and hydroxyurea backbone. Two trials applied induction chemotherapy, two trials tested simultaneous paclitaxel, and one trial used simultaneous cisplatin with hyperfractionated-accelerated radiotherapy. 56 % of patients had a neck dissection before treatment, and about 70 % of patients had N2a/N2b disease. The outcome was very favorable, only one patient developed a locoregional nodal relapse, and 5-year progression-free and overall survival were 75 and 83 %. There was one treatment-related death. Nutritional support via gastrostomy beyond 1 year after treatment was required in 16 % of patients. Xerostomy was reported in 44 % of cases.

Shehadeh et al. reported their experience on adjuvant platinum-based chemoradiotherapy in 37 patients with cervical CUP after neck dissection [51]. Most patients received 3 concurrent cycles of cisplatinum. The stage was N1–N2b in about 60 % of patients. There were only 2 regional failures, both in patients with N3 disease and extracapsular extension. Four patients developed distant metastases. Toxicity was acceptable with 3 cases of esophageal stricture. There were no long-term feeding tube dependencies.

In a retrospective, single-institution study, Chen et al. failed to show a benefit of the addition of concurrent cisplatin to radiotherapy in 60 patients with cervical CUP [52]. Cisplatin improved neither local control nor overall survival. 70 % of patients were treated in an adjuvant setting after neck dissection, and about 80 % had N1–N2b disease. Both acute and chronic toxicities were significantly higher with the addition of cisplatin.

Ligey et al. and Hauswald et al. provided subgroup analyses in their retrospective publications that also showed no additional benefit with concurrent chemotherapy

[38, 39]. In the retrospective study of Fakhrian et al., there was a trend for improved overall survival ($p=0.051$), but recurrence-free survival was unchanged [37].

In summary, the rationale for the addition of concurrent chemotherapy to radiotherapy for cervical CUP is scarce. Available evidence suggests that toxicity is increased, while no study so far has shown a benefit in terms of local control or survival. Nonetheless, due to the low level of evidence with multiple retrospective publications and one pooled analysis of several prospective single-arm studies and the heterogeneity of chemotherapy and radiotherapy regimens, the risk of bias is high. We believe that concurrent chemotherapy should be used in patients with an acceptable performance status and without significant comorbidities in high-risk situations, especially in the case of advanced nodal stages with extracapsular extension and when definitive radiotherapy is planned.

9.1.2.4 Intensity-Modulated Radiotherapy (IMRT) in Cervical CUP

Radiotherapy delivery and planning technique have undergone a significant evolution during the past decades. With the growing use of IMRT, many publications have addressed its application in head and neck oncology. It allows for a substantial increase in conformality of dose delivery and thus an optimized target volume coverage. On the other hand, the generation of sharp dose gradients improves sparing of surrounding normal tissue.

An example of a bilateral treatment plan is shown in Fig. 9.2.

The randomized phase III PARSPORT trial comparing 3D conformal radiotherapy to IMRT in head and neck squamous cell carcinoma patients showed that the reduction of radiation dose to the parotid glands through the use of IMRT translated into a significant reduction of xerostomia and salivary flow impairment and an improvement in the related quality of life domains [53]. Grade 2 or worse xerostomia at 1 year after treatment was reduced from 74 to 38 %. Chen et al. retrospectively analyzed dosimetric parameters for 51 cervical CUP patients treated with 3D conformal or intensity-modulated radiotherapy and also found a significant reduction of the radiation dose to the parotid gland on the noninvolved side of the neck in a similar magnitude as in the PARSPORT results [54]. This also led to a reduction of significant late xerostomia from 58 to 11 %. Gastric feeding tube dependency was 42 % versus 11 %, while the overall incidence of grade 3 or worse toxicity was 63 % versus 29 %. Similar results were published by other groups [55].

The only study to show an impact of radiotherapy technique on clinical outcome was the publication by Ligey et al. 95 patients who were treated by 2D radiotherapy using either wedged lateral fields or parallel opposed fields with an anterior field for the lower neck or CT-planned 3D conformal radiotherapy/IMRT were studied retrospectively [39]. On multivariate analysis, radiation technique was an independent prognostic factor for both local control and overall survival.

Recently, Janssen et al. published their experience with a risk-adapted approach of radiotherapy with IMRT and 3 dose levels for different risks of involvement according to the nodal involvement [56]. Overall survival, disease-free survival, and

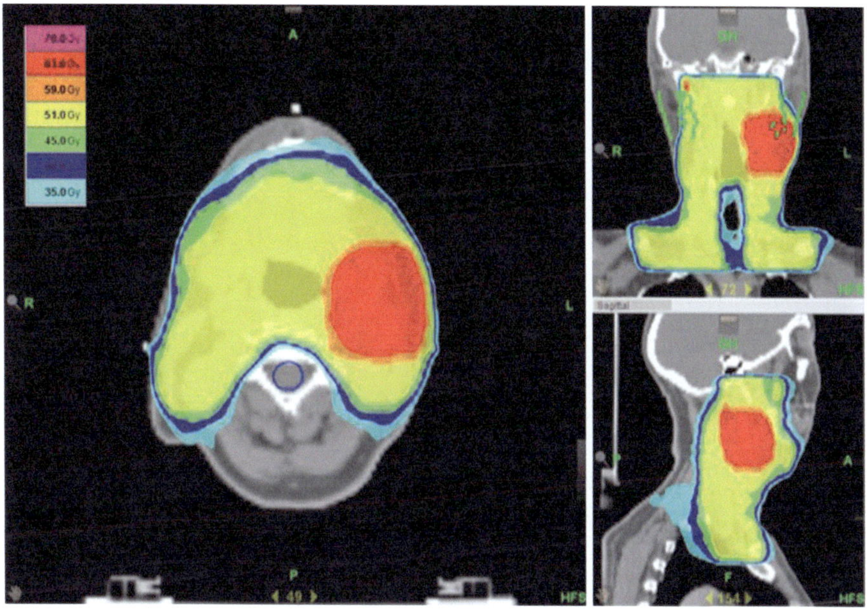

Fig. 9.2 Treatment of the bilateral neck and the mucosa in a patient with cervical CUP. The patient was initially treated with a neck dissection and had involvement of level II on the left side with extracapsular extension. Dose prescription was 66 Gy to the boost area (level II) and 54 Gy to the uninvolved neck and mucosa in 30 fractions. Optimal sparing of the parotid glands (*green*), the spinal cord (*blue*), and the trachea and cervical esophagus was provided

nodal control were 76, 81, and 93 % at 3 years. There were no late toxicities of grade II or higher.

Most reports of IMRT have shown very favorable clinical results (see Table 9.3); nonetheless, all of them are small, single-institutional studies, and the better outcome compared to historical reports might also represent a change in the underlying risk factors as well as changes in surgical approaches and chemotherapy use. While toxicity appears to be acceptable and significantly lower compared to 3D conformal radiotherapy, reports of increased rates of esophageal stenosis with IMRT and concurrent chemotherapy treatment warrant further investigation [57].

9.1.2.5 Conclusions

The treatment of patients with cervical CUP represents an interdisciplinary challenge in oncology. While surgery alone might represent an option for patients with N1 disease without extracapsular extension, patients with advanced nodal stages benefit from multimodal treatment approaches. The outcome of patients with cervical CUP has significantly improved over time, most likely due to advances in imaging leading to improved staging and detection of clinically occult primary tumors but also in radiotherapy delivery with reduction of late toxicity. From the standpoint

Table 9.3 Experience with IMRT in cervical CUP

Author	Study period	*n*	Follow-up	LC	DFS	OS	Details
Chen [54]	2001–2009	24	29 m	92 %	–	87 %	63 % Chemo, 70 % ND,
Janssen [56]	2006–2012	28	30.5 m	93 % (neck), 100 % (mucosa)	81 %	76 %	71 % Chemo, 71 % ND
Frank [92]	1998–2005	52	3.7 y	94.2 %	88 %	81 %	27 % Chemo, 25 % ND
Sher [57]	2004–2009	24	2.1 y	100 %	92 %	92 %	92 % Chemo, 13 % ND
Shoushtari [93]	2002–2008	27	41.9 m (surviving)	88.5 % (neck)	85.2 %	70.9 %	30 % Chemo, 80 % ND
Klem [94]	2002–2005	21	20 m	90 %	–	85 %	76 % Chemo, 67 % ND
Madani [55]	2003–2006	23	17 m	100 % (mucosa)	–	74.8 %	13 % Chemo, 83 % ND
Villeneuve [95]	2005–2008	25	38 m	100 %	100 %	100 %	72 % Chemo, 8 % ND

Adapted from Krug et al. [1]

LC local control, *DFS* disease-free survival, *OS* overall survival, *ND* neck dissection, *m* months, *y* years

of radiation oncology, the greatest challenge in the future will be the individualization of the target volume based on the results of contemporary imaging and molecular biology and pathology.

9.2 Palliative Treatment Concepts

9.2.1 Cerebral Metastases

In about 50 % of patients with cerebral metastases without a known primary tumor, adenocarcinoma is the underlying histology [27]. In a prospective study of 33 patients, 82 % later on developed a primary tumor, which was found in the lung in 78 % of patients. A population-based analysis from the Swedish Cancer Registry including 645 patients reported a median survival of 7 months for patients with cerebral metastases [27]. Survival for these patients was similar to that for patients with brain metastases from a known primary tumor with the exception of patients with colorectal cancer, who had a significantly lower risk of death [58].

The Graded Prognostic Assessment (GPA) score [59] was able to predict survival in a cohort of patients with rare causes of intracerebral metastases, including cerebral CUP patients on the basis of the Karnofsky Performance Index, number of brain metastases, patient age, and the presence of extracranial metastases [60]. Median survival of a mixed cohort including 39 CUP patients was 2.5, 4.5, 5.8, and 8.3

months for patients with a GPA score of 0–1, 1.5–2, 2.5–3, or 3.5–4, respectively. Bartelt et al. [61] and Rades et al. [62] described an improved survival of CUP patients corresponding to a recursive partitioning analysis (RPA) score [63] developed by the Radiation Therapy Oncology Group (RTOG). Other prognostic factors that have been described for patients with cerebral CUP are the number of brain metastases [64], resection, or stereotactic radiosurgery versus whole brain radiotherapy (WBRT) alone [60, 61, 64] and the presence of extracranial disease activity [62, 65].

9.2.1.1 Operation

Patients with a limited number of brain metastases (typically 1–3) should be evaluated for resection if they have a good performance status; if the extracranial disease extent is limited, especially if histological evaluation is not achievable otherwise; and if there is a long interval between the occurrence of brain metastases and the first diagnosis of the CUP. In solitary intracerebral lesions, differential diagnoses like high-grade gliomas or infectious conditions should be considered. Another indication for surgical resection is compression of sensitive structures like the brain stem, hydrocephalus, or herniation by mass effect of limited brain metastases in patients with an otherwise favorable prognosis.

As previously mentioned, resection emerged as a positive prognostic factor compared to whole brain radiotherapy alone in several studies. However, this most likely reflects a selection bias in terms of performance status, comorbidities, number of metastases, and potentially tumor location. In patients with a known primary tumor, a survival benefit compared to WBRT alone has only been shown for single brain metastases [66] (Table 9.4).

9.2.1.2 Radiosurgery

Another noninvasive treatment alternative for patients with limited brain metastases is stereotactic radiosurgery (SRS). This technique was first described by the Swedish neurosurgeon Lars Leksell, who later developed the Gamma Knife, a designated

Table 9.4 Prognostic scores for patients with brain metastases

Graded prognostic assessment (GPA [59])	0	0.5	1
Patient Age	>60	50–59	<50
KPS	<70	70–80	90–100
Number of intracerebral metastases	>3	2–3	1
Extracranial metastases	Present		None
Recursive partitioning analysis (RPA [63])			
I (patients <65 years, Karnofsky Performance Status [KPS] 70–100, controlled primary tumor, and no extracranial metastases)			
II neither group I nor group III			
III KPS <70			

radiosurgery tool using Cobalt-60 sources. Briefly, high radiation doses are applied in 1–5 fractions using a designated radiosurgery machine like the Gamma Knife or the Cyberknife or a modified linear accelerator. Historically, a coordinate system mounted to the treatment delivery machine was used for target localization. Today, most available systems do not use an external coordinate system but state-of-the-art-image guidance for high-precision target localization.

Figure 9.3 shows an example of a stereotactic radiosurgery in a patient with a single brain metastasis.

SRS was first developed as a boost treatment for patients receiving WBRT. A Cochrane Review of 3 randomized controlled trials comparing WBRT alone to WBRT and SRS showed comparable overall survival [67], although one trial found an overall survival benefit of 6.5 versus 4.9 months for patients with single brain metastasis treated with WBRT plus SRS [68]. Furthermore, local control was significantly improved by the addition of SRS to WBRT [67].

Researchers from the University of Pittsburgh reported their experience on SRS using a Gamma Knife in patients with cerebral CUP [65]. 31 tumors were treated in 15 patients with 80 % of patients receiving SRS to a single brain metastasis. All but one patient had additional WBRT. SRS was mostly used as a boost after WBRT; in some patients, it was a salvage treatment after initial resection and WBRT. Median survival after SRS was 15 months. Prognosis was significantly worse in patients with extracranial tumor activity and metastases located in the brain stem.

The group from Pittsburgh updated their experience in a later publication including 29 patients with 87 lesions [69]. Median overall survival was reported to be 12 months after SRS and 57.2 % at 1 year. Only 10 % of patients died from known intracerebral tumor progression. After a median imaging follow-up of 18.6 months, the local control rate was 88.5 %. Again, brain stem metastasis location was of negative prognostic impact.

The number of metastases amenable for stereotactic radiosurgery and the optimal criteria for patient selection for SRS remain an area of constant debate. Recently, feasibility of SRS in patients with up to 10 brain metastases was shown in a prospective observational study [70]. Survival for patients with 2–4 and 5–10 metastases was identical with 10.8 months, whereas patients with a single brain metastasis

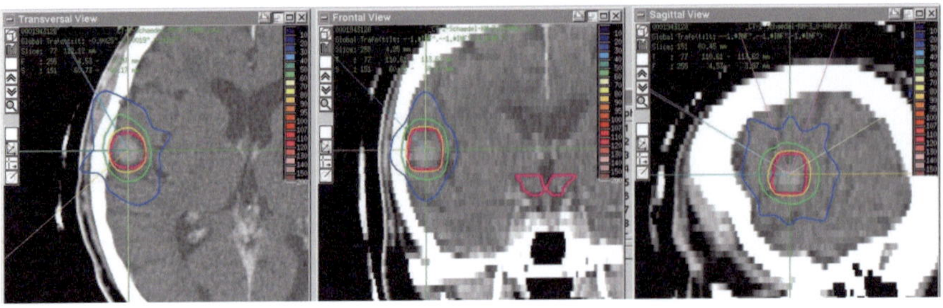

Fig. 9.3 Stereotactic radiosurgery of a brain metastasis in the right temporal lobe. Dose prescription was 20 Gy to the circumference of the lesion with a maximum of 25 Gy in the isocenter

had a better median overall survival of 13.9 months. Only 8 % of patients died of neurological death. However, this study has been criticized for its design, because the maximum tumor size was limited to 3 cm and the maximum cumulative volume of all metastases to 15 ml or less. The cumulative volume was 3.5 ml for patients with 5–10 metastases compared to 3.1 ml for patients with 2–4 metastases. The amount of patients with symptomatic metastases was similar which implies that there might have been a selection bias.

9.2.1.3 Whole Brain Radiotherapy

WBRT remains the treatment standard for patients with multiple intracerebral metastases. Survival after WBRT alone in patients with cerebral CUP ranges between 4.8 and 6 months [61, 64].

Since the risk of intracerebral failure after resection or SRS is high, WBRT is often used as an additional treatment in patients with a limited number of brain metastases. Two randomized trials failed to demonstrate an overall survival improvement by the addition of WBRT to resection or SRS in patients with up to 4 brain metastases but showed a significant improvement in local and distant intracerebral control [71, 72]. Distant intracranial failure occurred in 48 and 42 % at 2 years after SRS or resection alone as compared to 33 and 23 % with additional WBRT in the EORTC trial [72]. In the JROSG trial, 64 % of patients had a distant intracranial recurrence at 1 year after SRS alone compared to 42 % with SRS + WBRT [71].

Although the general assumption has been that intracranial failure is the most frequent reason for neurological decline in patients with brain metastases, negative neurocognitive effects of WBRT have gained growing attention in the absence of a survival benefit by its addition to surgery or SRS. Chang et al. reported a significant decline in neurocognitive function 4 months after treatment as determined by the Hopkins Verbal Learning Test – Revised in patients with 1–3 metastases treated with SRS and additional WBRT [73]. Data from the EORTC trial showed significantly impaired health-related quality of life compared to patients having surgery or SRS alone. Analysis was limited to 1 year after treatment due to limited compliance, but differences in several subdomains including physical functioning, cognitive functioning, and fatigue were judged to be clinically relevant during this period [74].

Thus, omission of WBRT after SRS or surgery of up to 4 brain metastases might be reasonable [75].

The most commonly used fractionation regimen for WBRT is 30 Gy delivered in 10 fractions over 2 weeks. Rades et al. performed a retrospective comparison of patients receiving either 10 × 3 Gy or 20 × 2 Gy over 4 weeks and patients treated with 5 × 4 Gy over 1 week [62]. There was no difference in overall survival or intracranial control between the long-course or short-course treatments. Nevertheless, short-course treatment should be reserved for patients with a limited prognosis due to the potentially deleterious neurocognitive effects of high fraction doses.

9.2.1.4 Conclusion

Patients with cerebral metastases from an unknown primary tumor have a prognosis that is similar to those with cerebral metastases from a known primary tumor. Patients with single brain metastasis should be considered for surgical resection, especially in the absence of extracerebral disease or if a mass effect is present. For patients with a limited number of brain metastases (usually defined as up to 4 metastases), SRS is an attractive, noninvasive treatment option. WBRT is used for patients with widespread intracranial disease as well as for patients with limited brain metastases with a poor performance index. Whether WBRT should be used after surgery or SRS in patients with limited intracranial disease is an area of debate as it is associated with significant neurocognitive impairment.

9.2.2 Bone Metastases

Bone metastases are a common source of pain, impairment of physical and social activities, and morbidity in cancer patients. Palliative radiotherapy is associated with an overall pain response rate of about 75 % and a complete response rate of 30 % [76].

In patients with CUP, presence of bone metastases was described as a negative prognostic factor [77]. The most frequent histology in bone metastases from CUP is adenocarcinoma in two thirds of the cases [27]. In a population-based analysis from the Swedish Cancer Registry, survival of CUP patients with bone metastases was inferior to patients with bone metastases from a known primary, but this difference was mainly driven by the long-term prognosis of breast and prostate cancer patients with bone metastases [58]. Similarly, men with osteoblastic bone metastases and an elevated PSA value have been described as a favorable subset of CUP patients [78].

Patients with painful bone metastases should be referred for palliative radiotherapy regardless of the underlying histology. Different fractionation regimens have been used in the past. Although abundant evidence exists that single fraction treatment with 8 Gy or a 1-week course of 5 × 4 Gy yields similar rates in pain response to longer treatment courses such as 10 × 3 Gy or 20 × 2 Gy, treatment with 10 × 3 Gy over 2 weeks still remains the most commonly used regimen [79]. Shorter treatment courses are associated with higher rates of retreatment, but even retreatment with 1 × 8 Gy after previous radiotherapy has been shown to be safe and effective [80].

A surgical referral should be considered in patients with impaired stability of the spine or long bones or a metastatic spinal cord compression with a good performance status, limited bone involvement, and limited extraosseous disease activity.

Metastatic spinal cord compression (MSCC) is a complication of bone metastases that occurs in 5–10 % of cancer patients [81]. In a retrospective study of 143 CUP patients receiving radiotherapy for MSCC, improvement of motor function was achieved in 10 %, while 57 % had a stable motor function [81]. Positive prognostic factors for motor function were the absence of visceral or further bone metastases and an interval from developing symptoms to the initiation of treatment of more than 7 days. Median survival was 4 months, while 76 % of patients died within 6 months. For overall survival, an ambulatory status before initiation of radiotherapy was an additional prognostic factor on multivariate analysis. Similar to radiotherapy for painful bone metastases, the fractionation regimen was prognostic neither for motor function nor for local control or survival [81, 82]. Nevertheless, it should be mentioned that longer fractionation regimens had a significant positive impact on local control but not motor function in another larger study not including CUP patients by the same authors [83].

Douglas et al. published a prognostic index on the basis of the performance status, the ambulatory status before radiotherapy, the presence of visceral metastases, and the time from developing motor deficits to the initiation of treatment [84]. Three prognostic groups were developed with corresponding 6-month survival rates of 5, 41, and 92 % (see Table 9.5). The score was tested on a validation set and provided reliable results.

9.3 Conclusion

Radiotherapy is an effective palliative treatment for patients with bone metastases and metastatic spinal cord compression. Short-term fractionation regimens offer comparable rates of pain response compared to longer fractionation regimens, but are associated with higher rates of retreatment and potentially of local failure. Thus, patients with a limited life expectancy should be treated with 1 × 8 Gy or 5 × 4 Gy, while patients with a favorable prognosis should be treated with 10 × 3 Gy or 20 × 2 Gy.

Table 9.5 Prognostic index for patients with MSCC from CUP [84]

ECOG performance status	
1–2	6
3–4	2
Ambulatory status before radiotherapy	
Not ambulatory	2
Ambulatory	4
Visceral metastases	
No	5
Yes	0
Time since developing motor deficits	
1–7 days	1
>7 days	5
Group A	<14 points – 6-month survival rate 5 %
Group B	14–16 points – 6-month survival rate 41 %
Group C	>16 points – 6-month survival rate 92 %

9.4 Radiotherapeutic Developments in Oligometastatic Disease

Stereotactic body radiotherapy (SBRT) is a method of external beam irradiation (photons or particles) that accurately delivers a high dose of irradiation in one or few fractions to an extracranial target [85]. There is an increasing body of literature of using this technique in an oligometastatic setting with excellent local control rates of more than 90 % after 2 years and minimal toxicity. The percentage of patients with CUP in the available studies is quite low. Nevertheless, SBRT presents a valid and important alternative to surgical approaches for both lung and liver metastases [86, 87]. There is also good evidence for using this technique in adrenal gland metastases [88]. It is important to remember that many of these patients will develop more metastases and require further treatment. This strongly argues for minimally or noninvasive strategies that can easily be fitted into a multidisciplinary approach including systemic therapy without long treatment delays, breaks, or interactions.

In a palliative setting, the most common treatment indication is pain or impaired stability of osseous lesions. These sites are clearly a domain of conventional techniques that can be planned and delivered very efficiently [89]. Single fraction or

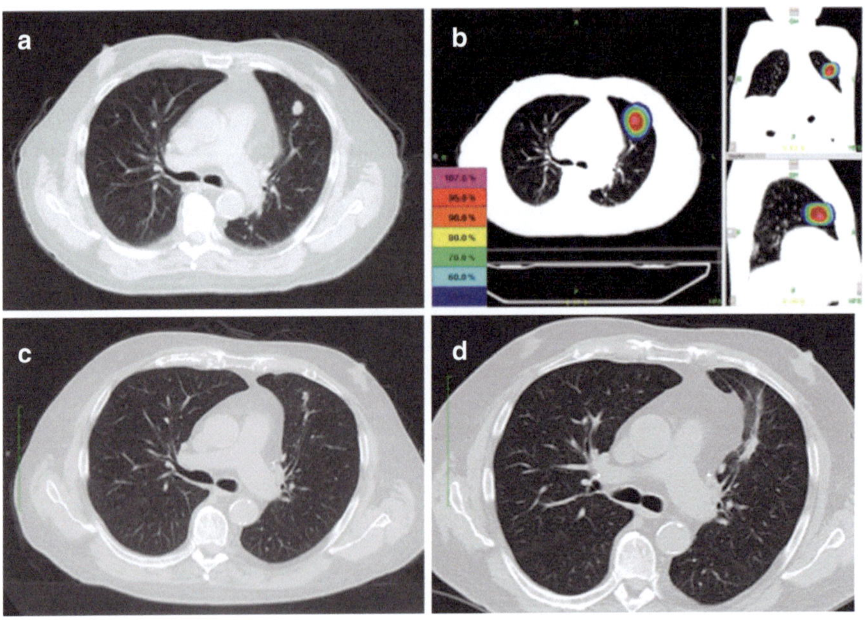

Fig. 9.4 A single lung metastasis (**a**) was treated with SBRT in a patient with carcinoma of the bladder who refused systemic therapy due to toxicities of prior treatments and comorbidities. The lesion was treated using SBRT after 4D CT-based treatment planning with a circumferential dose of 45 Gy in 3 fractions and a maximum dose of 60 Gy in the center of the lesion (**b**). The lesion showed an excellent partial remission 2 months after treatment (**c**). Fibrotic changes appeared 6 months later (**d**)

hypofractionated treatment can achieve pain relief and recalcification for a high percentage of patients. For reirradiation, another application of 8 Gy single dose can be an effective option [80]. To escalate the delivered dose for patients with a longer life expectancy, modern methods like IMRT and SBRT offer good options with high rates of long-term pain relief and local control [90].

Generally, SBRT for spine lesions plays an emerging role and has the potential to apply radiotherapy in one or few fractions with minimal side effects and longlasting local effects [91].

Figure 9.4 depicts a case study of a patient with a single lung metastasis in the left lung treated by SBRT.

References

1. Krug D, Debus J, Sterzing F. Radiotherapeutic concepts in cancer of unknown primary site. Radiologe. 2014;54(2):145–51. PubMed Epub 2013/12/18. Strahlentherapeutische Konzepte beim CUP-Syndrom.
2. Pentheroudakis G, Lazaridis G, Pavlidis N. Axillary nodal metastases from carcinoma of unknown primary (CUPAx): a systematic review of published evidence. Breast Cancer Res Treat. 2010;119(1):1–11. PubMed PMID: 19771506.
3. de Bresser J, de Vos B, van der Ent F, Hulsewe K. Breast MRI in clinically and mammographically occult breast cancer presenting with an axillary metastasis: a systematic review. Eur J Surg Oncol. 2010;36(2):114–9. PubMed.
4. Khandelwal AK, Garguilo GA. Therapeutic options for occult breast cancer: a survey of the American Society of Breast Surgeons and review of the literature. Am J Surg. 2005;190(4):609–13. PubMed PMID: 16164933. Epub 2005/09/17.
5. Barton SR, Smith IE, Kirby AM, Ashley S, Walsh G, Parton M. The role of ipsilateral breast radiotherapy in management of occult primary breast cancer presenting as axillary lymphadenopathy. Eur J Cancer. 2011;47(14):2099–106. PubMed PMID: 21658935.
6. Foroudi F, Tiver KW. Occult breast carcinoma presenting as axillary metastases. Int J Radiat Oncol Biol Phys. 2000;47(1):143–7. PubMed PMID: 10758316.
7. Ellerbroek N, Holmes F, Singletary E, Evans H, Oswald M, McNeese M. Treatment of patients with isolated axillary nodal metastases from an occult primary carcinoma consistent with breast origin. Cancer. 1990;66(7):1461–7. PubMed PMID: 2207996.
8. Masinghe SP, Faluyi OO, Kerr GR, Kunkler IH. Breast radiotherapy for occult breast cancer with axillary nodal metastases--does it reduce the local recurrence rate and increase overall survival? Clin Oncol. 2011;23(2):95–100. PubMed PMID: 21115330.
9. Shannon C, Walsh G, Sapunar F, A'Hern R, Smith I. Occult primary breast carcinoma presenting as axillary lymphadenopathy. Breast. 2002;11(5):414–8. PubMed PMID: 14965705.
10. Wang X, Zhao Y, Cao X. Clinical benefits of mastectomy on treatment of occult breast carcinoma presenting axillary metastases. Breast J. 2010;16(1):32–7. PubMed Epub 2010/05/15.
11. Blanchard DK, Farley DR. Retrospective study of women presenting with axillary metastases from occult breast carcinoma. World J Surg. 2004;28(6):535–9. PubMed PMID: 15366740. Epub 2004/09/16.
12. Campana F, Fourquet A, Ashby MA, Sastre X, Jullien D, Schlienger P, et al. Presentation of axillary lymphadenopathy without detectable breast primary (T0 N1b breast cancer): experience at Institut Curie. Radiother Oncol. 1989;15(4):321–5. PubMed PMID: 2552505. Epub 1989/08/01.
13. Early Breast Cancer Trialists' Collaborative Group, Darby S, McGale P, Correa C, Taylor C, Arriagada R, et al. Effect of radiotherapy after breast-conserving surgery on 10-year recur-

rence and 15-year breast cancer death: meta-analysis of individual patient data for 10,801 women in 17 randomised trials. Lancet. 2011;378(9804):1707–16. PubMed PMID: 22019144. Pubmed Central PMCID: 3254252. Epub 2011/10/25.
14. Sohn G, Son BH, Lee SJ, Kang EY, Jung SH, Cho SH, et al. Treatment and survival of patients with occult breast cancer with axillary lymph node metastasis: a nationwide retrospective study. J Surg Oncol. 2014;110(3):270–4. PubMed PMID: 24863883. Epub 2014/05/28.
15. Rueth NM, Black DM, Limmer AR, Gabriel E, Huo L, Fornage BD, et al. Breast conservation in the setting of contemporary multimodality treatment provides excellent outcomes for patients with occult primary breast cancer. Ann Surg Oncol. 2015;22(1):90–5. PubMed PMID: 25249256. Epub 2014/09/25.
16. Walker GV, Smith GL, Perkins GH, Oh JL, Woodward W, Yu TK, et al. Population-based analysis of occult primary breast cancer with axillary lymph node metastasis. Cancer. 2010;116(17):4000–6. PubMed PMID: 20564117.
17. Fehm T, Souchon R. Axilläre Lymphknotenmetastasen bei CUP. Onkologe. 2013;19:40–3.
18. Vlastos G, Jean ME, Mirza AN, Mirza NQ, Kuerer HM, Ames FC, et al. Feasibility of breast preservation in the treatment of occult primary carcinoma presenting with axillary metastases. Ann Surg Oncol. 2001;8(5):425–31.
19. Haviland JS, Owen JR, Dewar JA, Agrawal RK, Barrett J, Barrett-Lee PJ, et al. The UK Standardisation of Breast Radiotherapy (START) trials of radiotherapy hypofractionation for treatment of early breast cancer: 10-year follow-up results of two randomised controlled trials. Lancet Oncol. 2013;14(11):1086–94. PubMed Epub 2013/09/24.
20. Whelan TJ, Pignol JP, Levine MN, Julian JA, MacKenzie R, Parpia S, et al. Long-term results of hypofractionated radiation therapy for breast cancer. N Engl J Med. 2010;362(6):513–20. PubMed PMID: 20147717. Epub 2010/02/12.
21. Bartelink H, Horiot JC, Poortmans PM, Struikmans H, Van den Bogaert W, Fourquet A, et al. Impact of a higher radiation dose on local control and survival in breast-conserving therapy of early breast cancer: 10-year results of the randomized boost versus no boost EORTC 22881–10882 trial. J Clin Oncol. 2007;25(22):3259–65. PubMed PMID: 17577015. Epub 2007/06/20.
22. Sautter-Bihl ML, Sedlmayer F, Budach W, Dunst J, Feyer P, Fietkau R, et al. DEGRO practical guidelines: radiotherapy of breast cancer III--radiotherapy of the lymphatic pathways. Strahlenther Onkol. 2014;190(4):342–51. PubMed PMID: 24638236. Epub 2014/03/19.
23. EBCTCG (Early Breast Cancer Trialists' Collaborative Group), McGale P, Taylor C, Correa C, Cutter D, Duane F, et al. Effect of radiotherapy after mastectomy and axillary surgery on 10-year recurrence and 20-year breast cancer mortality: meta-analysis of individual patient data for 8135 women in 22 randomised trials. Lancet. 2014;383(9935):2127–35. PubMed PMID: 24656685. Epub 2014/03/25.
24. Uhl M, Sterzing F, Habl G, Schubert K, Holger H, Debus J, et al. Breast cancer and funnel chest. Comparing helical tomotherapy and three-dimensional conformal radiotherapy with regard to the shape of pectus excavatum. Strahlenther Onkol. 2012;188(2):127–35. PubMed PMID: 22218501. Epub 2012/01/06.
25. Caudrelier JM, Morgan SC, Montgomery L, Lacelle M, Nyiri B, Macpherson M. Helical tomotherapy for locoregional irradiation including the internal mammary chain in left-sided breast cancer: dosimetric evaluation. Radiother Oncol. 2009;90(1):99–105. PubMed PMID: 18977546. Epub 2008/11/04.
26. Kiebert GM, de Haes JC, van de Velde CJ. The impact of breast-conserving treatment and mastectomy on the quality of life of early-stage breast cancer patients: a review. J Clin Oncol. 1991;9(6):1059–70. PubMed PMID: 2033420. Epub 1991/06/01.
27. Hemminki K, Bevier M, Hemminki A, Sundquist J. Survival in cancer of unknown primary site: population-based analysis by site and histology. Ann Oncol. 2012;23(7):1854–63. PubMed PMID: 22115926.
28. Tribius S, Hoffmann AS, Bastrop S, Gorogh T, Haag J, Rocken C, et al. HPV status in patients with head and neck of carcinoma of unknown primary site: HPV, tobacco smoking, and outcome. Oral Oncol. 2012;48(11):1178–84. PubMed PMID: 22739067.

29. Park GC, Lee M, Roh JL, Yu MS, Choi SH, Nam SY, et al. Human papillomavirus and p16 detection in cervical lymph node metastases from an unknown primary tumor. Oral Oncol. 2012;48(12):1250–6. PubMed PMID: 22728322. Epub 2012/06/26.
30. Zengel P, Assmann G, Mollenhauer M, Jung A, Sotlar K, Kirchner T, et al. Cancer of unknown primary originating from oropharyngeal carcinomas are strongly correlated to HPV positivity. Virchows Arch. 2012;461(3):283–90. PubMed PMID: 22855133. Epub 2012/08/03.
31. Wong WL, Sonoda LI, Gharpurhy A, Gollub F, Wellsted D, Goodchild K, et al. 18F-fluorodeoxyglucose positron emission tomography/computed tomography in the assessment of occult primary head and neck cancers--an audit and review of published studies. Clin Oncol. 2012;24(3):190–5. PubMed PMID: 22183080.
32. Beldi D, Jereczek-Fossa BA, D'Onofrio A, Gambaro G, Fiore MR, Pia F, et al. Role of radiotherapy in the treatment of cervical lymph node metastases from an unknown primary site: retrospective analysis of 113 patients. Int J Radiat Oncol Biol Phys. 2007;69(4):1051–8. PubMed PMID: 17716824.
33. Grau C, Johansen LV, Jakobsen J, Geertsen P, Andersen E, Jensen BB. Cervical lymph node metastases from unknown primary tumours. Results from a national survey by the Danish Society for Head and Neck Oncology. Radiother Oncol. 2000;55(2):121–9. PubMed PMID: 10799723.
34. Wallace A, Richards GM, Harari PM, Kirwan JM, Morris CG, Katakam H, et al. Head and neck squamous cell carcinoma from an unknown primary site. Am J Otolaryngol. 2011;32(4):286–90. PubMed PMID: 20719404.
35. Erkal HS, Mendenhall WM, Amdur RJ, Villaret DB, Stringer SP. Squamous cell carcinomas metastatic to cervical lymph nodes from an unknown head-and-neck mucosal site treated with radiation therapy alone or in combination with neck dissection. Int J Radiat Oncol Biol Phys. 2001;50(1):55–63. PubMed PMID: 11316546. Epub 2001/04/24.
36. Coster JR, Foote RL, Olsen KD, Jack SM, Schaid DJ, DeSanto LW. Cervical nodal metastasis of squamous cell carcinoma of unknown origin: indications for withholding radiation therapy. Int J Radiat Oncol Biol Phys. 1992;23(4):743–9. PubMed PMID: 1618667. Epub 1992/01/01.
37. Fakhrian K, Thamm R, Knapp S, Molls M, Pigorsch S, Haller B, et al. Radio(chemo)therapy in the management of squamous cell carcinoma of cervical lymph nodes from an unknown primary site. A retrospective analysis. Strahlenther Onkol. 2012;188(1):56–61. PubMed PMID: 22189437. Epub 2011/12/23.
38. Hauswald H, Lindel K, Rochet N, Debus J, Harms W. Surgery with complete resection improves survival in radiooncologically treated patients with cervical lymph node metastases from cancer of unknown primary. Strahlenther Onkol. 2008;184(3):150–6. PubMed PMID: 18330511. Epub 2008/03/12.
39. Ligey A, Gentil J, Crehange G, Montbarbon X, Pommier P, Peignaux K, et al. Impact of target volumes and radiation technique on loco-regional control and survival for patients with unilateral cervical lymph node metastases from an unknown primary. Radiother Oncol. 2009;93(3):483–7. PubMed PMID: 19892420.
40. Christiansen H, Hermann RM, Martin A, Nitsche M, Schmidberger H, Pradier O. Neck lymph node metastases from an unknown primary tumor retrospective study and review of literature. Strahlenther Onkol. 2005;181(6):355–62. PubMed PMID: 15925977. Epub 2005/06/01.
41. Issing WJ, Taleban B, Tauber S. Diagnosis and management of carcinoma of unknown primary in the head and neck. Eur Arch Otorhinolaryngol. 2003;260(8):436–43. PubMed PMID: 12684829.
42. Balaker AE, Abemayor E, Elashoff D, St John MA. Cancer of unknown primary: does treatment modality make a difference? Laryngoscope. 2012;122(6):1279–82. PubMed PMID: 22538837.
43. Hamoir M, Ferlito A, Schmitz S, Hanin FX, Thariat J, Weynand B, et al. The role of neck dissection in the setting of chemoradiation therapy for head and neck squamous cell carcinoma with advanced neck disease. Oral Oncol. 2012;48(3):203–10. PubMed PMID: 22104248.

44. Nieder C, Gregoire V, Ang KK. Cervical lymph node metastases from occult squamous cell carcinoma: cut down a tree to get an apple? Int J Radiat Oncol Biol Phys. 2001;50(3):727–33. PubMed PMID: 11395241.
45. Reddy SP, Marks JE. Metastatic carcinoma in the cervical lymph nodes from an unknown primary site: results of bilateral neck plus mucosal irradiation vs. ipsilateral neck irradiation. Int J Radiat Oncol Biol Phys. 1997;37(4):797–802. PubMed PMID: 9128954. Epub 1997/03/01.
46. Perkins SM, Spencer CR, Chernock RD, Haughey BH, Nussenbaum B, Adkins DR, et al. Radiotherapeutic management of cervical lymph node metastases from an unknown primary site. Arch Otolaryngol Head Neck Surg. 2012;138(7):656–61. PubMed PMID: 22801890.
47. Glynne-Jones RG, Anand AK, Young TE, Berry RJ. Metastatic carcinoma in the cervical lymph nodes from an occult primary: a conservative approach to the role of radiotherapy. Int J Radiat Oncol Biol Phys. 1990;18(2):289–94. PubMed PMID: 2303361. Epub 1990/02/01.
48. Pignon JP, le Maitre A, Maillard E, Bourhis J, Group M-NC. Meta-analysis of chemotherapy in head and neck cancer (MACH-NC): an update on 93 randomised trials and 17,346 patients. Radiother Oncol. 2009;92(1):4–14. PubMed PMID: 19446902. Epub 2009/05/19.
49. Bernier J, Cooper JS, Pajak TF, van Glabbeke M, Bourhis J, Forastiere A, et al. Defining risk levels in locally advanced head and neck cancers: a comparative analysis of concurrent post-operative radiation plus chemotherapy trials of the EORTC (#22931) and RTOG (# 9501). Head Neck. 2005;27(10):843–50. PubMed PMID: 16161069.
50. Argiris A, Smith SM, Stenson K, Mittal BB, Pelzer HJ, Kies MS, et al. Concurrent chemoradiotherapy for N2 or N3 squamous cell carcinoma of the head and neck from an occult primary. Ann Oncol. 2003;14(8):1306–11. PubMed PMID: 12881397. Epub 2003/07/26.
51. Shehadeh NJ, Ensley JF, Kucuk O, Black C, Yoo GH, Jacobs J, et al. Benefit of postoperative chemoradiotherapy for patients with unknown primary squamous cell carcinoma of the head and neck. Head Neck. 2006;28(12):1090–8. PubMed PMID: 16933316. Epub 2006/08/26.
52. Chen AM, Farwell DG, Lau DH, Li BQ, Luu Q, Donald PJ. Radiation therapy in the management of head-and-neck cancer of unknown primary origin: how does the addition of concurrent chemotherapy affect the therapeutic ratio? Int J Radiat Oncol Biol Phys. 2011;81(2):346–52. PubMed PMID: 20933340.
53. Nutting CM, Morden JP, Harrington KJ, Urbano TG, Bhide SA, Clark C, et al. Parotid-sparing intensity modulated versus conventional radiotherapy in head and neck cancer (PARSPORT): a phase 3 multicentre randomised controlled trial. Lancet Oncol. 2011;12(2):127–36. PubMed PMID: 21236730. Pubmed Central PMCID: 3033533. Epub 2011/01/18.
54. Chen AM, Li BQ, Farwell DG, Marsano J, Vijayakumar S, Purdy JA. Improved dosimetric and clinical outcomes with intensity-modulated radiotherapy for head-and-neck cancer of unknown primary origin. Int J Radiat Oncol Biol Phys. 2011;79(3):756–62. PubMed PMID: 20421143.
55. Madani I, Vakaet L, Bonte K, Boterberg T, De Neve W. Intensity-modulated radiotherapy for cervical lymph node metastases from unknown primary cancer. Int J Radiat Oncol Biol Phys. 2008;71(4):1158–66. PubMed PMID: 18258383.
56. Janssen S, Glanzmann C, Huber G, Studer G. Individualized IMRT treatment approach for cervical lymph node metastases of unknown primary. Strahlenther Onkol. 2014;190(4):386–93. PubMed PMID: 24638240. Epub 2014/03/19.
57. Sher DJ, Balboni TA, Haddad RI, Norris Jr CM, Posner MR, Wirth LJ, et al. Efficacy and toxicity of chemoradiotherapy using intensity-modulated radiotherapy for unknown primary of head and neck. Int J Radiat Oncol Biol Phys. 2011;80(5):1405–11. PubMed PMID: 21177045.
58. Riihimaki M, Thomsen H, Hemminki A, Sundquist K, Hemminki K. Comparison of survival of patients with metastases from known versus unknown primaries: survival in metastatic cancer. BMC Cancer. 2013;13:36. PubMed PMID: 23356713. Pubmed Central PMCID: 3565900.
59. Sperduto PW, Berkey B, Gaspar LE, Mehta M, Curran W. A new prognostic index and comparison to three other indices for patients with brain metastases: an analysis of 1,960 patients

in the RTOG database. Int J Radiat Oncol Biol Phys. 2008;70(2):510–4 PubMed PMID: 17931798. Epub 2007/10/13.
60. Nieder C, Andratschke NH, Geinitz H, Grosu AL. Use of the Graded Prognostic Assessment (GPA) score in patients with brain metastases from primary tumours not represented in the diagnosis-specific GPA studies. Strahlenther Onkol. 2012;188(8):692–5. PubMed PMID: 22526229.
61. Bartelt S, Lutterbach J. Brain metastases in patients with cancer of unknown primary. J Neurooncol. 2003;64(3):249–53. PubMed PMID: 14558600.
62. Rades D, Bohlen G, Lohynska R, Veninga T, Stalpers LJ, Schild SE, et al. Whole-brain radiotherapy with 20 Gy in 5 fractions for brain metastases in patients with cancer of unknown primary (CUP). Strahlenther Onkol. 2007;183(11):631–6. PubMed PMID: 17960339.
63. Gaspar L, Scott C, Rotman M, Asbell S, Phillips T, Wasserman T, et al. Recursive partitioning analysis (RPA) of prognostic factors in three Radiation Therapy Oncology Group (RTOG) brain metastases trials. Int J Radiat Oncol Biol Phys. 1997;37(4):745–51. PubMed PMID: 9128946. Epub 1997/03/01.
64. Ruda R, Borgognone M, Benech F, Vasario E, Soffietti R. Brain metastases from unknown primary tumour: a prospective study. J Neurol. 2001;248(5):394–8. PubMed PMID: 11437161.
65. Maesawa S, Kondziolka D, Thompson TP, Flickinger JC, Dade L. Brain metastases in patients with no known primary tumor. Cancer. 2000;89(5):1095–101. PubMed PMID: 10964340.
66. Patchell RA, Tibbs PA, Walsh JW, Dempsey RJ, Maruyama Y, Kryscio RJ, et al. A randomized trial of surgery in the treatment of single metastases to the brain. N Engl J Med. 1990;322(8):494–500. PubMed PMID: 2405271. Epub 1990/02/22.
67. Patil CG, Pricola K, Garg SK, Bryant A, Black KL. Whole brain radiation therapy (WBRT) alone versus WBRT and radiosurgery for the treatment of brain metastases. Cochrane Database Syst Rev. 2010;6:CD006121. PubMed PMID: 20556764. Epub 2010/06/18.
68. Andrews DW, Scott CB, Sperduto PW, Flanders AE, Gaspar LE, Schell MC, et al. Whole brain radiation therapy with or without stereotactic radiosurgery boost for patients with one to three brain metastases: phase III results of the RTOG 9508 randomised trial. Lancet. 2004;363(9422):1665–72. PubMed PMID: 15158627. Epub 2004/05/26.
69. Niranjan A, Kano H, Khan A, Kim IY, Kondziolka D, Flickinger JC, et al. Radiosurgery for brain metastases from unknown primary cancers. Int J Radiat Oncol Biol Phys. 2010;77(5):1457–62. PubMed PMID: 20056342. Epub 2010/01/09.
70. Yamamoto M, Serizawa T, Shuto T, Akabane A, Higuchi Y, Kawagishi J, et al. Stereotactic radiosurgery for patients with multiple brain metastases (JLGK0901): a multi-institutional prospective observational study. Lancet Oncol. 2014;15(4):387–95. PubMed PMID: 24621620. Epub 2014/03/14.
71. Aoyama H, Shirato H, Tago M, Nakagawa K, Toyoda T, Hatano K, et al. Stereotactic radiosurgery plus whole-brain radiation therapy vs stereotactic radiosurgery alone for treatment of brain metastases: a randomized controlled trial. JAMA. 2006;295(21):2483–91. PubMed Epub 2006/06/08.
72. Kocher M, Soffietti R, Abacioglu U, Villa S, Fauchon F, Baumert BG, et al. Adjuvant whole-brain radiotherapy versus observation after radiosurgery or surgical resection of one to three cerebral metastases: results of the EORTC 22952–26001 study. J Clin Oncol. 2011;29(2):134–41. PubMed PMID: 21041710. Pubmed Central PMCID: 3058272. Epub 2010/11/03.
73. Chang EL, Wefel JS, Hess KR, Allen PK, Lang FF, Kornguth DG, et al. Neurocognition in patients with brain metastases treated with radiosurgery or radiosurgery plus whole-brain irradiation: a randomised controlled trial. Lancet Oncol. 2009;10(11):1037–44. PubMed PMID: 19801201. Epub 2009/10/06.
74. Soffietti R, Kocher M, Abacioglu UM, Villa S, Fauchon F, Baumert BG, et al. A European Organisation for Research and Treatment of Cancer phase III trial of adjuvant whole-brain radiotherapy versus observation in patients with one to three brain metastases from solid tumors after surgical resection or radiosurgery: quality-of-life results. J Clin Oncol. 2013;31(1):65–72. PubMed PMID: 23213105. Epub 2012/12/06.

75. Kocher M, Wittig A, Piroth MD, Treuer H, Seegenschmiedt H, Ruge M, et al. Stereotactic radiosurgery for treatment of brain metastases. A report of the DEGRO Working Group on Stereotactic Radiotherapy. Strahlenther Onkol. 2014;190(6):521–32. PubMed PMID: 24715242. Epub 2014/04/10.
76. Chow E, Harris K, Fan G, Tsao M, Sze WM. Palliative radiotherapy trials for bone metastases: a systematic review. J Clin Oncol. 2007;25(11):1423–36. PubMed PMID: 17416863.
77. Kodaira M, Takahashi S, Yamada S, Ueda K, Mishima Y, Takeuchi K, et al. Bone metastasis and poor performance status are prognostic factors for survival of carcinoma of unknown primary site in patients treated with systematic chemotherapy. Ann Oncol. 2010;21(6):1163–7. PubMed PMID: 20019088.
78. Pavlidis N, Petrakis D, Golfinopoulos V, Pentheroudakis G. Long-term survivors among patients with cancer of unknown primary. Crit Rev Oncol Hematol. 2012;84(1):85–92. PubMed PMID: 22386806.
79. Fairchild A, Barnes E, Ghosh S, Ben-Josef E, Roos D, Hartsell W, et al. International patterns of practice in palliative radiotherapy for painful bone metastases: evidence-based practice? Int J Radiat Oncol Biol Phys. 2009;75(5):1501–10. PubMed PMID: 19464820. Epub 2009/05/26.
80. Chow E, van der Linden YM, Roos D, Hartsell WF, Hoskin P, Wu JS, et al. Single versus multiple fractions of repeat radiation for painful bone metastases: a randomised, controlled, non-inferiority trial. Lancet Oncol. 2014;15(2):164–71. PubMed PMID: 24369114. Epub 2013/12/27.
81. Rades D, Fehlauer F, Veninga T, Stalpers LJ, Basic H, Hoskin PJ, et al. Functional outcome and survival after radiotherapy of metastatic spinal cord compression in patients with cancer of unknown primary. Int J Radiat Oncol Biol Phys. 2007;67(2):532–7. PubMed PMID: 17084539.
82. Douglas S, Huttenlocher S, Bajrovic A, Rudat V, Schild SE, Rades D. Prognostic factors for different outcomes in patients with metastatic spinal cord compression from cancer of unknown primary. BMC Cancer. 2012;12:261. PubMed PMID: 22720880. Pubmed Central PMCID: 3411458.
83. Rades D, Lange M, Veninga T, Stalpers LJ, Bajrovic A, Adamietz IA, et al. Final results of a prospective study comparing the local control of short-course and long-course radiotherapy for metastatic spinal cord compression. Int J Radiat Oncol Biol Phys. 2011;79(2):524–30. PubMed PMID: 20452136. Epub 2010/05/11.
84. Douglas S, Schild SE, Rades D. Metastatic spinal cord compression in patients with cancer of unknown primary. Estimating the survival prognosis with a validated score. Strahlenther Onkol. 2012;188(11):1048–51. PubMed PMID: 23053138.
85. Guckenberger M, Andratschke N, Alheit H, Holy R, Moustakis C, Nestle U, et al. Definition of stereotactic body radiotherapy: principles and practice for the treatment of stage I non-small cell lung cancer. Strahlenther Onkol. 2014;190(1):26–33. PubMed PMID: 24052011. Pubmed Central PMCID: 3889283. Epub 2013/09/21.
86. Navarria P, Ascolese AM, Tomatis S, Cozzi L, De Rose F, Mancosu P, et al. Stereotactic body radiotherapy (sbrt) in lung oligometastatic patients: role of local treatments. Radiat Oncol. 2014;9(1):91. Pubmed Central PMCID: 3999881. Epub 2014/04/04.
87. Sterzing F, Brunner TB, Ernst I, Baus WW, Greve B, Herfarth K, et al. Stereotactic body radiotherapy for liver tumors: principles and practical guidelines of the DEGRO Working Group on Stereotactic Radiotherapy. Strahlenther Onkol. 2014;190(10):872–81. PubMed PMID: 25091267. Epub 2014/08/06.
88. Gunjur A, Duong C, Ball D, Siva S. Surgical and ablative therapies for the management of adrenal 'oligometastases' - A systematic review. Cancer Treat Rev. 2014;40(7):838–46. PubMed PMID: 24791623. Epub 2014/05/06.
89. Chow E, Hoskin P, Mitera G, Zeng L, Lutz S, Roos D, et al. Update of the international consensus on palliative radiotherapy endpoints for future clinical trials in bone metastases. Int J Radiat Oncol Biol Phys. 2012;82(5):1730–7. PubMed PMID: 21489705. Epub 2011/04/15.
90. Sterzing F, Hauswald H, Uhl M, Herm H, Wiener A, Herfarth K, et al. Spinal cord sparing reirradiation with helical tomotherapy. Cancer. 2010;116(16):3961–8. PubMed PMID: 20564110. Epub 2010/06/22.

91. Bydon M, De la Garza-Ramos R, Bettagowda C, Gokaslan ZL, Sciubba DM. The use of stereotactic radiosurgery for the treatment of spinal axis tumors: a review. Clin Neurol Neurosurg. 2014;125:166–72. PubMed PMID: 25156410. Epub 2014/08/27.
92. Frank SJ, Rosenthal DI, Petsuksiri J, Ang KK, Morrison WH, Weber RS, et al. Intensity-modulated radiotherapy for cervical node squamous cell carcinoma metastases from unknown head-and-neck primary site: M. D. Anderson Cancer Center outcomes and patterns of failure. Int J Radiat Oncol Biol Phys. 2010;78(4):1005–10. PubMed PMID: 20207504.
93. Shoushtari A, Saylor D, Kerr KL, Sheng K, Thomas C, Jameson M, et al. Outcomes of patients with head-and-neck cancer of unknown primary origin treated with intensity-modulated radiotherapy. Int J Radiat Oncol Biol Phys. 2011;81(3):e83–91. PubMed PMID: 21377283.
94. Klem ML, Mechalakos JG, Wolden SL, Zelefsky MJ, Singh B, Kraus D, et al. Intensity-modulated radiotherapy for head and neck cancer of unknown primary: toxicity and preliminary efficacy. Int J Radiat Oncol Biol Phys. 2008;70(4):1100–7. PubMed PMID: 17980501.
95. Villeneuve H, Despres P, Fortin B, Filion E, Donath D, Soulieres D, et al. Cervical lymph node metastases from unknown primary cancer: a single-institution experience with intensity-modulated radiotherapy. Int J Radiat Oncol Biol Phys. 2012;82(5):1866–71. PubMed PMID: 21497452. Epub 2011/04/19.

Chapter 10
Favorable Subsets Among Cancers of Unknown Primary

Kanwal Raghav and Gauri R. Varadhachary

10.1 Introduction

Cancers of unknown primary origin (CUP) are defined as metastatic cancers with no primary anatomic site of origin despite an adequate evaluation [1]. This "adequate" evaluation includes a detailed history and physical examination, a complete blood count and biochemical analysis (including urinalysis and stool test for occult blood (where indicated)), an in-depth pathological review, and imaging using computerized tomography of the chest, abdomen, and pelvis directed toward identifying a primary origin [1–3]. Therefore, by definition CUP is a heterogeneous group of histologically confirmed metastatic neoplasms without an overt primary site. Despite several trials of empiric chemotherapy regimens in CUP, the overall prognosis remains poor with median survivals ranging between 6 and 13 months [4–7].

Although there is no overt primary in CUP, certain distinct clinicopathological phenotypes are observable amidst these diverse neoplasms, which suggest a specific primary origin and a more favorable prognosis [8]. These favorable CUP subsets have been well described in the literature, and about 15–20 % of all CUP patients present with these distinct clinicopathological phenotypes [8]. Panel 10.1 lists the favorable subsets of CUP documented in the literature.

Panel 10.1 Favorable subsets of cancers of unknown primary

- Solitary metastatic disease
- Men with osteoblastic metastases and elevated prostate-specific antigen
- Adenocarcinoma with isolated axillary lymph node involvement in women
- Women with papillary carcinoma of the peritoneal cavity
- Poorly differentiated carcinoma with midline distribution

K. Raghav • G.R. Varadhachary (✉)
Department of Gastrointestinal Medical Oncology,
The University of Texas MD Anderson Cancer Center, Houston, TX, USA
e-mail: kpraghav@mdanderson.org; gvaradha@mdanderson.org

A. Krämer, H. Löffler (eds.), *Cancer of Unknown Primary*,
DOI 10.1007/978-3-319-22581-4_10

- Neuroendocrine carcinomas
- Squamous cell carcinoma involving cervical lymph nodes
- Adenocarcinoma with immunophenotype consistent with a gastrointestinal primary

With the emerging recognition that putative primary site-directed therapy may be more effective strategy than empiric therapy, recognizing these subtypes can guide oncologists in formulating a tailored therapeutic strategy, and patients with these can expect a prolonged survival compared to CUP patients who do not fit into these specific subgroups. The current chapter reviews the evidence behind contemporary management of these favorable subsets of CUP. Neuroendocrine carcinomas of unknown primary are not discussed in details in this chapter and should be managed as per guidelines used for neuroendocrine tumors [9]. Poorly differentiated neuroendocrine tumors, irrespective of tumor of origin, are treated with systemic chemotherapy according to the guidelines for small cell lung cancer [9]. Table 10.1 summarizes all the favorable subsets of CUP with regard to diagnostic workup and treatment strategies.

Table 10.1 Favorable subsets of cancers of unknown primary (CUP)

CUP subset	Diagnostics[a]	Pathology	Treatment options
Solitary metastatic disease	Positron emission tomography (PET)	Variable	Surgery followed by radiotherapy or chemoradiotherapy adjuvant chemotherapy Neoadjuvant chemotherapy + surgery Definitive radiotherapy or chemoradiotherapy
Osteoblastic metastases in men with elevated serum PSA (prostate-specific antigen)	Serum PSA	*Immunostains*: PSA, p63, P501S, prostate-specific acid phosphatase (PSAP), prostein, prostate-specific membrane antigen (PSMA), Androgen receptor (AR)	*Per guidelines for advanced/ metastatic prostate cancer* Androgen deprivation therapy or chemotherapy
Adenocarcinoma with isolated axillary lymphadenopathy in women	Mammography Breast ultrasound Breast magnetic resonance imaging (MRI)	*Immunostains:* mammaglobin, GCDFP-15, GATA-3, ER, PR, HER2/neu	*Per guidelines for TX or T0/N + (node-positive) breast cancer* Ipsilateral mastectomy/ breast-conserving surgery with axillary lymph node dissection Radiotherapy Adjuvant/neoadjuvant chemotherapy ± hormonal therapy

Table 10.1 (continued)

CUP subset	Diagnostics[a]	Pathology	Treatment options
Papillary carcinoma of the peritoneal cavity in women	Serum CA 125	*Immunostains:* CK7, P53, WT-1, ER, PAX-8, Ber-EP4, MOC-31	*Per guidelines for stage III/IV epithelial ovarian cancer* Chemotherapy (platinum/taxane) only for distant metastases excluding peritoneal disease Cytoreductive surgery + chemotherapy (platinum/taxane)
Poorly differentiated carcinoma with midline distribution	Testicular ultrasound Serum AFP and βHCG	*Immunostains*: AFP, βHCG, OCT-4	*Per guidelines for poor-risk germ cell tumors* Cisplatin-based combination chemotherapy
Squamous cell carcinoma with cervical lymphadenopathy	CT head/neck + PET/CT Laryngoscopy with directed biopsies Bilateral tonsillectomy	No specific immunohisto chemistry	*Per guidelines for head and neck squamous cell carcinoma* Lymph node dissection Radiotherapy or chemoradiotherapy
Adenocarcinoma with immunophenotype consistent with gastrointestinal primary	Colonoscopy (if clinically indicated)	*Immunoprofile*: CDX2 positive, CK20 positive, CK7 variable	Chemotherapy FOLFOX or FOLFIRI Targeted agents (bevacizumab, cetuximab/panitumumab in RAS wild-type tumors)
Neuroendocrine cancer of unknown primary	Well differentiated: Octreoscan Urinary 5-HIAA Poorly differentiated: PET Brain MRI	*Immunostains*: Synaptophysin, chromogranin, CD56, Ki-67	*Per guidelines for neuroendocrine tumors* Well differentiated: Local therapy (surgery, embolization) Systemic therapy (somatostatin analog, cytotoxic, sunitinib, everolimus) Poorly differentiated: Chemotherapy (cisplatin/carboplatin + etoposide or irinotecan)

Abbreviations: *AFP* alpha fetoprotein, *βHCG* beta-human chorionic gonadotropin, *CT* computerized tomography, *5-HIAA* 5-hydroxyindoleacetic acid

[a]Investigations in addition to those considered as initial evaluation per guidelines [9, 10]

10.2 Solitary Metastatic Disease

Case Study

A 72-year-old lady presented with pneumonia. Chest X-ray (Fig. 10.1a) showed a right lung mass. CT-guided biopsy showed moderately differentiated adenocarcinoma. Immunohistochemistry was strongly and diffusely positive for CDX2, cytokeratin (CK) 20, villin, and carcinoembryonic antigen (CEA) and negative for CK7 and TTF-1. CT chest showed a right upper lobe mass (Fig. 10.1b). PET showed an intensely FDG-avid lung mass but no evidence of distant metastases (Fig. 10.1c, d). Colonoscopy and upper gastrointestinal endoscopy were performed and were normal. The patient received four cycles of mFOLFOX6 chemotherapy in neoadjuvant setting and had a partial response (Fig. 10.1e). The patient then underwent en bloc right upper lobe lobectomy with mediastinal lymph node dissection. Pathology showed poorly differentiated adenocarcinoma with 11 lymph nodes without any evidence of malignancy. The patient was then followed closely with surveillance scans, and PET-CT 4-year status postsurgery showed no evidence of recurrent or metastatic disease (Fig. 10.1f).

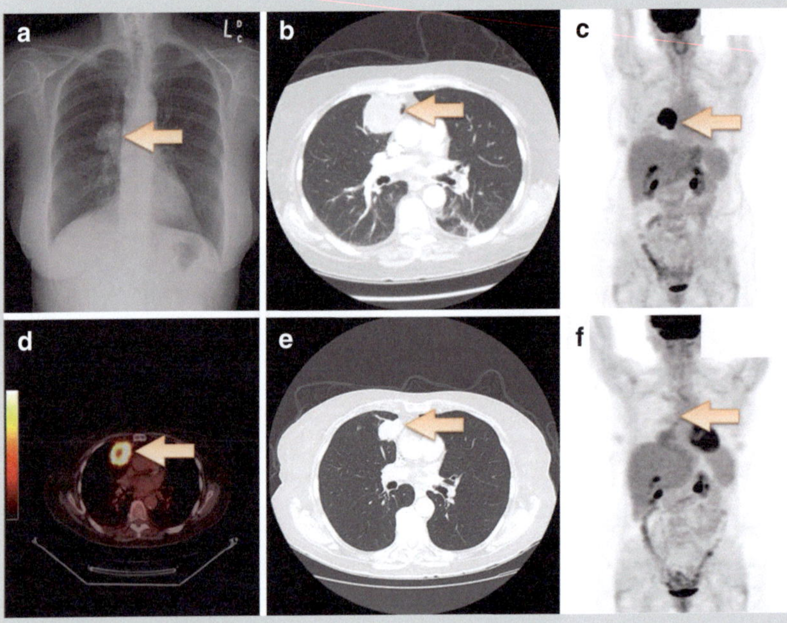

Fig. 10.1 Chest X-Ray (**a**), CT Chest (**b**) and PET Scan (**c** and **d**) showing a solitary intensely FDGavid right lung mass. CT Chest after 4 cycles of chemotherapy (**e**) showing partial response. Surveillance PET Scan (**f**) 4 years after surgery showed no evidence of recurrent or metastatic disease

In several studies involving CUP patients, the number of metastatic sites has been identified as a significant prognostic factor [11, 12]. A small proportion of CUP patients present with isolated or oligometastatic disease. Aggressive management with a combination of systemic chemotherapy and radical local therapy using surgical resection and/or radiotherapy or chemoradiotherapy is a reasonable option in such patients, and long-term survival in these patients has been reported [13].

Patients should be carefully selected to undergo aggressive and definite management. Exhaustive imaging should be performed to rule out any other sites of distant metastases, and positron emission tomography (PET) imaging can be useful in this regard. In a retrospective analysis of 42 CUP patients with localized disease examined by PET with fluorine-18-fluorodeoxyglucose, disseminated disease was detected only by PET in 16 (38 %) patients [14].

Multidisciplinary management of these patients can be facilitated by early engagement of surgeons, medical oncologists, and radiation oncologists. Since the role of adjuvant chemotherapy in such patients is unclear, neoadjuvant systemic chemotherapy can be attempted to help with chemical cytoreduction. Furthermore, a short period of neoadjuvant systemic chemotherapy can also aid in selecting patients for a more radical local approach, since in most patients, other metastatic sites may become evident within this time. With localized disease not amenable to surgery, definitive radiation or chemoradiation can offer palliative benefit and a prolonged disease-free interval.

With isolated cutaneous adenocarcinoma, the possibility of an unusual primary site such as an apocrine neoplasm should be considered. These rare indolent tumors can be managed with a wide local excision and are associated with a median survival of over 4 years [15]. These tumors cannot always be distinguished from metastatic breast carcinoma using immunohistochemistry, and this distinction is made on the basis of clinical presentation and careful pathological review [16, 17].

With isolated liver lesions, cholangiocarcinoma must always be considered in the differential diagnosis. Cholangiocarcinomas present as peripherally enhanced hypodense lesions and can be associated with biliary ductal dilatation (Fig. 10.2;

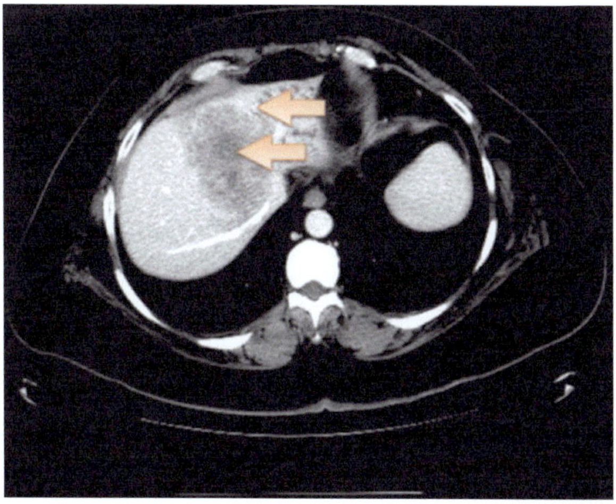

Fig. 10.2 Multiphasic contrast-enhanced CT showing hypodense mass lesion (*arrows*) in the liver with peripheral (*rim*) enhancement (*arrows*) suggestive of cholangiocarcinoma

Ref. [18]). The pathology is nonspecific though a majority of these are adenocarcinomas and express CK7. The management depends largely on the resectability of the tumor and presence of distant metastases.

Within this subset presenting with solitary metastatic disease, it should be recognized that patients with soft tissue and nodal sites fare better than visceral solitary metastatic presentations, especially those with brain and liver metastases.

Summary

Select patients with CUP who present with a solitary site of disease represent a unique favorable subset that benefit substantially from aggressive therapy involving systemic chemotherapy, radiation, and surgery and can attain prolonged disease-free intervals with multidisciplinary care. Comprehensive pathological evaluation can help with neoadjuvant or adjuvant therapy planning, and given the unknown biology of CUP, a detailed discussion with the patients regarding the rationale for this approach is necessary.

10.3 Osteoblastic Metastases with Elevated Prostate-Specific Antigen in Men

Osteoblastic lesions are predominantly seen in metastases from prostate, breast, and lung cancer. Prostate-specific antigen (PSA) is a glycoprotein which is expressed in both normal and neoplastic prostate tissues and is a highly sensitive marker of prostate cancer. All patients with known prostate cancer and bone metastases have elevation of serum PSA [19, 20]. Conversely, serum PSA also has a high negative predictive value of 99.7 % for bony metastatic disease [19]. The International Society of Urological Pathology (ISUP) recommends routine use of immunohistochemistry with PSA, and positive staining is considered diagnostic for prostate cancer [21].

Men presenting with blastic bone metastases should have serum PSA evaluation and immunophenotyping performed on the pathology specimen with prostate markers such as PSA and prostein [22]. In fact, the utility of all common serum tumor markers such as CEA, CA 19-9, and CA-125 with the exception of PSA is limited in the diagnostic workup of CUP [3]. CT pelvis should be reviewed with special attention toward prostate enlargement. Multiple core biopsies using transrectal ultrasound (TRUS) guidance can be performed although a negative biopsy does not rule out the prostate cancer subset of CUP.

Men with osteoblastic lesions, elevated serum PSA, and pathology suggestive of prostate cancer should be treated as metastatic prostate cancer with androgen deprivation therapy and subsequently systemic chemotherapy for castration-resistant disease [9, 23, 24].

Summary

Men presenting with adenocarcinoma of unknown primary with predominant osteoblastic metastases, elevated serum PSA, and immunophenotypic expression of prostate-specific tumor markers should be considered a favorable subset of CUP given the ease of management with initial hormonal therapy and expected benefit with treatment. Treatment guidelines for advanced prostate cancer are followed for the course of the disease.

10.4 Adenocarcinoma with Isolated Axillary Lymph Node Involvement in Women

Although the incidence of occult breast cancer is less than 0.5 %, breast cancer is the most common cause of malignant axillary lymphadenopathy in women [25–27]. Therefore, the probability of occult breast cancer should be considered high in the differential diagnosis in women presenting with CUP and isolated axillary lymph node(s) involvement. Patients with such a presentation should be managed on the lines of breast cancer and undergo a complete physical examination, mammography, ultrasound, and if these are negative, MRI of the breasts to look for any indication of a breast primary.

The immunophenotype of this subset is typically CK7 positive and CK20 negative. Breast cancer-specific markers include mammaglobin, GCDFP15, and GATA3 [28]. The sensitivity of these markers in breast cancer is 26 %, 14 %, and 86 %, respectively [29]. However, the expression frequency of any of these markers is variable and depends on morphology and grade of breast cancer, making interpretation of negative markers difficult [30]. Although staining for estrogen receptor (ER), progesterone receptor (PR), and HER2/neu supports a diagnosis of occult breast cancer and can be used to tailor therapy, they have low sensitivity and specificity to be used for diagnostic purposes. Breast magnetic resonance imaging (MRI) should be performed in addition to mammography and breast ultrasound due to its enhanced sensitivity. In patients with clinically occult breast cancer, breast MRI detects mammographically occult cancer in 50 % of cases with axillary metastases, regardless of breast density [31]. Any suspicious findings should be biopsied. MRI has a very low false-negative rate. Of approximately 40 women reported in the literature with isolated axillary adenocarcinoma and negative breast MRI findings, only 4 were found to have breast cancer at surgery or during follow-up [32].

With multimodality management involving breast surgery (mastectomy or breast-conserving surgery) with axillary lymph node dissection (ALND), chemotherapy, and radiation, such patients are potentially curable [33]. These patients have a 10-year survival of approximately 65 %, making this one of the most favorable subsets in CUP [24]. Although a negative MRI can identify patients for whom ALND with radiation may be sufficient, in the absence of a primary breast cancer, the management of the ipsilateral breast is unclear [9, 32]. In a population-based analysis, surgery or radiation of the ipsilateral breast showed improved survival compared with ALND alone [27]. Also, in retrospective studies, the actuarial freedom from appearance of a primary in the untreated breast was significantly lowered with radiation [34]. ALND followed by breast radiotherapy appears to be equivalent to mastectomy with respect to locoregional recurrence-free survival, recurrence/metastasis-free survival, and breast cancer-specific survival [35]. These studies should be evaluated with caution given their retrospective nature, and only a limited number of patients included in the series underwent breast MRI prior to therapy decision. An appropriately powered prospective study in this setting is unlikely; albeit knowing the limitations, breast radiation is often offered to CUP patients with a negative breast MRI. Likewise, although there are no prospective trials for use of adjuvant systemic therapy in this setting, retrospective data indicate that it is reasonable to treat these patients similarly to patients with corresponding nodal stage breast cancer [9, 36].

This management paradigm is changing as molecular profiling complements pathology as a diagnostic tool in this subset of patients. Not all women with axillary adenopathy do have occult breast cancer. Profiling for tissue of origin can help with treatment decisions especially if the immunohistochemistry does not correlate with breast cancer and ER, PR, and Her-2 status is negative.

Summary

Women presenting with CUP and isolated axillary lymphadenopathy are a unique favorable subset of CUP, in whom management should be designed in accordance with treatment of locally advanced breast cancer. When breast markers are not positive on immunohistochemistry, especially in patients with poorly differentiated carcinoma, it can present a challenge for management and most would treat it as breast cancer in the absence of an identifiable putative primary with additional studies. With aggressive local management (breast surgery and ALND with or without radiation) and chemotherapy, these patients are expected to have prolonged survival.

10.5 Papillary Carcinoma of the Peritoneal Cavity in Women

Case Study

A 54-year-old lady presented with progressively worsening abdominal pain for the past 3 weeks. She had no significant medical history, and total abdominal hysterectomy and bilateral salpingo-oophorectomy was performed 12 years ago for uterine fibroids. CT abdomen and pelvis showed a 3.8×6 cm mass in the omentum, left of midline in the lower abdomen with some nonspecific lymphadenopathy (Fig. 10.3a, b). Mammography, upper GI endoscopy, and colonoscopy were performed and were normal. An ultrasound-guided biopsy of this omental mass showed a poorly differentiated carcinoma. The immunohistochemical profile was not specific and showed malignant cells positive for CK7 and ER (about 90 %) and negative for synaptophysin, CK20, TTF-1, CD56, PR, GCDFP15, P63, P40, mammaglobin, and CK5/CK6. Due to the presence of peritoneal carcinomatosis, additional staining was performed and showed tumor cells to be positive for WT-1 and PAX-8 and negative for inhibin. The histopathology and immunophenotype was most consistent with a high-grade serous carcinoma of Mullerian origin (peritoneal/ovary). CA 125 was found to be 220.5 U/ml (reference range: 0.0–35.0) (Fig. 10.3d). Preoperative PET scan showed FDG-avid disease in the peritoneum without any evidence of distant metastases (Fig. 10.3c). The patient underwent diagnostic laparoscopy, exploratory laparotomy, omentectomy, and resection of the anterior abdominal wall mass with optimal tumor reductive surgery. No additional metastatic disease was noted in the peritoneum. Pathology showed high-grade serous carcinoma. Postoperatively, CA 125 decreased to 89.1 U/ml (Fig. 10.3d). She was then treated with systemic chemotherapy with carboplatin and paclitaxel, but chemotherapy was held after two cycles due to poor tolerance. The patient has since been on surveillance for the past 1.5 years without any signs of local or distant recurrence.

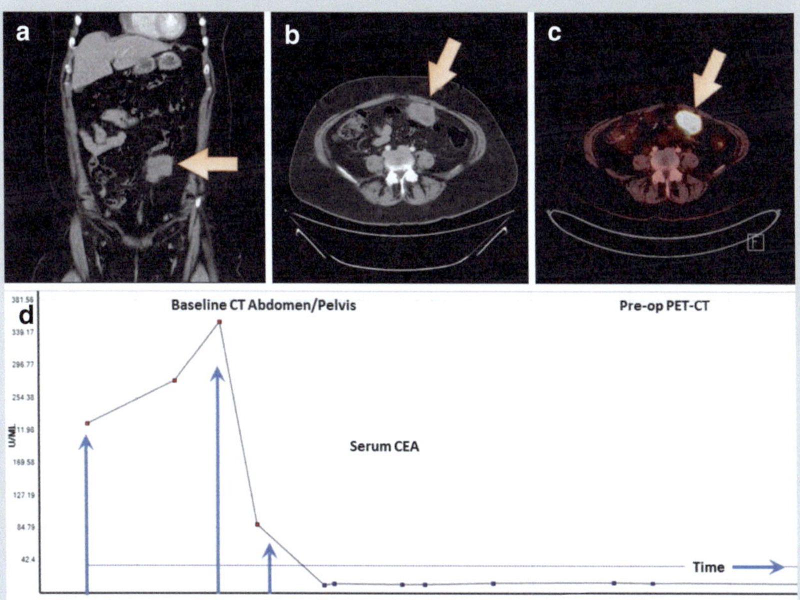

Fig. 10.3 CT abdomen and pelvis (**a** and **b**) showing omental mass. PET Scan (**c**) showing solitary FDG-avid disease in the peritoneum. CA-125 trends (**d**) over the course of treatment

Peritoneal serous papillary carcinoma has been recognized as a phenotypic variant of familial ovarian cancer and is seen in patients with increased risk of ovarian cancer such as those with germline BRCA1 and BRCA2 mutations [37]. These tumors have also been seen to occur after prophylactic oophorectomy [38]. Therefore, in women presenting with serous papillary peritoneal carcinoma, primary peritoneal carcinoma should be suspected [39, 40]. The clinical characteristics and treatment outcome of patients with primary peritoneal serous papillary carcinomas are similar to those of stage III–IV papillary serous ovarian carcinoma [41].

Pathological review may show a heterogeneous appearance with complex papillary or glandular architecture. Psammoma bodies may be present. The key feature is prominent mitotic activity, and many tumors can present as poorly differentiated carcinomas. The immunophenotype of this subset is typically positive for CK7, P53, WT-1, ER, and PAX-8 in most cases and negative for calretinin [42–45]. These tumors need to be distinguished from peritoneal mesotheliomas which are negative for Ber-EP4 and MOC-31 and positive for calretinin and D2-40 [46].

Combining optimal debulking with a platinum-based chemotherapy similar to that used for ovarian cancer is the most effective treatment. The median disease-free interval in these patients is about 15 months, and the median survival is about 21–23 months with a 5-year survival of 18 %, making the prognosis more favorable compared to the unfavorable CUP subset [40, 41]. The extent of cytoreduction is the most important prognostic indicator of survival in these patients, with median survival time of 20 months with residual tumor equal to or greater than 2 cm compared to 24 months with residual tumor less than 2 cm [41, 47]. Patients with this primary peritoneal adenocarcinoma presentation and widespread disease can also be given induction chemotherapy with paclitaxel-cisplatin/carboplatin as first-line chemotherapy [47]. Overall, the management for this subgroup should follow the guidelines for stage III–IV ovarian cancer with surgical cytoreduction and chemotherapy (platinum based and taxane based; Refs. [9, 48]).

Unfortunately, the majority of women with peritoneal carcinomatosis and CUP have disease without serous and Mullerian features and rather show mucin-producing or non-mucinous adenocarcinoma, some with signet ring cells. The primary site in these instances is most likely the GI tract (i.e., stomach, small bowel, appendix, colon, or pancreaticobiliary).

Summary

Poorly differentiated carcinoma/adenocarcinoma of unknown primary presenting with peritoneal involvement in women and having clinicopathological features suggestive of serous ovarian neoplasms represent a favorable subset of CUP similar to primary peritoneal carcinoma with long-term remission seen in about 15 % of cases. This subset should be treated as stage III–IV ovarian cancer using cytoreductive surgery and platinum-taxane-based chemotherapy.

10.6 Poorly Differentiated Carcinoma with Midline Distribution

Midline nodal CUP is thought to represent a subset of CUP with relatively favorable prognosis [49]. However, the definition of this entity varies considerably from one series to another, making this a group of heterogeneous disorders comprising multiple tumors types, especially germ cell tumors and lymphoma [50]. With progress in immunohistochemical techniques, the relevance of this subset is uncertain. Immunohistochemical stainings such as OCT4 are highly sensitive and specific for the diagnosis of germ cell tumors [51]. Similarly, antibodies to leukocyte common antigen (LCA) very reliably differentiate lymphomas from non-hematological malignancies [52]. Furthermore, the presence of 12p chromosomal gain (isochromosome 12p) is a diagnostic feature of extragonadal germ cell tumors [53].

Young patients presenting with poorly differentiated carcinoma in midline distribution should always be investigated for the possibility of extragonadal germ cell tumors and if they have features suggestive of germ cell tumors should be treated as having poor-risk germ cell tumor with platinum-based combination chemotherapy [9, 49]. In all these patients, the presence of a primary testicular tumor must be excluded using testicular ultrasound [54]. Serum tumor markers such as human chorionic gonadotropin (hCG) and alpha fetoprotein (AFP) can be helpful in suggesting the diagnosis of extragonadal germ cell tumor in these patients.

Due to traditionally high responses to platinum-based chemotherapy in germ cell tumors, these patients are expected to have favorable prognosis. The median survival in midline nodal CUP ranges from 8 to 23 months in literature, highlighting the heterogeneity of this subset [49]. In a series of 64 patients with poorly differentiated carcinoma or adenocarcinoma with predominantly midline nodal involvement, response rates of 48 % were seen with platinum-based chemotherapy [49]. Median survival of 12 months was reported for all patients [49]. However, in a subgroup of 15 male patients selected with more stringent clinical definition with the following criteria: age less than 50 years, tumor involving primarily midline nodal areas, rapid tumor growth, and histopathological diagnosis of undifferentiated or poorly differentiated carcinoma, median survival was reported to be 18 months [49].

Summary

Young patients with poorly differentiated carcinoma predominantly involving mediastinal, retroperitoneal lymph nodes should be evaluated for the possibility of extragonadal germ cell cancer syndrome with tumor markers, immunohistochemistry, and if needed chromosomal analysis and can be treated as per guidelines for poor-risk germ cell tumors with platinum-based combination chemotherapy.

10.7 Squamous Cell Carcinoma Involving Cervical Lymph Nodes

Squamous cell carcinomas constitute 5 % of all diagnosed CUP [2]. The clinical presentation can vary, but patients with cervical lymphadenopathy appear to have a favorable prognosis. Patients with cervical lymphadenopathy are managed as squamous cell carcinoma of head and neck, while those with inguinal lymphadenopathy need an approach similar to those for anogenital primaries. In patients with squamous cell carcinoma involving cervical lymph nodes with an initial occult primary, a primary will emerge in about 20 % of cases after definitive treatment [55, 56]. Although most patients with this subset are smokers, a small subset of these patients is HPV positive [57].

Workup should include CT of the head and neck, panendoscopy (laryngoscopy and nasopharyngoscopy) with multiple random mucosal biopsies, and bilateral tonsillectomies. PET scanning has emerged as an integral part of imaging in these patients if a primary site cannot be identified by CT or endoscopy [58]. In a prospective study of 60 patients, FDG-PET detected a primary missed by other modalities in 29 % cases [58]. Additionally, PET done before panendoscopy demonstrated fewer false-positive pathological foci [58]. An integrated PET-CT is superior to PET in the detection of the primary site with a higher overall detection rate (55.2 % vs. 30.8 %) and positive prediction value (93.3 % vs. 46.1 %; Ref. [59]). Surgical workup should include bilateral tonsillectomy as this increases the likelihood of finding occult tonsillar tumors (40 %) compared to tonsil biopsy (3 %; Ref. [60]).

Patients with squamous cell carcinoma of unknown primary with cervical lymph nodes should be treated according to the guidelines for locally advanced head and neck cancer [9, 61]. The management involves multidisciplinary care with surgery (lymph node dissection) and radiotherapy or chemoradiotherapy. Outcomes improve with multimodality therapy [62]. In a study with 52 patients with squamous cell carcinoma metastatic to cervical lymph nodes from an unknown primary site, 5-year disease-free survival rate was better (61 %) for patients who had lymph node dissection and irradiation compared to those who had radiation alone (37 %; Ref. [62]). Furthermore, in this study, tumor control in the contralateral side was better and emergence of occult primary was lower in patients who received radiotherapy to bilateral neck regions [62].

With aggressive multimodality therapy, 5-year locoregional recurrence-free survival approaches 65 %, and 5-year overall survival rate ranges from 50 to 70 % [55, 63]. The prognosis in these patients, similar to the prognosis in head and neck squamous cell carcinoma patients, is linked to the number of lymph nodes involved [55].

Summary

CUP patients presenting with squamous cell carcinoma of unknown primary with cervical lymphadenopathy represent a favorable subset of CUP and should be treated according to guidelines for locally advanced head and neck cancer with multimodality therapy involving surgery and radiation with or without chemotherapy.

10.8 Adenocarcinoma with Immunohistochemical Profile Consistent with Gastrointestinal Primary

Case Study

A 61-year-old lady presented with mild postmenopausal vaginal bleeding for past 1 month. The patient underwent total abdominal hysterectomy and bilateral salpingo-oophorectomy in 2000 for uterine fibroids. Physical examination showed a 3×6 cm mass lesion at the apex of the vaginal cuff. Biopsy of this mass showed a poorly differentiated adenocarcinoma with immunohistochemistry showing tumor cells strongly and diffusely positive for CK20 and CDX2 and negative for CK7. Baseline CT chest, abdomen, and pelvis showed multiple peritoneal implants (Fig. 10.4a, b). A mass was also seen around the cecal wall and

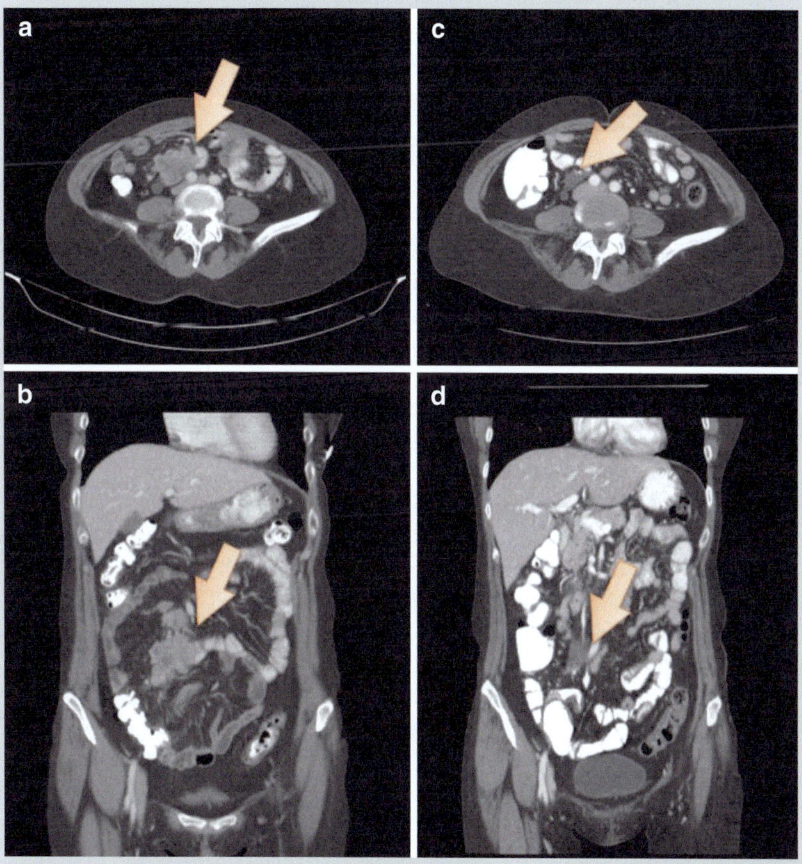

Fig. 10.4 CT abdomen and pelvis (**a** and **b**) showing multiple peritoneal implants but no evidence of a primary. CT after 4 cycles of chemotherapy (**c** and **d**) showing significant interval decrease in peritoneal disease

vaginal cuff and appeared more like a serosal implant rather than a colon primary. Upper GI endoscopy was normal. Colonoscopy showed an extrinsic compressing mass at the level of the cecum but no evidence of a primary. PET-CT showed significant FDG-avid disease in the peritoneum. The patient was treated with systemic chemotherapy with 5-fluorouracil and oxaliplatin. Restaging scans after four cycles of therapy showed significant interval decrease in the peritoneal disease and near complete metabolic response on PET-CT (Fig. 10.4c, d).

Immunohistochemistry has become the mainstay in the current management of CUP. The concordance of expression for tumor-specific antigens between the primary and the metastatic site seen in tumors has led investigators to believe that the immunophenotypic profile of CUP tumors can predict the putative primary tissue of origin [64]. Several panels of immunohistochemical markers have been developed to allow for recognition of patterns suggestive of specific tumor types [65]. One such immunohistochemical phenotype characterized by markers commonly seen in colon cancer is increasingly being recognized as a distinct favorable subset of CUP [66].

This subset is identified by expression of cytokeratin (CK) 20 and CDX2 (a nuclear transcription factor and product of a homeobox gene necessary for intestinal organogenesis) and absence of staining for CK7 [66]. CK20 expression is seen in 70–100 % of colon cancer [67, 68]. CK20-positive and CK7-negative immunophenotype is seen in 64 % of colorectal cancers and has a specificity of 97 % in predicting colorectal adenocarcinomas [69]. Similarly, CDX2 is a reliable, specific, and sensitive marker of normal and neoplastic intestinal epithelium and is expressed in nearly 97 % of colorectal cancers [70].

In a retrospective analysis of 32 CUP patients with this colon immunoprofile, the median survival was reported to be 37 months [71]. Nearly 80 % of these patients were treated with colon cancer regimens such as 5-fluorouracil-oxaliplatin and 5-fluorouracil-irinotecan chemotherapy. The authors also reported a second cohort of CDX2-positive tumors irrespective of CK20 or CK7 status ($n=36$), called "probable lower GI profile CUP," with a median survival of 21 months [71]. In a second study using a 92-gene real-time polymerase chain reaction (RT-PCR) molecular profiling assay performed on 1544 CUP cases, the investigators found 125 (12 %) cases with diagnosis of colorectal cancer predicted with greater than 80 % probability [72]. In the 42 patients with available clinical data, response rate to colon cancer regimens was 50 % compared to 17 % for empiric chemotherapy. The median survival of 32

(76 %) patients treated with site-specific therapy was 27 months [72]. Nearly 54 % of these patients had CK7−/CK20+ and/or CDX2+ immunophenotype.

Apart from the retrospective nature and small size of these studies, one must keep in mind that both CDX2-negative and CK20-negative phenotypes of colorectal cancer have been reported in the literature, especially associated with microsatellite instable or poorly differentiated tumors [73]. Prospective validation of the therapeutic effectiveness of colon cancer regimens in this immunohistochemical subset of CUP is needed.

Summary

Patients with carcinoma of unknown primary with an immunohistochemical phenotype consistent with gastrointestinal profile (CK7−/CK20+/CDX2+) is a unique favorable subset of CUP which appears to derive substantial benefit from site-specific chemotherapy with regimens used in colon cancer and is associated with improved survival.

10.9 Neuroendocrine Cancers

Case Study

A 65-year-old lady presented with abdominal pain, and CT abdomen and pelvis showed peritoneal carcinomatosis and liver metastases. CT-guided biopsy showed a high-grade carcinoma (Ki-67: 80 %) with diffuse and strong expression of CD56, chromogranin, and synaptophysin. Past medical history was significant for a diagnosis of high-grade serous carcinoma involving the peritoneal cavity 5 years ago. The patient was treated with cytoreductive surgery followed by adjuvant chemotherapy with carboplatin and paclitaxel. PET scan showed multiple, intensely FDG-avid hepatic, mesenteric, pulmonary metastases (Fig. 10.5a, b). Laboratory data showed elevated lactate dehydrogenase (LDH), 2941 IU/L (reference range: 313–618) and neuron-specific enolase (NSE), 95 ng/ml (reference range: <15), but normal CA 125. The patient was treated with cisplatin and irinotecan for three cycles. Restaging scans showed normalization of LDH and NSE and morphological and metabolic response to therapy (Fig. 10.5c, d).

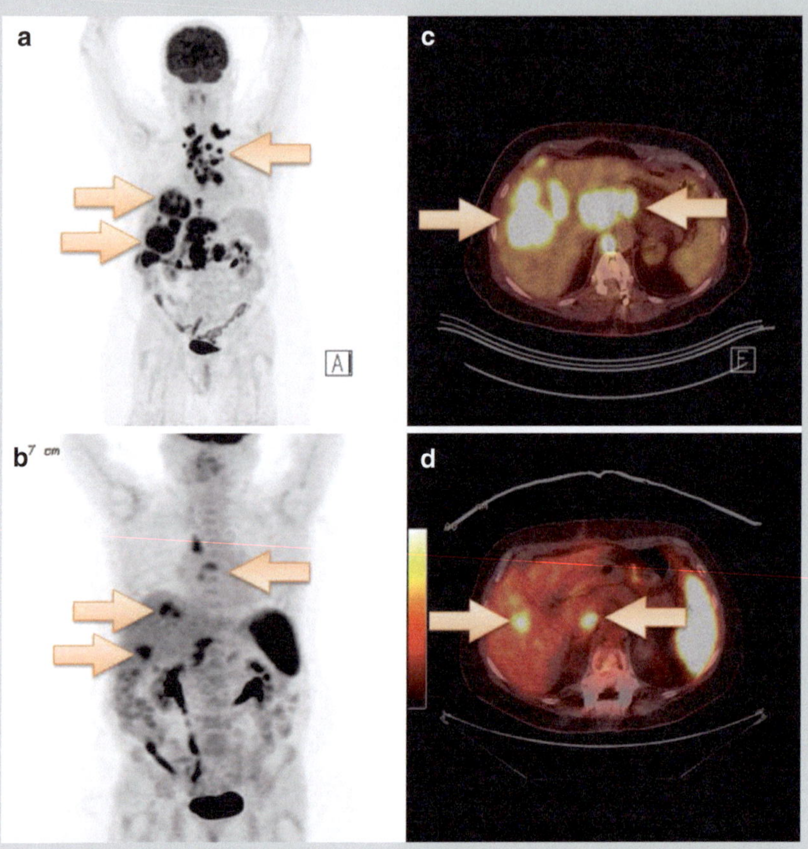

Fig. 10.5 PET Scan (**a** and **b**) showing multiple, intensely FDG-avid hepatic, mesenteric, pulmonary metastases. Restaging PET Scan showing metabolic response to systemic chemotherapy (**c** and **d**)

Neuroendocrine tumors compose about 4 % of all CUPs and commonly present with diffuse liver or bone metastases [74]. Neuroendocrine tumors are heterogeneous tumors whose clinical presentation, treatment, and prognosis depend uniquely on the grade or differentiation of the tumor. The novel classification of these tumors by the World Health Organization categorizes them into a well-differentiated group, composed of low- and intermediate-grade tumors, and a poorly differentiated group, composed of high-grade tumors [75]. Immunohistochemical markers most useful in the diagnosis of these tumors include CD56, chromogranin, and synaptophysin [76]. Well-differentiated neuroendocrine tumors are indolent and should be managed based on the same principles as used for the treatment of advanced carcinoid tumors [9]. In patients with limited disease, treatment includes local therapies such as surgery, radio-frequency ablation, or hepatic arterial embolization [9]. In more advanced disease, where local therapies are not an option, systemic therapy can be used and includes somatostatin analogs such as octreotide, targeted therapies such as sunitinib and everolimus, and cytotoxic chemotherapy such as temozolomide and capecitabine [9]. Poorly differentiated neuroendocrine tumors, irrespective of site of origin, should be managed as per guidelines for small cell lung cancer with cytotoxic chemotherapy including platinum agents, etoposide, irinotecan, and topotecan [9].

10.10 Additional Considerations

In the context of favorable subsets and for all cancers of unknown primary, per se, three important points should always be deliberated upon.

- Due to significant advances in immunohistochemistry, the diagnosis of putative primaries in CUP has come to rely heavily on pathology. However, it is important to understand the limits of immunohistochemistry given that several of the favorable subset designations depend on immunophenotypic patterns that fit a putative primary cancer. The sensitivity and specificity of immunohistochemistry can vary depending on type and number of immunostains used, grade of tumor, and biological subtypes of cancers [29, 77, 78]. Therefore, although pathology supersedes radiology in CUP therapy decisions, in select patients, especially those with poorly differentiated carcinomas, immunohistochemical differentiation can be challenging and clinical acumen is the key.
- Application of tissue of origin testing in favorable subsets of CUP is as yet unclear. Concordance of gene expression profiling with the favorable subset, although reassuring, is rarely helpful in management. However, discordant findings should raise a certain level of suspicion regarding the validity of the provisional diagnosis.
- Role of mutational profiling in favorable subsets needs further evaluation. Broadly, there is an extensive push toward personalizing cancer care through the use of genomic tools to identify driver mutations in an individual tumor. For CUP cancers, if this approach works and novel drugs are effective against specific mutations, additional subtypes of favorable subsets may emerge which are mutation specific and histology agnostic (e.g., ALK mutation-positive subset, BRAF V600E mutation subset, and others). For this, novel drugs effective against specific mutations are necessary and patients should be encouraged to enter well-designed biomarker-enriched clinical trials.

References

1. Varadhachary GR, Raber MN. Cancer of unknown primary site. N Engl J Med. 2014;371(8):757–65. PubMed PMID: 25140961.
2. Pavlidis N, Pentheroudakis G. Cancer of unknown primary site. Lancet. 2012;379(9824):1428–35. PubMed PMID: 22414598.

3. Fizazi K, Greco FA, Pavlidis N, Pentheroudakis G, ESMO Guidelines Working Group. Cancers of unknown primary site: ESMO Clinical Practice Guidelines for diagnosis, treatment and follow-up. Ann Oncol Off J Eur Soc Med Oncol ESMO. 2011;22(Suppl 6):vi64–8. PubMed PMID: 21908507.
4. Culine S, Lortholary A, Voigt JJ, Bugat R, Theodore C, Priou F, et al. Cisplatin in combination with either gemcitabine or irinotecan in carcinomas of unknown primary site: results of a randomized phase II study--trial for the French Study Group on Carcinomas of Unknown Primary (GEFCAPI 01). J Clin Oncol Off J Am Soc Clin Oncol. 2003;21(18):3479–82. PubMed PMID: 12972523.
5. Golfinopoulos V, Pentheroudakis G, Salanti G, Nearchou AD, Ioannidis JP, Pavlidis N. Comparative survival with diverse chemotherapy regimens for cancer of unknown primary site: multiple-treatments meta-analysis. Cancer Treat Rev. 2009;35(7):570–3. PubMed PMID: 19539430.
6. Hainsworth JD, Daugaard G, Lesimple T, Hubner G, Greco FA, Stahl MJ, et al. Paclitaxel/carboplatin with or without belinostat as empiric first-line treatment for patients with carcinoma of unknown primary site: a randomized, phase 2 trial. Cancer. 2015;121(10):1654–61. PubMed PMID: 25611313.
7. Hainsworth JD, Spigel DR, Thompson DS, Murphy PB, Lane CM, Waterhouse DM, et al. Paclitaxel/carboplatin plus bevacizumab/erlotinib in the first-line treatment of patients with carcinoma of unknown primary site. Oncologist. 2009;14(12):1189–97. PubMed PMID: 19965914.
8. Pavlidis N, Briasoulis E, Hainsworth J, Greco FA. Diagnostic and therapeutic management of cancer of an unknown primary. Eur J Cancer. 2003;39(14):1990–2005. PubMed PMID: 12957453.
9. NCCN. National comprehensive cancer network clinical practice guidelines in oncology (NCCN Guidelines®) 2015. Available from: http://www.nccn.org/professionals/physician_gls/f_guidelines.asp.
10. Briasoulis E, Tolis C, Bergh J, Pavlidis N, Force EGT. ESMO Minimum Clinical Recommendations for diagnosis, treatment and follow-up of cancers of unknown primary site (CUP). Ann Oncol Off J Eur Soc Med Oncol ESMO. 2005;16 Suppl 1:i75–6. PubMed PMID: 15888766.
11. Culine S. Prognostic factors in unknown primary cancer. Semin Oncol. 2009;36(1):60–4. PubMed PMID: 19179189.
12. Hainsworth JD, Johnson DH, Greco FA. Cisplatin-based combination chemotherapy in the treatment of poorly differentiated carcinoma and poorly differentiated adenocarcinoma of unknown primary site: results of a 12-year experience. J Clin Oncol Off J Am Soc Clin Oncol. 1992;10(6):912–22. PubMed PMID: 1375284.
13. Levy A, Massard C, Gross-Goupil M, Fizazi K. Carcinomas of an unknown primary site: a curable disease? Ann Oncol Off J Eur Soc Med Oncol ESMO. 2008;19(9):1657–8. PubMed PMID: 18647966.
14. Rades D, Kuhnel G, Wildfang I, Borner AR, Schmoll HJ, Knapp W. Localised disease in cancer of unknown primary (CUP): the value of positron emission tomography (PET) for individual therapeutic management. Ann Oncol Off J Eur Soc Med Oncol ESMO. 2001;12(11):1605–9. PubMed PMID: 11822762.
15. Hollowell KL, Agle SC, Zervos EE, Fitzgerald TL. Cutaneous apocrine adenocarcinoma: defining epidemiology, outcomes, and optimal therapy for a rare neoplasm. J Surg Oncol. 2012;105(4):415–9. PubMed PMID: 21913192.
16. Mentrikoski MJ, Wick MR. Immunohistochemical distinction of primary sweat gland carcinoma and metastatic breast carcinoma: can it always be accomplished reliably? Am J Clin Pathol. 2015;143(3):430–6. PubMed PMID: 25696802.
17. Rollins-Raval M, Chivukula M, Tseng GC, Jukic D, Dabbs DJ. An immunohistochemical panel to differentiate metastatic breast carcinoma to skin from primary sweat gland carcinomas with a review of the literature. Arch Pathol Lab Med. 2011;135(8):975–83. PubMed PMID: 21809988.

18. Kim SH, Lee CH, Kim BH, Kim WB, Yeom SK, Kim KA, et al. Typical and atypical imaging findings of intrahepatic cholangiocarcinoma using gadolinium ethoxybenzyl diethylenetriamine pentaacetic acid-enhanced magnetic resonance imaging. J Comput Assist Tomogr. 2012;36(6):704–9. PubMed PMID: 23192208.
19. Chybowski FM, Keller JJ, Bergstralh EJ, Oesterling JE. Predicting radionuclide bone scan findings in patients with newly diagnosed, untreated prostate cancer: prostate specific antigen is superior to all other clinical parameters. J Urol. 1991;145(2):313–8. PubMed PMID: 1703240.
20. Katagiri H, Takahashi M, Inagaki J, Sugiura H, Ito S, Iwata H. Determining the site of the primary cancer in patients with skeletal metastasis of unknown origin: a retrospective study. Cancer. 1999;86(3):533–7. PubMed PMID: 10430264.
21. Epstein JI, Egevad L, Humphrey PA, Montironi R; Members of the ISUP Immunohistochemistry in Diagnostic Urologic Pathology Group.. Best practices recommendations in the application of immunohistochemistry in the prostate: report from the International Society of Urologic Pathology consensus conference. Am J Surg Pathol. 2014;38(8):e6–19. PubMed PMID: 25029122
22. Queisser A, Hagedorn SA, Braun M, Vogel W, Duensing S, Perner S. Comparison of different prostatic markers in lymph node and distant metastases of prostate cancer. Mod Pathol Off J U S Can Acad Pathol Inc. 2015;28(1):138–45. PubMed PMID: 24925052.
23. Horwich A, Hugosson J, de Reijke T, Wiegel T, Fizazi K, Kataja V, et al. Prostate cancer: ESMO Consensus Conference Guidelines 2012. Ann Oncol Off J Eur Soc Med Oncol ESMO. 2013;24(5):1141–62. PubMed PMID: 23303340.
24. Iwamura H, Hatakeyama S, Tanaka Y, Tanaka T, Tokui N, Yamamoto H, et al. A case of metastatic cancer with markedly elevated PSA level that was not detected by repeat prostate biopsy. BMC Res Notes. 2014;7:64. PubMed PMID: 24476098. Pubmed Central PMCID: 3909476.
25. Foroudi F, Tiver KW. Occult breast carcinoma presenting as axillary metastases. Int J Radiat Oncol Biol Phys. 2000;47(1):143–7. PubMed PMID: 10758316.
26. Walsh R, Kornguth PJ, Soo MS, Bentley R, DeLong DM. Axillary lymph nodes: mammographic, pathologic, and clinical correlation. AJR Am J Roentgenol. 1997;168(1):33–8. PubMed PMID: 8976915.
27. Walker GV, Smith GL, Perkins GH, Oh JL, Woodward W, Yu TK, et al. Population-based analysis of occult primary breast cancer with axillary lymph node metastasis. Cancer. 2010;116(17):4000–6. PubMed PMID: 20564117. Pubmed Central PMCID: 4329781.
28. Sangoi AR, Shrestha B, Yang G, Mego O, Beck AH. The Novel Marker GATA3 is Significantly More Sensitive Than Traditional Markers Mammaglobin and GCDFP15 for Identifying Breast Cancer in Surgical and Cytology Specimens of Metastatic and Matched Primary Tumors. Appl Immunohistochem Mol Morphol AIMM Off Publ Soc Appl Immunohistochem. 2015;21. PubMed PMID: 25906123.
29. Braxton DR, Cohen C, Siddiqui MT. Utility of GATA3 immunohistochemistry for diagnosis of metastatic breast carcinoma in cytology specimens. Diagn Cytopathol. 2015;43(4):271–7. PubMed PMID: 25088841.
30. Huo L, Gong Y, Guo M, Gilcrease MZ, Wu Y, Zhang H, et al. GATA-binding protein 3 enhances the utility of gross cystic disease fluid protein-15 and mammaglobin A in triple-negative breast cancer by immunohistochemistry. Histopathology. 2015;67(2):245–54. PubMed PMID: 25564996.
31. Buchanan CL, Morris EA, Dorn PL, Borgen PI, Van Zee KJ. Utility of breast magnetic resonance imaging in patients with occult primary breast cancer. Ann Surg Oncol. 2005;12(12):1045–53. PubMed PMID: 16244803.
32. Olson Jr JA, Morris EA, Van Zee KJ, Linehan DC, Borgen PI. Magnetic resonance imaging facilitates breast conservation for occult breast cancer. Ann Surg Oncol. 2000;7(6):411–5. PubMed PMID: 10894136.
33. Rueth NM, Black DM, Limmer AR, Gabriel E, Huo L, Fornage BD, et al. Breast conservation in the setting of contemporary multimodality treatment provides excellent outcomes for patients with occult primary breast cancer. Ann Surg Oncol. 2015;22(1):90–5. PubMed PMID: 25249256.

34. Ellerbroek N, Holmes F, Singletary E, Evans H, Oswald M, McNeese M. Treatment of patients with isolated axillary nodal metastases from an occult primary carcinoma consistent with breast origin. Cancer. 1990;66(7):1461–7. PubMed PMID: 2207996.
35. He M, Tang LC, Yu KD, Cao AY, Shen ZZ, Shao ZM, et al. Treatment outcomes and unfavorable prognostic factors in patients with occult breast cancer. Eur J Surg Oncol J Eur Soc Surg Oncol Br Assoc Surg Oncol. 2012;38(11):1022–8. PubMed PMID: 22959166.
36. Senkus E, Kyriakides S, Penault-Llorca F, Poortmans P, Thompson A, Zackrisson S, et al. Primary breast cancer: ESMO Clinical Practice Guidelines for diagnosis, treatment and follow-up. Ann Oncol Off J Eur Soc Med Oncol ESMO. 2013;24 Suppl 6:vi7–23. PubMed PMID: 23970019.
37. Karlan BY, Baldwin RL, Lopez-Luevanos E, Raffel LJ, Barbuto D, Narod S, et al. Peritoneal serous papillary carcinoma, a phenotypic variant of familial ovarian cancer: implications for ovarian cancer screening. Am J Obstet Gynecol. 1999;180(4):917–28. PubMed PMID: 10203660.
38. Finch A, Beiner M, Lubinski J, Lynch HT, Moller P, Rosen B, et al. Salpingo-oophorectomy and the risk of ovarian, fallopian tube, and peritoneal cancers in women with a BRCA1 or BRCA2 mutation. JAMA. 2006;296(2):185–92. PubMed PMID: 16835424.
39. Killackey MA, Davis AR. Papillary serous carcinoma of the peritoneal surface: matched-case comparison with papillary serous ovarian carcinoma. Gynecol Oncol. 1993;51(2):171–4. PubMed PMID: 8276289.
40. Strnad CM, Grosh WW, Baxter J, Burnett LS, Jones 3rd HW, Greco FA, et al. Peritoneal carcinomatosis of unknown primary site in women. A distinctive subset of adenocarcinoma. Ann Intern Med. 1989;111(3):213–7. PubMed PMID: 2502058.
41. Ben-Baruch G, Sivan E, Moran O, Rizel S, Menczer J, Seidman DS. Primary peritoneal serous papillary carcinoma: a study of 25 cases and comparison with stage III-IV ovarian papillary serous carcinoma. Gynecol Oncol. 1996;60(3):393–6. PubMed PMID: 8774644.
42. Attanoos RL, Webb R, Dojcinov SD, Gibbs AR. Value of mesothelial and epithelial antibodies in distinguishing diffuse peritoneal mesothelioma in females from serous papillary carcinoma of the ovary and peritoneum. Histopathology. 2002;40(3):237–44. PubMed PMID: 11895489.
43. Ozcan A, Shen SS, Hamilton C, Anjana K, Coffey D, Krishnan B, et al. PAX 8 expression in non-neoplastic tissues, primary tumors, and metastatic tumors: a comprehensive immunohistochemical study. Mod Pathol Off J U S Can Acad Pathol Inc. 2011;24(6):751–64. PubMed PMID: 21317881.
44. Matsuo K, Sheridan TB, Mabuchi S, Yoshino K, Hasegawa K, Studeman KD, et al. Estrogen receptor expression and increased risk of lymphovascular space invasion in high-grade serous ovarian carcinoma. Gynecol Oncol. 2014;133(3):473–9. PubMed PMID: 24674832. Pubmed Central PMCID: 4170217.
45. Liu Q, Lin JX, Shi QL, Wu B, Ma HH, Sun GQ. Primary peritoneal serous papillary carcinoma: a clinical and pathological study. Pathol Oncol Res POR. 2011;17(3):713–9. PubMed PMID: 21647781.
46. Ordonez NG. The diagnostic utility of immunohistochemistry and electron microscopy in distinguishing between peritoneal mesotheliomas and serous carcinomas: a comparative study. Mod Pathol Off J U S Can Acad Pathol Inc. 2006;19(1):34–48. PubMed PMID: 16056246.
47. Piver MS, Eltabbakh GH, Hempling RE, Recio FO, Blumenson LE. Two sequential studies for primary peritoneal carcinoma: induction with weekly cisplatin followed by either cisplatin-doxorubicin-cyclophosphamide or paclitaxel-cisplatin. Gynecol Oncol. 1997;67(2):141–6. PubMed PMID: 9367697.
48. Ledermann JA, Raja FA, Fotopoulou C, Gonzalez-Martin A, Colombo N, Sessa C, et al. Newly diagnosed and relapsed epithelial ovarian carcinoma: ESMO Clinical Practice Guidelines for diagnosis, treatment and follow-up. Ann Oncol Off J Eur Soc Med Oncol ESMO. 2013;24 Suppl 6:vi24–32. PubMed PMID: 24078660.
49. Pentheroudakis G, Stoyianni A, Pavlidis N. Cancer of unknown primary patients with midline nodal distribution: midway between poor and favourable prognosis? Cancer Treat Rev. 2011;37(2):120–6. PubMed PMID: 20673701.

50. Hainsworth JD, Greco FA. Poorly differentiated carcinoma and germ cell tumors. Hematol Oncol Clin North Am. 1991;5(6):1223–31. PubMed PMID: 1663941.
51. Cheng L. Establishing a germ cell origin for metastatic tumors using OCT4 immunohistochemistry. Cancer. 2004;101(9):2006–10. PubMed PMID: 15386301.
52. Michels S, Swanson PE, Frizzera G, Wick MR. Immunostaining for leukocyte common antigen using an amplified avidin-biotin-peroxidase complex method and paraffin sections. A study of 735 hematopoietic and nonhematopoietic human neoplasms. Arch Pathol Lab Med. 1987;111(11):1035–9. PubMed PMID: 2444189.
53. Motzer RJ, Rodriguez E, Reuter VE, Bosl GJ, Mazumdar M, Chaganti RS. Molecular and cytogenetic studies in the diagnosis of patients with poorly differentiated carcinomas of unknown primary site. J Clin Oncol Off J Am Soc Clin Oncol. 1995;13(1):274–82. PubMed PMID: 7799031.
54. Sakai N, Yamada T, Asao T, Murayama T. Sonographically-detected impalpable testicular cancer with retroperitoneal bulky metastases: a case report. Int J Urol Off J Jpn Urol Assoc. 1997;4(5):533–4. PubMed PMID: 9354963.
55. Lu X, Hu C, Ji Q, Shen C, Feng Y. Squamous cell carcinoma metastatic to cervical lymph nodes from an unknown primary site: the impact of radiotherapy. Tumori. 2009;95(2):185–90. PubMed PMID: 19579864.
56. Grau C, Johansen LV, Jakobsen J, Geertsen P, Andersen E, Jensen BB. Cervical lymph node metastases from unknown primary tumours. Results from a national survey by the Danish Society for Head and Neck Oncology. Radiother Oncol J Eur Soc Ther Radiol Oncol. 2000;55(2):121–9. PubMed PMID: 10799723.
57. Compton AM, Moore-Medlin T, Herman-Ferdinandez L, Clark C, Caldito GC, Wang XI, et al. Human papillomavirus in metastatic lymph nodes from unknown primary head and neck squamous cell carcinoma. Otolaryngol Head Neck Surg Off J Am Acad Otolaryngol Head Neck Surg. 2011;145(1):51–7. PubMed PMID: 21493313.
58. Johansen J, Buus S, Loft A, Keiding S, Overgaard M, Hansen HS, et al. Prospective study of 18FDG-PET in the detection and management of patients with lymph node metastases to the neck from an unknown primary tumor. Results from the DAHANCA-13 study. Head Neck. 2008;30(4):471–8. PubMed PMID: 18023031.
59. Keller F, Psychogios G, Linke R, Lell M, Kuwert T, Iro H, et al. Carcinoma of unknown primary in the head and neck: comparison between positron emission tomography (PET) and PET/CT. Head Neck. 2011;33(11):1569–75. PubMed PMID: 21990221.
60. Waltonen JD, Ozer E, Schuller DE, Agrawal A. Tonsillectomy vs. deep tonsil biopsies in detecting occult tonsil tumors. Laryngoscope. 2009;119(1):102–6. PubMed PMID: 19117304.
61. Gregoire V, Lefebvre JL, Licitra L, Felip E, Group E-E-EGW. Squamous cell carcinoma of the head and neck: EHNS-ESMO-ESTRO Clinical Practice Guidelines for diagnosis, treatment and follow-up. Ann Oncol Off J Eur Soc Med Oncol ESMO. 2010;21 Suppl 5:v184–6. PubMed PMID: 20555077.
62. Reddy SP, Marks JE. Metastatic carcinoma in the cervical lymph nodes from an unknown primary site: results of bilateral neck plus mucosal irradiation vs. ipsilateral neck irradiation. Int J Radiat Oncol Biol Phys. 1997;37(4):797–802. PubMed PMID: 9128954.
63. Klop WM, Balm AJ, Keus RB, Hilgers FJ, Tan IB. [Diagnosis and treatment of 39 patients with cervical lymph node metastases of squamous cell carcinoma of unknown primary origin, referred to Netherlands Cancer Institute/Antoni van Leeuwenhoek Hospital, 1979-98]. Nederlands tijdschrift voor geneeskunde. 2000;144(28):1355–60. PubMed PMID: 10923158. Diagnostiek en behandeling van 39 patienten met halskliermetastasen van plaveiselcelcarcinoom van onbekende primaire origine, verwezen naar het Nederlands Kanker Instituut/Antoni van Leeuwenhoek Ziekenhuis, 1979/'98.
64. Dennis JL, Hvidsten TR, Wit EC, Komorowski J, Bell AK, Downie I, et al. Markers of adenocarcinoma characteristic of the site of origin: development of a diagnostic algorithm. Clin Cancer Res Off J Am Assoc Cancer Res. 2005;11(10):3766–72. PubMed PMID: 15897574.
65. Brown RW, Campagna LB, Dunn JK, Cagle PT. Immunohistochemical identification of tumor markers in metastatic adenocarcinoma. A diagnostic adjunct in the determination of primary site. Am J Clin Pathol. 1997;107(1):12–9. PubMed PMID: 8980361.

66. Varadhachary GR, Raber MN, Matamoros A, Abbruzzese JL. Carcinoma of unknown primary with a colon-cancer profile-changing paradigm and emerging definitions. Lancet Oncol. 2008;9(6):596–9. PubMed PMID: 18510991.
67. Chu P, Wu E, Weiss LM. Cytokeratin 7 and cytokeratin 20 expression in epithelial neoplasms: a survey of 435 cases. Mod Pathol Off J U S Can Acad Pathol Inc. 2000;13(9):962–72. PubMed PMID: 11007036.
68. Blumenfeld W, Turi GK, Harrison G, Latuszynski D, Zhang C. Utility of cytokeratin 7 and 20 subset analysis as an aid in the identification of primary site of origin of malignancy in cytologic specimens. Diagn Cytopathol. 1999;20(2):63–6. PubMed PMID: 9951598.
69. Bayrak R, Haltas H, Yenidunya S. The value of CDX2 and cytokeratins 7 and 20 expression in differentiating colorectal adenocarcinomas from extraintestinal gastrointestinal adenocarcinomas: cytokeratin 7-/20+ phenotype is more specific than CDX2 antibody. Diagn Pathol. 2012;7:9. PubMed PMID: 22268990. Pubmed Central PMCID: 3331835.
70. Barbareschi M, Murer B, Colby TV, Chilosi M, Macri E, Loda M, et al. CDX-2 homeobox gene expression is a reliable marker of colorectal adenocarcinoma metastases to the lungs. Am J Surg Pathol. 2003;27(2):141–9. PubMed PMID: 12548159.
71. Varadhachary GR, Karanth S, Qiao W, Carlson HR, Raber MN, Hainsworth JD, et al. Carcinoma of unknown primary with gastrointestinal profile: immunohistochemistry and survival data for this favorable subset. Int J Clin Oncol. 2014;19(3):479–84. PubMed PMID: 23813044.
72. Hainsworth JD, Schnabel CA, Erlander MG, Haines 3rd DW, Greco FA. A retrospective study of treatment outcomes in patients with carcinoma of unknown primary site and a colorectal cancer molecular profile. Clin Colorectal Cancer. 2012;11(2):112–8. PubMed PMID: 22000811.
73. Kim JH, Rhee YY, Bae JM, Cho NY, Kang GH. Loss of CDX2/CK20 expression is associated with poorly differentiated carcinoma, the CpG island methylator phenotype, and adverse prognosis in microsatellite-unstable colorectal cancer. Am J Surg Pathol. 2013;37(10):1532–41. PubMed PMID: 24025523.
74. Spigel DR, Hainsworth JD, Greco FA. Neuroendocrine carcinoma of unknown primary site. Semin Oncol. 2009;36(1):52–9. PubMed PMID: 19179188.
75. Anlauf M, Gerlach P, Schott M, Raffel A, Krausch M, Knoefel WT, et al. Pathology of neuroendocrine neoplasms. Chirurg Z Alle Geb Oper Med. 2011;82(7):567–73. PubMed PMID: 21487814. Pathologie neuroendokriner Neoplasien.
76. Mlika M, Zendah I, Braham E, El Mezni F. CD56 antibody: old-fashioned or still trendy in endocrine lung tumors. J Immunoassay Immunochem. 2015;36(4):414–9. PubMed PMID: 25140506.
77. Johnson H, Cohen C, Fatima N, Duncan D, Siddiqui MT. Thyroid transcription factor 1 and Napsin A double stain: utilizing different vendor antibodies for diagnosing lung adenocarcinoma. Acta Cytol. 2012;56(6):596–602. PubMed PMID: 23207437.
78. Surrey LF, Frank R, Zhang PJ, Furth EE. TTF-1 and Napsin-A are expressed in a subset of cholangiocarcinomas arising from the gallbladder and hepatic ducts: continued caveats for utilization of immunohistochemistry panels. Am J Surg Pathol. 2014;38(2):224–7. PubMed PMID: 24418856.

Chapter 11
Novel Diagnostic and Therapeutic Strategies in the Management of Patients with Cancers of Unknown Primary Site

F. Anthony Greco and John D. Hainsworth

11.1 Introduction

Cancer of unknown primary site (CUP) is a syndrome characterized by the presence of metastatic cancer in the absence of a clinically detectable anatomical primary site. Patients with this syndrome are heterogeneous, since many different occult primary sites are represented. Estimates of the incidence of CUP range from 2 to 8 % of cancer diagnoses in various countries [1]; in the Unites States, this syndrome affects 90,000 patients/year. The diagnosis of CUP has frustrated physicians, patients, and their families for decades, since an anatomical primary tumor site cannot be identified, despite the presence of metastatic tumor. Most of these patients were particularly difficult to treat in the past; the precise type of cancer or tissue of origin was unknown, and for many advanced cancers, even with most known primary tumor sites, there were no effective therapies.

The evaluation and therapy of CUP patients have changed with the development of improved diagnostic technology and the ongoing improvement of therapies for many types of advanced solid tumors. Examination of the biopsy specimen can now accurately diagnose the tissue of origin in most CUP patients, providing the basis for potentially improved site-specific therapies [2–26], despite the failure to identify the anatomical primary tumor site.

F.A. Greco, MD (✉) • J.D. Hainsworth, MD
Department of Medical Oncology, Sarah Cannon Cancer Center and Research Institute, Tennessee Oncology, PLLC,
250 25th Avenue North, Suite 100, Nashville, TN 37203, USA
e-mail: fgreco@tnonc.com

A. Krämer, H. Löffler (eds.), *Cancer of Unknown Primary*,
DOI 10.1007/978-3-319-22581-4_11

11.1.1 Epidemiology

CUP is among the ten most frequently diagnosed advanced cancers in Europe and the United States [27]. In the United States, the exact incidence is very difficult to determine since many of these patients are "assigned" a specific primary site based on the sites of metastasis, histologic appearance, or the physician's clinical opinion [1, 2]. The median age at diagnosis is about 60 years; the syndrome occurs with equal frequency in men and women. The majority of these cancers are carcinomas and most of these adenocarcinomas, but sarcomas, melanomas, and lymphomas are occasionally eventually diagnosed. Multiple metastatic sites are usually present at the time of diagnosis; common metastatic sites include the liver, lymph nodes, lung, and bone. During the past 40 years, several favorable subsets of patients have been recognized based on clinical and pathologic features; however, these patients represent only about 20 % of the CUP population [28] (see Chap. 10).

11.1.2 Pathogenesis

The pathogenesis of CUP remains a mystery; autopsy series have identified small, clinically undetectable, invasive primary tumors in about 75 % of patients [29]. Therefore, most CUP patients have a primary site, albeit too small to detect by clinical evaluation. Unique nonrandom acquired somatic genetic and/or epigenetic alterations are very likely the cause of the CUP syndrome, explaining the small clinically occult invasive primaries with detectable metastasis [30]. However, such alterations have not yet been discovered. Despite the clinically occult anatomical primaries, the clinical biology of the specific cancer types within the CUP syndrome appears similar to corresponding metastatic cancers with known primary sites [1, 2].

11.2 Diagnosis

The diagnostic approach for patients with possible CUP has evolved in the last several years (Tables 11.1, 11.2, and 11.3 and Fig. 11.1). The clinical evaluation begins as always with a history and physical examination followed by reviewing/obtaining clinical data (Tables 11.1 and 11.2). Biopsy of a metastatic site and review of the histologic features complete the initial evaluation. The goal is to find the anatomical primary site. If an anatomical primary site is identified, regardless of the size of the primary tumor, the patient does not have CUP and treatment proceeds in a standard fashion for that type of metastatic cancer. The patient has CUP if an anatomical primary site is not detected. Immunohistochemical (IHC) staining (Table 11.3) and, if necessary, gene expression profiling (molecular cancer classifier assay testing) of the biopsy specimen are performed to determine the cancer type or tissue of origin.

Prior to 2008, the precise cancer type for the majority of CUP patients could not be determined, but was presumed in a minority of patients within several subsets

Table 11.1 Initial evaluation of a possible CUP patient

History and physical examination
Laboratory tests: CBC, CMP, LDH, urine analysis, PSA in men
Computerized tomographic (CT) scans of the chest, abdomen, pelvis
Positron emission tomography (PET) scan in selected patients (squamous carcinoma in cervical/inguinal nodes and others with a single site of involvement)
Mammography in women
Pathology evaluation: including screening immunohistochemical stains of the biopsy on carcinomas (CK7, CK20, TTF-1, CDX-2)
Additional clinical and pathologic evaluation based on details from history, physical examination, laboratory testing, medical imaging, and specialized pathology (Table 11.4)
If an anatomical primary site found the patients do not have CUP
Molecular cancer classifier assay on very small biopsy/aspiration/cytology specimens or when immunohistochemical stains not diagnostic of a single cancer type or tissue of origin

Table 11.2 Additional evaluation determined by findings from initial diagnostic evaluation

	Additional evaluation	
Results of initial diagnostic evaluation	Clinical	IHC staining/other testing
Features of lung carcinoma (hilar/mediastinal adenopathy; biopsy positive for CK7 and TTF-1)	Bronchoscopy	EGFR mutation, FISH for ALK, ROS1 rearrangement
Features of colorectal carcinoma (liver/peritoneal metastasis; biopsy positive for CK20 and CDX2)	Colonoscopy	KRAS mutation test
Features of breast cancer in women (axillary nodes, lung, bone, liver metastasis; biopsy positive for CK7)	Breast MRI	ER, GCDFP-15, mammoglobin, GATA3, FISH for HER2
Features of ovarian cancer in women (pelvic/peritoneal metastases; CK7+)	Pelvic/intravaginal ultrasound	WT-1, PAX8, ER
Mediastinal/retroperitoneal mass in young adults	Testicular ultrasound, serum AFP, HCG, LDH	PLAP, OCT4; FISH for i(12)p
Poorly differentiated carcinoma, with or without clear cell features	Serum AFP if Hepar1+; octreotide scan if neuroendocrine stains+	Chromogranin, synaptophysin, RCC, PAX8, Hepar1, MelanA, HMB-45
Liver metastasis predominant (CK7-,CK20-)	Serum AFP	Hepar1
Any histology without a single cancer site or tissue of origin predicted by IHC		Molecular cancer classifier assay

which were recognized over many years as favorable subsets. (For example, women with metastatic adenocarcinoma involving axillary lymph nodes were presumed to have breast cancer; patients with metastatic squamous carcinoma involving upper or mid-cervical lymph nodes were presumed to have a head/neck primary site; etc.) However, the use of IHC stains and molecular cancer classifier assays performed on the biopsy specimen now results in a diagnosis of the tissue of origin/type of cancer for most CUP cancers.

Table 11.3 Immunohistochemical staining patterns of a biopsy characteristic of a single cancer or tissue of origin

Prostate	CK7–, CK20–, PSA+
Lung adenocarcinoma and large cell	CK7+, CK20+ TTF-1+, Napsin A+
Lung neuroendocrine (small cell/large cell)	Chromogranin+, synaptophysin+, CD56+, TTF-1+
Thyroid carcinoma (papillary/follicular)	Thyroglobin+, TTF-1+
Melanoma	MelanA+, HMB45+, S100+
Adrenal carcinoma	Alpha-inhibin+, Melan-A+(A103)
Renal cell carcinoma	RCC+, PAX8+
Germ cell carcinoma	PLAP+, OCT4+
Ovary carcinoma	CK7+, WT-1+, PAX8+, ER+
Hepatocellular carcinoma	Hepar-1+, CD10+, CD13+
Breast carcinoma	ER+, GCDFP-15+, mammaglobin+, GATA-3+

In the appropriate clinical and pathologic setting, the staining profiles may be diagnostic of the cancer type or tissue of origin. There are many overlapping stains, and not all the stains are always positive or negative as indicated above

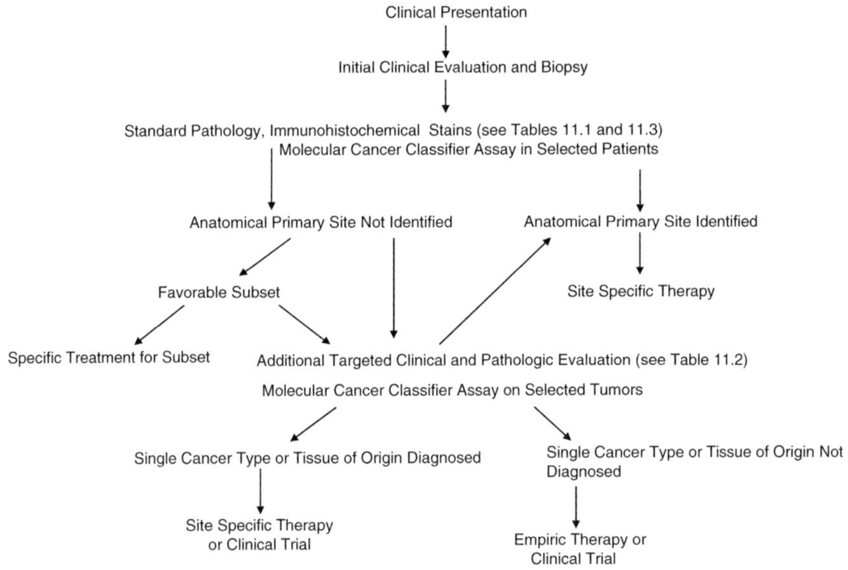

Fig. 11.1 Evaluation of a possible CUP patient

11.2.1 Immunohistochemical Staining

Immunohistochemistry has improved over the past several years with the discovery of increasingly specific cellular proteins. In addition, panels of IHC stains have been useful (Table 11.3) in diagnosing a number of cancers based on relatively specific tumor staining profiles [3, 4]. False-negative and false-positive stains are relatively common, and the characteristic staining patterns shown in Table 11.3 are not always observed in those cancer types; positive and negative staining may overlap in

Table 11.4 Comparison of the accuracy of IHC versus molecular cancer classifier assays in identification of metastatic tumors of known primary site

	Handorf et al. [21]			Weiss et al. [19]		
	Number of	Accuracy (%)		Number of	Accuracy (%)	
Known Primary site	specimens	[a]IHC	MCCA	specimens	[a]IHC	MCCA
All	157	83	89	122	69	79
Poorly differentiated histology	33	71	91	——	[a]NR	NR
Lung	6	100	83	24	67	75
Colon	25	92	100	17	94	94
Breast	25	84	100	11	55	73
Kidney	14	100	86	13	77	77
Bladder	10	43	60	11	45	82
Ovary	8	75	88	5	100	100
Stomach/esophagus	7	29	29	5	60	60
Prostate	5	56	100	4	50	100
Pancreaticobiliary	3	73	60	4	75	50

[a]*IHC* immunohistochemistry, *MCCA* molecular cancer classifier assay, *NR* not reported

different tumors. The prediction of a single-specific cancer type or tissue of origin by IHC staining is much more reliable than several years ago, but such a prediction is still not possible in about 60 % of CUP cancers [3, 6, 17].

The role of IHC staining in the management of CUP has developed over many years, and certain results are now accepted and used to make treatment decisions. For example, IHC stains are used to evaluate poorly differentiated neoplasms, and when a lineage is established (e.g., lymphoma, germ cell tumor, neuroendocrine carcinoma, thyroid carcinoma, melanoma), appropriate treatments are instituted. Although the clinical validity of this practice has been supported by small, retrospective trials, the use of IHC staining results to direct therapy has never been evaluated or validated in prospective studies. Paradoxically, several common epithelial cancers (e.g., lung, colorectal, breast, kidney) now have rather specific diagnostic IHC staining patterns (Table 11.3), yet these IHC results have not been widely used to direct treatment for these CUP subsets. We call attention to these inconsistencies not to minimize the contribution of IHC but to provide a backdrop for the current controversies regarding the studies required to establish molecular profiling results as integral in directing CUP treatment (see below).

11.2.2 *Molecular Cancer Classifier Assays*

Molecular cancer classifier assays, based on tissue-specific patterns of gene expression, have been developed to diagnose the specific tissue of origin by testing the biopsy from a metastatic site. These molecular assays complement IHC staining [16–21] and are particularly useful when IHC stains are not conclusive [3, 14,

17–19, 21, 31]. Several molecular cancer classifier assays have been studied in CUP [3, 5, 11–15, 22–26, 31], but most information has been reported from three assays [92-gene RT-PCR assay, CancerTYPE ID [7]; microarray for microRNAs, Cancer Origin Test [9]; microarray for mRNA, Tissue of Origin Test [8]].

There have been no direct comparisons of these assays, but their ability to diagnose the specific tissue of origin in CUP is now well documented [3, 5–21, 31]. Since the occult anatomical primary sites could not serve as a gold standard of reference, the accuracy and diagnostic utility of molecular assays have been evaluated by indirect methods (clinicopathologic comparisons). In one study of 171 CUP patients, the accuracy of the 92-gene RT-PCR assay was evaluated by three separate methods [17]: (1) direct comparison to latent primary sites found months to years later, (2) comparison to single IHC staining diagnoses, and (3) obtaining additional confirmatory/supportive IHC staining based on the molecular assay diagnosis. An accuracy rate of about 80 % was determined using each of these 3 evaluative methods [17].

Molecular cancer classifier assays are therefore not 100 % accurate, and the limitations of their ability to make precise diagnoses are now well recognized [17]. All data, including clinical information (age, gender, imaging studies, laboratory values, sites of metastasis), tumor histology, and IHC staining results (initially and if necessary as confirmatory/supportive testing after a molecular assay diagnosis), should be considered in concert with the molecular assay result to determine the specific cancer type or tissue of origin. When all available data are considered, the tissue of origin can be identified or highly suspected in about 95 % of patients with CUP.

11.2.3 Comparisons of IHC Staining and Molecular Cancer Classifier Assays

Two relatively large studies have compared molecular cancer classifier assays and IHC staining in their respective abilities to diagnose a cancer type or tissue of origin [19, 21]. Both studies were performed on biopsies from patients with metastatic cancer of known origin; pathologists were given biopsy specimens and informed of the site of the biopsy and the gender of the patient. The specimens were large, and the pathologists could perform as many IHC stains as felt necessary for an optimal diagnosis. They were asked to predict a single cancer or primary site even if the IHC staining results were not completely characteristic or diagnostic. A molecular cancer classifier assay, the 92 gene RT-PCR (CancerTYPE ID) in one study [19] and the microarray mRNA assay (tissue of origin) in the second study [21], was performed on each biopsy specimen.

The results of these two studies are illustrated in Table 11.4. The primary sites of most tumors were correctly identified by both IHC staining and the molecular assays. In the study using the 92 gene RT-PCR assay, a median of 7.9 IHC stains/tumor were used, and 84 of 122 tumors (69 %) were correctly diagnosed compared to 96 of 122 tumors (79 %) for the molecular assay [19]. In the study using the microarray mRNA assay, the median number of IHC stains was 8.3 stains/tumor;

IHC staining correctly diagnosed 83 % of 157 tumors versus 89 % for the molecular assay [21]. The molecular assay was more accurate in diagnosing poorly differentiated carcinomas (91 % vs. 71 %). In both studies, the diagnostic accuracy of IHC decreased (to about 70 %) once greater than 8 stains were performed.

In both of these comparative studies, the spectrum of tumor types included may have influenced the results in favor of IHC staining. The majority of cancers originated in the lung, breast, ovary, kidney, or colon, all sites with relatively specific IHC staining patterns. In contrast, several tumor types lacking specific IHC staining patterns but common in the CUP population (e.g., stomach, biliary tract, pancreas, gastrointestinal junction, urothelial carcinoma) were not well represented.

The use of IHC staining and molecular assays has also been reported in a few studies in patients with CUP [3]. In 5 reported studies, biopsies from a total of 117 patients were evaluated with IHC and molecular profiling [12, 14, 17, 32, 33]. In approximately 50 % of cases, IHC staining led to prediction of a single tissue of origin. In 78 % of these cases, molecular profiling yielded an identical prediction. However, molecular profiling gave a tissue of origin prediction in 96 % of all patients and was therefore useful in many of the tumors that were not characterized by IHC.

11.3 Treatment of Patients with CUP

11.3.1 Background

Patients who are classified within several recognized favorable CUP subsets (about 20 % of all CUP) are treated with specific regimens based upon their presumed tissues of origin (see Chap. 10). In general, these treatments are site specific, based on the probable site of tumor origin in these patient subsets. Examples include treatment of women with adenocarcinoma involving axillary lymph nodes as breast cancer, and treatment of patients with squamous carcinoma in cervical lymph nodes as head/neck cancer. Such treatments have resulted in improved survival in these patient subsets.

The majority of the remaining CUP patients (approximately 80 % of all CUP) have received empiric chemotherapy regimens; prognosis for most of these patients has remained poor. Empiric chemotherapy regimens (i.e., paclitaxel/carboplatin, gemcitabine/cisplatin, others) were developed because the specific cancer type or tissue of origin was not known and for most patients could not be determined. Empiric chemotherapy became the standard of care in the mid-1990s after clinical trials showed benefit at least for some patients [34]. At that time, CUP was considered by many as a single entity with a similar clinical biology, rather than a heterogeneous group comprising many types of cancer with varying behavior. Large trials (100 or more patients) of empiric chemotherapy for the unfavorable group of CUP patients have invariably resulted in median survivals of about 9 months and 2-year survivals of 10–20 % [34]. Those patients with benefit likely harbored more sensitive cancer types (such as breast or ovarian cancer), while treatment was ineffective for those with unresponsive cancers types (such as biliary tract, pancreas).

A few clinical trials several years [1, 2] ago incorporated a few targeted type drugs (first-generation drugs) alone (bevacizumab, erlotinib) or combined with chemotherapy (paclitaxel/carboplatin) but without any knowledge at that time of specific targets within the cancer cells. These endeavors, although producing some tumor responses, were essentially empirical approaches based on activity and benefit seen in a few known advanced solid tumors (non-small cell lung, colorectal).

Recent improvements in therapy have resulted in improved survival for patients with many types of known advanced cancers. These therapies have also become more individualized or specific for each particular cancer type. Furthermore, genetic alterations are now recognized in many cancers and provide the basis for effective precision or targeted therapies for selected patients. Therefore, the recognition or diagnosis of the specific cancer type or tissue of origin in each CUP patient may have critical therapeutic implications. The optimal treatment today for patients with advanced cancers requires the identification of the site of origin or specific type of cancer.

11.3.2 Site-Specific Therapies Based on Tissue of Origin in CUP

The ability to diagnose the tissue of origin in the majority of CUP patients has inaugurated an era of site-specific therapies rather than the continued use of empiric chemotherapy. Three critical questions needed to be addressed and resolved in order to confidently change the standard of care. First, can molecular cancer classifier assays accurately provide a specific tissue of origin diagnosis? Second, can molecular assays complement standard pathology? Finally, do patients have a better survival if they are treated with site-specific therapies based on a tissue of origin diagnosis versus empiric chemotherapy?

As previously reviewed in this chapter, the accuracy of molecular cancer classifier assays and their ability to complement standard pathology are firmly established. Molecular cancer classifier assays, when used with IHC and the clinical features, facilitate a specific/single tissue of origin diagnosis in 95 % of patients, and about 80 % of these diagnoses are accurate [1–3, 17]. The molecular assays complement IHC staining and frequently make a single diagnosis when IHC is inconclusive [3, 19–21, 25, 26, 31].

Conclusive demonstration of the superiority of site-specific versus empiric therapy in CUP patients is difficult for a number of reasons. There are at least 30 different types/subtypes of metastatic cancers within the CUP population. About half of these are relatively resistant to therapy (e.g., pancreas, biliary tract, liver, others) and can be expected to do poorly regardless of the treatment administered. Many of the CUP patients with more responsive cancers (e.g., breast, ovary, lung) would derive some benefit from empiric taxane/platinum regimens (although without the benefit of site-specific targeted agents and sequential useful therapies), while in only a small percentage (e.g., colorectal, renal) would site-specific and empiric CUP therapy diverge markedly. Given these considerations, a randomized trial comparing empiric chemotherapy versus assay-directed site-specific therapy, as advocated by some, would require a minimum of several hundred patients. Fewer patients would be required if enrollment was limited to potentially responsive subtypes, but enrolling these patients may pose an ethical dilemma for some physicians.

Although data from randomized trials do not exist, the efficacy of site-specific therapy has been addressed in several retrospective studies and a large prospective phase II study; results of these studies merit a brief review here.

11.3.2.1 Retrospective Studies

Several retrospective studies have focused on CUP patients with molecular profiling diagnoses in which site-specific treatment differs markedly from empiric CUP therapy (and would be expected to improve treatment results).

Colorectal Cancer

Modern treatment for patients with metastatic colorectal cancer produces a median survival of approximately 2 years. Treatment includes chemotherapy combinations (FOLFOX, FOLFIRI, others) that differ from empiric CUP regimens, as well as targeted therapy (anti-angiogenesis agents, EGFR inhibitors) not approved for use in CUP patients.

The initial suggestion that a CUP colorectal subset may have a better outcome treated with colorectal site-specific therapies came from a retrospective study of CUP patients who had molecular profiling of their biopsy specimens [11]. In this study, 23 patients had a colorectal molecular diagnosis; 7 evaluable patients received empiric chemotherapy (paclitaxel/carboplatin), and 8 evaluable patients received colorectal site-specific therapies (FOLFOX or variants). Only 1 of 7 (14 %) patients had an objective response from empiric chemotherapy, while all 8 responded to colorectal site-specific regimens.

Two subsequent retrospective studies reported treatment results in CUP patients who were predicted to have a colorectal site of origin by molecular profiling [23, 24]. In these two studies, containing 42 and 32 patients, respectively, the median survivals were 27 and 21 months following site-specific treatment for colorectal cancer. Most patients in these series had clinical features typical of metastatic colon cancer (metastases predominantly in the liver, peritoneal cavity, abdominal lymph nodes); however, an anatomical primary site could not be identified by colonoscopy.

Patients with CUP and a "colorectal profile" have also been identified on the basis of typical clinical features and IHC staining (CK20+/CK7− or CDX2+), and this group is now recognized as a favorable subset [35, 36]. In a recent publication, 68 patients with CUP diagnosed as the colorectal subset with IHC staining (no molecular profiling used) had a median survival of about 30 months following treatment with colorectal chemotherapy regimens [36].

Taken together, data from these retrospective studies strongly suggest that (1) CUP patients with a colorectal site of origin can be identified by molecular profiling or IHC stains and (2) such patients respond well to treatment for metastatic colon cancer. Most of these patients have clinical findings typical of metastatic colon cancer, although the anatomical primary sites are not detectable with colonoscopy. If IHC staining reveals a characteristic colorectal pattern, there is no need for a molecular assay. However, a substantial minority of patients identified by molecular profiling had atypical IHC staining. Treatment for patients identified by either method should mirror treatment for metastatic colon cancer; at present, testing for KRAS mutations is important, but additional molecular abnormalities are likely to be important in the future.

Renal Cell Carcinoma

Treatment of advanced renal cell carcinoma has changed markedly during the last 10 years. Traditional cytotoxic agents (including empiric regimens for CUP) are completely inactive, but several agents targeting angiogenesis or the mTOR pathway have improved the survival of these patients. Therefore, the ability to recognize a renal site of origin in patients with CUP could greatly impact the treatment of these patients.

In evaluating a biopsy specimen from a patient with CUP (i.e., no kidney masses present on CT scan), the pathologist considers renal cell carcinoma if clear cell elements are present. In this situation, IHC staining (PAX8 and RCC stains) is quite specific and can confirm the diagnosis. However, the possibility of renal cell carcinoma is often not considered when the histology is adenocarcinoma [25], and relatively specific IHC stains may not be performed. A retrospective report presented data better characterizing this CUP renal cell subset [26].

A few years ago, the authors saw a patient with CUP who was diagnosed with renal cell carcinoma by a molecular cancer classifier assay. The diagnosis was subsequently supported by IHC staining, and the patient responded favorably to targeted renal cell therapy [25]. We subsequently reviewed the records of 488 CUP patients seen between 2008 and 2012 at the Sarah Cannon Cancer Center and clinics of Tennessee Oncology in whom molecular profiling (92-gene RT-PCR [CancerTYPE ID] assay) had been performed [26]. Twenty-two patients (4.5 %) had renal cell carcinoma diagnosed; the histologic subtypes predicted by the assay included clear cell carcinoma (7), papillary adenocarcinoma (8), and unknown subtype (7). Abdominal computed tomography did not reveal a primary renal lesion in any patient, and the sites of metastasis most often involved the retroperitoneum (63 %), mediastinum (31 %), lung (22 %), and bone (18 %). Histopathologic examination of these tumors showed adenocarcinoma in 7 (4 papillary, 1 clear cell, 2 otherwise not specified) and poorly differentiated carcinoma in 15. Since renal cell carcinoma was not initially suspected, IHC staining looking for renal cell carcinoma was performed initially in only 3 tumors (14 %), but staining done (usually PAX8 and RCC) after the molecular cancer classifier diagnosis was supportive of the molecular diagnoses in 7 of 9 tumors. All 22 patients received site-specific targeted therapies for renal cell carcinoma at some time during their course (16 received first-line targeted therapy). Four patients (18 %) had an objective response and 10 patients (82 %) had stable disease; the median survival for the total group of 22 patients was 13.4 months. These survival data are similar to known advanced renal cell carcinoma patients receiving standard targeted therapies.

A renal primary site can be diagnosed in CUP patients by IHC staining and/or a molecular cancer classifier assay. In our retrospective series, the percentage of papillary adenocarcinomas was high, possibly because clear cell features on biopsy raised suspicion of a renal primary site and led to confirmatory IHC stains. Whether identified by IHC or molecular assay, these patients should be treated with site-specific treatment; although experience is currently limited, targeted renal cell carcinoma therapies appear active in these patients.

Poorly Differentiated Neoplasms

A difficult and challenging subset of CUP patients has very poorly differentiated or anaplastic neoplasms otherwise not characterized. In these patients, the general cancer type or lineage (carcinoma, sarcoma, melanoma, lymphoma) remains in doubt. Accurate diagnosis is important since it has been known for many years that some of these patients have highly treatable and potentially curable cancers [1, 2]. Modern IHC staining can define the lineage in most tumors and generally has been accepted for planning treatment for lymphoma, neuroendocrine carcinoma, melanoma, thyroid carcinoma, sarcoma, and germ cell tumors [1, 2, 37]. However, a small minority of tumors remain without a recognized general cancer type even after extensive standard pathological study.

A retrospective review of 751 CUP patients seen over a 12-year period revealed 30 patients (4 %) who retained the nonspecific diagnosis of “poorly differentiated neoplasm” after standard pathologic evaluation [38]. Biopsies had been extensively evaluated with IHC stains (median 18 stains; range 9–46). A molecular cancer classifier assay (92 gene RT-PCR) proved to be useful in diagnosing the tumor lineage in 25 of 30 patients; in several of these patients, a specific tissue of origin was also identified. The molecular assay diagnoses included 8 sarcomas (3 mesotheliomas, 5 others), 5 melanomas, 2 lymphomas, and 10 carcinomas (3 germ cell tumors, 2 neuroendocrine tumors, 5 others). Additional IHC staining and genetic testing [BRAF, i(12)p] performed after the molecular assay diagnoses supported the molecular diagnoses in 12 of the 16 patients with adequate remaining biopsy specimens. Although the study was retrospective, 7 patients were tested at the time of initial diagnosis and received site-specific therapies based on their molecular diagnoses (germ cell tumors 2, neuroendocrine tumors 2, mesotheliomas 2, lymphoma 1). All 7 patients responded favorably to therapy and remain alive (5 without progression) after 25+–72+ months.

The molecular cancer classifier assay provided a specific lineage diagnosis and precise tissue of origin in most of these poorly differentiated neoplasms that were unclassifiable by standard IHC evaluation. Molecular diagnosis in this challenging subset of patients is useful for planning therapy and is particularly important for several highly treatable and potentially curable cancers. The utility of IHC staining in the diagnosis and subsequent therapy in this setting is generally already universally accepted when these responsive/treatable tumors are diagnosed. Molecular testing now adds further to the appropriate recognition of the cancer types and subtypes in these patients.

11.3.2.2 Prospective Study of Assay-Directed Site-Specific Therapy

A large prospective nonrandomized phase II study was designed, completed, and published [22] to compare the outcome of CUP patients treated with assay-directed, site-specific therapy to 396 historical control CUP patients treated with empiric chemotherapy by the same cooperative group [1, 34]. Patients in the control group were enrolled and treated in several sequential clinical trials using identical entry criteria; the median survival for all 396 patients was 9.1 months. In addition to assessing the survival of the entire group, a secondary objective was to compare the results of site-specific therapy in patients diagnosed with responsive versus less responsive tumor types. (For the purposes of this analysis, responsive tumor types were defined as having an expected median survival of >1 year when treated with standard therapies; less responsive tumor types had median survival <1 year with standard therapy.)

The molecular assay made a single diagnosis in 194 patients; each received standard site-specific therapy for this diagnosis [22]. The overall median survival of these 194 patients was 12.5 months, compared to 9.1 months for the 396 historical control patients ($P=0.045$). The molecularly diagnosed patients with responsive tumor types (ovary, breast, kidney, prostate, colorectal, bladder, non-small cell lung, germ cell, poorly differentiated neuroendocrine tumors, lymphoma, and small-cell lung cancer) had a median survival of 13.4 months versus 7.6 months ($p=0.040$) for those patients with molecularly diagnosed less responsive tumor types (pancreas, biliary tract, liver, melanoma, gastroesophageal, sarcoma, cervix, endometrium, mesothelioma, skin, thyroid, head and neck, and adrenal). The survival observed in the molecularly diagnosed patient subsets was similar to known advanced cancers of the same type, but small numbers in each subset precluded adequate statistical comparisons. The median survivals of the subsets were as follows: ovary (29.6 months), breast (not reached but greater than 24 months), pancreas (8.2 months), biliary tract (6.8 months), and non-small cell lung (15.9 months).

The results of this prospective trial support the use of site-directed therapies based upon tissue of origin diagnoses in CUP patients. In patients with treatment-sensitive cancer types, identification of the tissue of origin is not only useful in selection of first-line therapy but also allows the use of second- and third-line therapies known to further improve survival. Many CUP patients have tumor types that are relatively insensitive to all known forms of therapy. Therefore, accurate identification of the tissue of origin does not have much impact on the current therapeutic outcomes in these patient groups. The diagnosis of a relatively insensitive or unresponsive cancer type does not detract from the value of the molecular assay or IHC staining as diagnostic tests. In the future, when more effective therapies are developed for these currently refractory tumors, their specific diagnosis within the CUP syndrome will assume greater clinical importance.

11.3.3 Arguments for a Paradigm Change to Site-Specific Therapy in CUP

The management of CUP patients is continuing to evolve. The aim of clinical and pathologic evaluation in any patient with metastatic cancer has always been to find the anatomical primary tumor site and proceed with therapy for that specific cancer. In CUP, the anatomical primary site is occult and not found despite a search, and up until the last 6 years, the determination of the tissue of origin for most patients was not possible. With improved diagnostic technologies including IHC and molecular cancer classifier assays, the tissue of origin can now be determined in the majority of CUP patients, despite the fact that the anatomical primary site is not detected. The accuracy of these predictions, although not 100 %, is generally accepted to be high, based on the cumulative data already reviewed.

In spite of agreement concerning the accuracy of the new diagnostic technologies, there remains disagreement as to whether these primary site predictions should be used to direct treatment for CUP patients. If the accuracy is accepted, the only conceivable reason for hesitation is the belief that cancers presenting as CUP will respond differently to site-specific therapy than do their counterparts with manifest primary sites. In addition to data from prospective and retrospective clinical trials already discussed (which are uniformly supportive of assay-directed therapy), several further considerations are pertinent.

The first data to consider have been appreciated for several years. Patients in several of the favorable subsets of CUP make a compelling argument for the effectiveness of site-specific therapy. Patients with squamous cell carcinoma in neck nodes and no detectable primary site have been treated with combined radiotherapy and chemotherapy for a presumed primary site in the head/neck, and their response and survival are very similar to head/neck primary cancers with cervical node metastasis [1]. Women with axillary carcinoma or peritoneal serous carcinoma without a detectable primary site are two additional examples in whom a presumed primary resides in the breast or ovary/fallopian tube/peritoneum, respectively. Once again, site-specific therapies for breast or ovarian cancer, respectively, produce results similar to those with known primary sites [1, 2]. The primary sites remain occult, yet these favorable subset CUP patients respond and survive very much like their counterparts with anatomically defined primaries.

The more recent recognition of the colorectal subset of CUP based on characteristic IHC staining patterns or molecular cancer classifier assays has resulted in site-specific treatment of this subgroup. Prolonged median survival (>20 months) has been repeatedly documented, regardless of whether IHC or molecular profiling was used to define the subset. In all of these examples, response to treatment and survival closely parallel the expected treatment results in corresponding advanced cancers of known primary site.

A second argument is a plea for consistency regarding diagnosis and therapy for CUP patients. The National Comprehensive Cancer Network (NCCN) guidelines are considered a reliable source in the United States to recommend the most appropriate evidence-based evaluation, treatment, and surveillance for cancer patients. Their most recent published guidelines for occult primary or CUP [37] recommend selected IHC stains and accept their reliability in the diagnoses and subsequent treatments for several specific cancers with initial presentations as CUP including lymphoma, thyroid carcinoma, melanoma, sarcoma, and germ cell tumors. These data are from small retrospective series of patients, and most oncologists accept these recommendations. Several other cancers are now well characterized by classic diagnostic IHC staining patterns (including colorectal, ovary, breast, renal, lung adenocarcinoma, others), but the NCCN did not recommend treatments for these CUP patients based on their IHC diagnoses. The NCCN panel of 25 expert members acknowledged the diagnostic accuracy of gene expression profiling (molecular cancer classifier assays) in CUP, but only 5 members believed the molecular assays should be used routinely in CUP. The concern of the majority of members was that a survival benefit from site-specific therapies based on molecular diagnoses has not been proven by phase III prospective randomized studies. However, the panel members accept IHC for selected diagnoses as listed above with only retrospective data from small series of patients. The disagreement and inconsistency within the NCCN regarding IHC and molecular assay diagnoses in CUP are of interest and illustrate the evolution now in process. A minority of the NCCN committee members accept the usefulness of IHC and molecular diagnoses in determining the tissue of origin and most appropriate therapy for each patient. The accuracy of IHC and molecular diagnoses and data now available regarding outcomes argue for no longer using empiric chemotherapy for most CUP patients, but treating according to the type of cancer each patient harbors.

A final clinical argument regarding the biologic similarity of CUP and their clinical counterparts with known primary sites can be made by considering the size of the primary site. In patients diagnosed with metastatic cancer and an identified anatomical primary site, systemic treatment is identical, and prognosis is similar regardless of the size of the primary. Autopsy series have documented that at least 75 % of CUP patients have identifiable small primary sites [29]. These small primary sites were clinically undetectable. It is very doubtful that there is a difference in biology or response to treatment between a clinically diagnosed primary site measuring 1.8 cm versus a clinically undetectable primary site measuring 0.6 cm. Based on this line of reasoning, it is logical to assume that advanced cancers with small, undetectable primary sites will respond to site-specific therapy in the same way as advanced cancers with larger, detectable primary sites.

The aggregate data, clinical experience, and general understanding of the CUP syndrome make a new management paradigm inescapable (Fig. 11.1). Oncologists should first determine the tissue of origin using all available information (clinical features, pathologic studies including selected IHC staining, and molecular cancer classifier assay if necessary) and then proceed with site-specific therapy for the type of cancer present. Unless a large-scale, adequately powered, randomized prospective phase III trial shows no advantage of site-specific therapies versus empiric chemotherapy (particularly in more responsive patient subsets), the new paradigm for management of CUP as illustrated in Fig. 11.1 should now be followed.

11.3.4 Potentially Actionable Genetic Alterations and Immunotherapy

Cancers are for the most part diseases of acquired/somatic genetic alterations. The altered genome of malignant cells and their therapeutic relevance is being more understood by the use of next-generation sequencing technology. Although many mutations and other alterations appear to be drivers of neoplastic development and growth/metastasis, it has become more evident that genetic alterations in subclones of neoplastic cells can change and vary within the same primary cancer and their metastasis over time. Most targeted precision therapies are directed at specific driver alterations (such as EGFR mutations in lung cancer, BRAF mutation in melanoma) and show remarkable tumor responses initially, but invariably resistance develops and tumors progress, often from new genetic alterations.

Optimism seems realistic for further detailed understanding of the processes involved [39, 40] and more successful targeted therapies (perhaps used in combination or sequentially) for many cancers. Targeted therapies are accepted and standard for several specific cancers containing genetic alterations/the target (such as chronic myeloid leukemia, GIST, subsets of breast, lung, colon, gastric cancers, and melanoma). As more precise genomic knowledge is revealed, many other targeted drugs are likely to be found beneficial.

The situation is even more complex in the CUP syndrome. Genetic and/or epigenetic alterations are likely at play to explain the existence of the small clinically undetectable invasive primary cancers which give rise to larger detectable metastasis, although no specific nonrandom genetic alterations unique to CUP have been reported. Other than the distinct biologic difference regarding the size of the primary, most clinical, pathologic, and genomic data support the biologic similarity of the specific tumors of CUP and their counterparts with known primary sites (i.e., larger, clinically detectable primary sites).

Given these considerations, it is reasonable to assume that actionable molecular abnormalities seen in specific cancer types will also appear in CUP with the same site of origin. For example, a CUP adenocarcinoma diagnosed as lung cancer on the basis of IHC/molecular assay may have an EGFR-activating mutation or an ALK or ROS1 rearrangement; these abnormalities would be expected to respond to appropriate targeted therapy. Currently, there are only a few case reports [41] to now support this assertion, but there are no other data to refute this reasoning. The same argument can be made in CUP found to be melanoma (BRAF mutated), breast cancer (HER 2 amplified), colorectal cancer (KRAS mutated), and several others.

The relevance of a more general question concerns the use of next-generation sequencing to search for "actionable" genetic alterations in CUP. Will precise targeting of these alterations benefit patients regardless of the primary site or tissue of origin? Several so-called basket trials are now in process, allowing patients with advanced cancers to be treated with a targeted drug if their cancer cells have the target found by next-generation sequencing, other genetic testing, or IHC, regardless of their cancer type.

The evaluation of CUP biopsies using next-generation sequencing is just the beginning, and the early data show many genetic alterations, similar to those found in large groups of known cancer types [42]. Further clinical studies are necessary to determine if targeting seemingly important alterations will benefit these patients. This same question is the subject of clinical trials in known cancer types with alterations found that are not common or typical for their cancers (e.g., BRAF mutations in lung, colorectal, and other cancers). The primary site or tissue of origin for now is an important element necessary for planning further evaluation and optimal therapy, but in the future may not be as important once the specific genetic lesions for each patient's cancer are fully elucidated and targeted.

The era of relatively successful immunotherapy has also begun [43–49] and, at least for the immune checkpoint inhibitors (CTLA-4, PD-1/PDL-1, others), clinical activity is likely related to specific genetic alterations (e.g., include PDL-1 expression in cancer cells and for CTLA-4 specific genetic neoepitopes) [44, 50]. The immune checkpoint inhibitors and genetically engineered T-cell therapies are promising [45–49] and may be components of combination and/or sequential therapies with targeted agents for several solid tumors in the future. These same considerations apply to the many different constituent cancers in the CUP syndrome.

References

1. Greco FA, Hainsworth JD. Cancer of unknown primary site. In: Devita VT, Lawrence TS, Rosenberg SA, editors. Cancer: principles and practice of oncology. 9th ed. Philadelphia: Lippincott, Williams, and Wilkins; 2011. p. 2033–51.
2. Greco FA, Hainsworth JD. Cancer of unknown primary site. In: DeVita VT, Lawrence TS, Rosenberg SA, editors. Cancer: principles and practice of oncology. 10th ed. Philadelphia: Lippincott, Wolters Kluwer; 2015. p. 1720–37.
3. Hainsworth JD, Greco FA. Gene expression profiling in patients with carcinoma of unknown primary site: from translational research to standard of care. Virchows Arch. 2014;464:393–402.
4. Oien KA. Pathologic evaluation of unknown primary cancer. Semin Oncol. 2009;36:8–37.
5. Greco FA, Erlander MG. Molecular classification of cancer of unknown primary site. Mol Diagn Ther. 2009;13:367–73.
6. Greco FA, Spigel DR, Yardley DA, Erlander MG, Ma XJ, Hainsworth JD. Molecular profiling in unknown primary cancer: accuracy of tissue of origin prediction. Oncologist. 2010;15:500–6.
7. Kerr SE, Schnabel CA, Sullivan PS, et al. Multisite validation study to determine performance characteristics of a 92-gene molecular cancer classifier. Clin Cancer Res. 2012;18:3953–60.

8. Monzon FA, Lyons-Weiler M, Burturovic LJ, et al. Multicenter validation of the 1,550-gene expression profile for identification of tumor tissue of origin. J Clin Oncol. 2009;27:2503–8.
9. Rosenfeld N, Aharonov R, Meiri E, et al. MicroRNAs accurately identified cancer tissue origin. Nat Biotechnol. 2008;26:462–9.
10. Ma XJ, Patel R, Wang X, et al. Molecular classification of human cancers using 92-gene real time quantitative polymerase chain reaction assay. Arch Pathol Lab Med. 2006;130:465–73.
11. Varadhachary GR, Talantov D, Raber MN, et al. Molecular profiling of carcinoma of unknown primary and correlation with clinical evaluation. J Clin Oncol. 2008;26:4442–8.
12. Horlings HM, van Laar RK, Kerst JM, et al. Gene expression profiling to identify the histogenic origin of metastatic adenocarcinoma of unknown primary. J Clin Oncol. 2008;26:4435–41.
13. Bridgewater J, van Laar RK, Floore A, et al. Gene expression profiling may improve diagnosis in patients with carcinoma of unknown primary. Br J Cancer. 2008;98:1425–30.
14. Varadhachary GR, Spector Y, Abbruzzese JL, et al. Prospective gene signature study using micro RNA to identify the tissue of origin in patients with carcinoma of unknown primary. Clin Cancer Res. 2011;17:4063–70.
15. Greco FA. Cancer of unknown primary site: Improved patient management with molecular and immunohistochemical diagnosis. Am Soc Clin Oncol Educ Book. 2013;33:175–81.
16. Greco FA. Cancer of unknown primary site: evolving understanding and management of patients. Clin Adv Hematol Oncol. 2012;10:518–24.
17. Greco FA, Lennington WJ, Spigel DR, et al. Molecular profiling diagnosis in unknown primary cancer: accuracy and ability to complement standard pathology. J Natl Cancer Inst. 2013;105:782–90.
18. Schwartz AM, Harpaz N. A primary approach to cancer of unknown primary. J Natl Cancer Inst. 2013;105:759–61.
19. Weiss LM, Chu P, Schroeder BE, et al. Blinded comparator study of immunohistochemical analysis versus a 92-gene classifier in the diagnosis of the primary site in metastatic tumors. J Mol Diagn. 2013;15:263–9.
20. Kulkarni A, Pillai R, Ezekiel AM, et al. Comparison of histology to gene expression profiling for the diagnosis of metastatic cancer. Diagn Pathol. 2012;7:1010–113.
21. Handorf CR, Kulkarni A, Grenert JR, et al. A multicenter study directly comparing the diagnostic accuracy of gene expression profiling and immunohistochemistry for primary site Identification in metastatic tumors. Am J Surg Pathol. 2013;37:1067–75.
22. Hainsworth JD, Ruben MS, Spigel DR, et al. Molecular gene expression profiling to predict the tissue of origin and direct site-specific therapy in patients with carcinoma of unknown primary site: a prospective trial of the Sarah Cannon Research Institute. J Clin Oncol. 2013;31:217–23.
23. Greco FA, Lennington WJ, et al. Carcinoma of unknown primary site: outcomes in patients with a colorectal molecular profile treated with site-specific chemotherapy. J Cancer Ther. 2012;33:337–43.
24. Hainsworth JD, Schnabel CA, Erlander MG, et al. A retrospective study of treatment outcomes in patients with carcinoma of unknown primary site and a colorectal cancer molecular profile. Clin Colorectal Cancer. 2012;11:112–8.
25. Sorscher SM, Greco FA. Papillary renal carcinoma presenting as a cancer of unknown primary (CUP) and diagnosed through gene expression profiling. Case Rep Oncol. 2012;5:229–32.
26. Hainsworth JD, Spigel DR, Greco FA. Renal cell carcinoma (RCC) presenting as cancer of unknown primary (CUP): Diagnosis by molecular tumor profiling (MTP). J Clin Oncol. 2013;31(Suppl):Abstract e 15501.
27. Kamposioras K, Pentheroudakis G, Pavlidis N. Exploring the biology of cancer of unknown primary: breakthroughs and drawbacks. Eur J Clin Invest. 2013;43:491–500.
28. Hainsworth JD, Fizazi K. Treatment for patients with unknown primary cancer and favorable prognostic factors. Semin Oncol. 2009;36:44–52.
29. Pentheroudakis G, Greco FA, Pavlidis N. Molecular assignment of tissue of origin in cancer of unknown primary may not predict response to therapy or outcome: a systematic literature review. Cancer Treat Rev. 2009;35:221–7.

30. Greco FA. Cancer of unknown primary site; still an entity, a biologic mystery and a metastatic model. Nat Rev Cancer. 2014;14(1):3–4.
31. Pentheroudakis G, Pavlidis N, Fountzilas G, et al. Novel microRNA-based assay demonstrates 92% agreement with diagnosis based on clinicopathologic and management data in a cohort of patients with carcinoma of unknown primary. Mol Cancer. 2013;12:57. doi:10.1186/1476-4598-12-57.
32. Monzon FA, Medeiras F, Lyons-Weiler M, et al. Identification of tissue of origin in carcinoma of unknown primary with a microarray-based gene expression test. Diagn Pathol. 2010;5:3.
33. Morawietz L, Floure A, Stark-Sloots L, et al. Comparison of histopathologic and gene expression-based typing of cancer of unknown primary. Virchows Arch. 2010;456:23–9.
34. Greco FA, Pavlidis N. Treatment for patients with unknown primary carcinoma and unfavorable prognostic factors. Semin Oncol. 2009;36:65–74.
35. Varadhachary GR, Raber MN, Matamorsa A, et al. Carcinoma of unknown primary with a colon- cancer profile- changing paradigm and emerging definitions. Lancet Oncol. 2008;9:596–608.
36. Varadhachary GR, Karanth S, Qiaow W, et al. Carcinoma of unknown primary with gastrointestinal profile: immunohistochemistry and survival data for this favorable subset. Int J Clin Oncol. 2014;19(3):479–84.
37. Ettinger DS, Handorf CR, Agulnik M, et al. Occult primary, version 3.2014 featured updates to the NCCN guidelines. J Natl Compr Canc Netw. 2014;12:969–74.
38. Greco FA, Spigel DR, Hainsworth JD. Molecular tumor profiling of poorly differentiated neoplasms of unknown primary site. J Clin Oncol. 2013;31(Suppl):681 s (abstract # 11102).
39. Hoadley KA, Yau C, Wolf DM, et al. Multiplatform analysis of 12 cancer types reveals classification within and across tissues of origin. Cell. 2014;158:929–44.
40. Meador CB, Micheel CM, Levy MA, et al. Beyond histology: translating tumor genotypes into clinically effective targeted therapies. Clin Cancer Res. 2014;20(9):2264–75.
41. Penley WC, Spigel DR, Greco FA, et al. Confirmation of non-small cell lung cancer diagnosis using ALK testing and genetic profiling in patients presenting with carcinoma of unknown primary site. J Clin Oncol. 2013;31(Suppl):Abstract e115004.
42. Gatalica Z, Millis S, Bender R, et al. Molecular profiling of cancers of unknown primary site (CUP): paradigm shift in management of CUP. EJC. 2011;47(Suppl 2):Abstract LBA39.
43. Brahmer JR, Tykodi SS, Chow LQ, et al. Safety and activity of anti-PD-L1 antibody in patients with advanced cancer. N Engl J Med. 2012;366:2455–65.
44. Taubo JM, Klein A, Brahmer JR, et al. Association of PD-1, PD-1 ligands, and other features of the tumor immune microenvironment with response to anti-PD-1 therapy. Clin Cancer Res. 2014;20(19):5064–74.
45. Tran E, Rosenberg SA. T-cell therapy against cancer mutations. Oncotarget. 2014;5(13):4579–80.
46. Rosenberg SA. Decade in review-cancer immunotherapy; entering the mainstream of cancer treatment. Nat Rev Clin Oncol. 2014;11(11):630–2.
47. Tran E, Turcotte S, Gros A, et al. Cancer immunotherapy based on mutation-specific CD4+ T cells in a patient with epithelial cancer. Science. 2014;344(6184):641–5.
48. Lu YC, Yao X, Crystal JS, et al. Efficient identification of mutated cancer antigens recognized by T cells associated with durable tumor regressions. Clin Cancer Res. 2014;20(13):3401–10.
49. Kochenderfer JN, Dudley ME, Kassim SH, et al. Chemotherapy-refractory diffuse large B-cell lymphoma and indolent B-cell malignancies can be effectively treated with autologous T cells expressing an anti-CD19 chimeric antigen receptor. J Clin Oncol. 2014;33:540–9. pii: JCO.2014.56.2025 (ahead of print).
50. Snyder A, Makarov V, Merghoub T, et al. Genetic basis for clinical response to CTLA-4 blockade in melanoma. N Engl J Med. 2014;371:2189–99.

Chapter 12
Future Directions

Alwin Krämer and Harald Löffler

12.1 Personalized Medicine and Precision Oncology

When thinking about possible future directions in the management of CUP, it seems worth to pay attention to the fact that the whole field of oncology (and even medicine in general) might face a paradigm shift in the near future. Terms that are being used in this context include "personalized cancer medicine" and "precision oncology," which are commonly defined as individualized treatment based on the molecular characteristics of a tumor from an individual patient [1–3]. What is the difference to current practice in clinical oncology? The central dogma of evidence-based medicine has taught us that any hypothesis regarding the effect of a medical intervention needs to be confirmed, if possible, in a prospectively randomized controlled trial. This implies that sufficiently large groups of patients are treated with standardized therapy protocols, thereby limiting individualization of treatment. With the advent of molecularly targeted drugs, this is predicted to become more and more problematic since patient groups benefiting from a given agent, or a given combination, become smaller and smaller. In addition, every targeted drug ideally needs to be connected to a molecular predictor, which must be validated. Currently, it is far from clear how this dilemma should be handled in the context of evidence-based medicine. Up to now, the impact of targeted therapies is therefore limited due to their, in many cases, broad-spectrum application in the absence of validated molecular predictors.

A. Krämer (✉) • H. Löffler
Clinical Cooperation Unit Molecular Hematology/Oncology, German Cancer Research Center (DKFZ) and University of Heidelberg, Heidelberg, Germany
e-mail: a.kraemer@Dkfz-Heidelberg.de; h.loeffler@Dkfz-Heidelberg.de

A. Krämer, H. Löffler (eds.), *Cancer of Unknown Primary*,
DOI 10.1007/978-3-319-22581-4_12

12.2 From Nonspecific Standards to Individualized Approaches?

Management of CUP is currently dictated by two approaches: Patients could either be treated according to uniform standards generally applicable to this entity, or individualized approaches could be applied. One such individualized approach is to tailor therapy according to the most likely site of origin, as traditionally incorporated into CUP management by the definition of "prognostically favorable" subgroups. Gene expression profiling has extended the possibilities to define a likely site of origin, raising the percentage of CUP cases where a reasonable working hypothesis can be defined from 10–30 % to 80 % or more. One obviously possible future direction may therefore be that uniform CUP therapy standards will gradually disappear, and instead, a likely site of origin will be defined in most cases, leading to assignment of site-specific therapies. However, as already discussed, there is still no high-level evidence that molecular site-of-origin assignment yields any therapeutic benefit in comparison to conventional standard treatments. Hence, it may still make sense to advance therapeutic standards applicable to CUP independently of site-of-origin assignment. Such therapeutic advances may include molecularly targeted therapies, which may become established for unselected patients as long as there are no suitable molecular predictors and exemplified by the use of bevacizumab/erlotinib in phase II trials [4, 5]. Another promising field of innovation is the recently established cancer immunotherapies, with antibodies to cytotoxic T-lymphocyte-associated antigen-4 (CTLA-4) and programmed death-1 (PD-1) or programmed death ligand-1 (PDL-1), whose mechanisms of action are fundamentally different from "traditional" targeted therapies since they do not target tumor cells but act on tumor-responsive immune cells instead [6–10]. Some of these novel antibodies have already been approved for the therapy of advanced malignant melanoma and are being tested in a wide range of other malignancies. They may be promising for CUP as well, although it should be noted that for these substances, validated molecular predictors are missing so far as well.

Apart from site-of-origin assignment, there might be another individualized approach to the management of CUP patients: Patients could be stratified according to molecular targets warranting targeted therapies, which may be efficient independently from the site of origin. For example, trastuzumab has been approved for both breast and gastric cancers, the relevant predictor for its efficacy being in both entities HER-2/neu overexpression [2, 11]. Since the field of oncology will likely see a growing number of molecular targets for which both suitable drugs and validated tests to predict their efficacy are available, it may be possible to transfer these relations from larger entities to CUP. Indeed, there is a, probably growing, trend that molecularly targeted drugs are tested in so-called basket studies where the eligibility for treatment with the respective drug solely depends on the molecular target, while the organ site is irrelevant [12]. With regard to CUP, this means that determining the site of origin might gradually become less relevant, although it has to be mentioned that there are examples where the predictive value of a therapeutic target depends on the organ site, e.g., BRAF inhibition, which has been proven beneficial in malignant melanomas while there seems to be no benefit in colorectal cancer [13–16].

In practice, the introduction of next-generation sequencing has facilitated studies on molecular targets including their practical application as therapeutic predictors. Tothill et al. [17] published a first study testing this concept, where they claimed that among 16 CUP cases examined by massively parallel sequencing, they identified 12 patients possibly benefiting from targeted treatment approaches, with strong clinical evidence supporting the efficacy of a targeted drug in five of these cases. We have discussed this study in greater detail in Sect. 3.6 of this book. Also given the fact that several abstracts regarding determination of molecular targets in CUP patients by next-generation sequencing have been released (as also discussed in Sect. 3.6), we prognosticate that molecular targets and their therapeutic application will be among the major directions of future research on CUP.

12.3 From Single Molecular Targets to a Unified Molecular Classification?

Beyond focusing on specific therapeutic targets, molecular studies might have a much more fundamental role in the future of cancer medicine, as demonstrated in a recent work published by the Cancer Genome Atlas Research Network [18]. In this study, 12 cancer types as defined by conventional means, i.e., the site of origin and histologic features, were included. A total of 3527 specimens were studied for their whole-exome DNA sequence, DNA copy-number variation, DNA methylation, genome-wide mRNA levels, microRNA levels, and protein levels for 131 proteins and/or phosphorylated proteins. Using a method termed cluster-of-cluster assignments, this information was integrated into a molecular classification which yielded 11 major molecular types. Interestingly, while five of these molecular types were nearly identical to classical entities as defined by tissue of origin, there were some discordant groups: Whereas some of the tissue-of-origin-based cancer types were, not unexpectedly, split into more than one group (e.g., breast cancer into a "luminal" and a "basal" group), there were also molecular groups which included tumors from more than one site of origin, e.g., a group composed of head and neck squamous cell carcinomas and lung squamous cell carcinomas and a subset of bladder cancers. On the other hand, significant proportions of bladder cancers were recruited to two other molecular groups, one being a unique "bladder cancer" group, while the rest of bladder cancers fell into a common group with lung adenocarcinomas and a minority of lung squamous cell carcinomas [18]. These examples demonstrate that eventually, tissue-of-origin-based and molecular cancer types might diverge from each other. One would intuitively think that molecular classification more closely reflects true biological tumor entities and is therefore a better predictor for therapy assignment. Although this assumption requires, of course, validation in clinical trials, we think that in the future, the relative weight of molecular classification will grow, and in the long run, the tissue of origin might become less relevant. With regard to CUP, this might finally be good news, since it opens up the prospect that in the distant future, searching for the site of origin may be simply dispensable, because therapy will be assigned according to molecular classifiers. It remains an exciting question how these classifiers might look like.

References

1. Wistuba II, Gelovani JG, Jacoby JJ, Davis SE, Herbst RS. Methodological and practical challenges for personalized cancer therapies. Nat Rev Clin Oncol. 2011;8(3):135–41. PubMed.
2. Stern HM. Improving treatment of HER2-positive cancers: opportunities and challenges. Sci Transl Med. 2012;4(127):127rv2. PubMed.
3. Shrager J, Tenenbaum JM. Rapid learning for precision oncology. Nat Rev Clin Oncol. 2014;11(2):109–18. PubMed.
4. Hainsworth JD, Spigel DR, Farley C, Thompson DS, Shipley DL, Greco FA. Phase II trial of bevacizumab and erlotinib in carcinomas of unknown primary site: the Minnie Pearl Cancer Research Network. J Clin Oncol. 2007;25(13):1747–52. PubMed.
5. Hainsworth JD, Spigel DR, Thompson DS, Murphy PB, Lane CM, Waterhouse DM, et al. Paclitaxel/carboplatin plus bevacizumab/erlotinib in the first-line treatment of patients with carcinoma of unknown primary site. Oncologist. 2009;14(12):1189–97. PubMed.
6. Antonia SJ, Larkin J, Ascierto PA. Immuno-oncology Combinations: a review of clinical experience and future prospects. Clin Cancer Res. 2014;20(24):6258–68. PubMed.
7. Robert C, Long GV, Brady B, Dutriaux C, Maio M, Mortier L, et al. Nivolumab in previously untreated melanoma without BRAF mutation. N Engl J Med. 2015;372(4):320–30. PubMed.
8. Wolchok JD, Kluger H, Callahan MK, Postow MA, Rizvi NA, Lesokhin AM, et al. Nivolumab plus ipilimumab in advanced melanoma. N Engl J Med. 2013;369(2):122–33. PubMed.
9. Pardoll DM. The blockade of immune checkpoints in cancer immunotherapy. Nat Rev Cancer. 2012;12(4):252–64. PubMed.
10. Hodi FS, O'Day SJ, McDermott DF, Weber RW, Sosman JA, Haanen JB, et al. Improved survival with ipilimumab in patients with metastatic melanoma. N Engl J Med. 2010;363(8):711–23. PubMed Pubmed Central PMCID: 3549297.
11. Martin V, Cappuzzo F, Mazzucchelli L, Frattini M. HER2 in solid tumors: more than 10 years under the microscope; where are we now? Future Oncol. 2014;10(8):1469–86. PubMed.
12. Willyard C. 'Basket studies' will hold intricate data for cancer drug approvals. Nat Med. 2013;19(6):655. PubMed.
13. Girotti MR, Saturno G, Lorigan P, Marais R. No longer an untreatable disease: how targeted and immunotherapies have changed the management of melanoma patients. Mol Oncol. 2014;8(6):1140–58. PubMed.
14. Finn L, Markovic SN, Joseph RW. Therapy for metastatic melanoma: the past, present, and future. BMC Med. 2012;10:23. PubMed Pubmed Central PMCID: 3308914.
15. Tie J, Desai J. Targeting BRAF mutant metastatic colorectal cancer: clinical implications and emerging therapeutic strategies. Target Oncol. 2015;10(2):179–88. PubMed.
16. Hall RD, Kudchadkar RR. BRAF mutations: signaling, epidemiology, and clinical experience in multiple malignancies. Cancer Control. 2014;21(3):221–30. PubMed.
17. Tothill RW, Li J, Mileshkin L, Doig K, Siganakis T, Cowin P, et al. Massively-parallel sequencing assists the diagnosis and guided treatment of cancers of unknown primary. J Pathol. 2013;4:413–23. PubMed.
18. Hoadley KA, Yau C, Wolf DM, Cherniack AD, Tamborero D, Ng S, et al. Multiplatform analysis of 12 cancer types reveals molecular classification within and across tissues of origin. Cell. 2014;158(4):929–44. PubMed Pubmed Central PMCID: 4152462.

MIX
Papier aus verantwortungsvollen Quellen
Paper from responsible sources
FSC® C105338

If you have any concerns about our products,
you can contact us on
ProductSafety@springernature.com

In case Publisher is established outside the EU,
the EU authorized representative is:
Springer Nature Customer Service Center GmbH
Europaplatz 3, 69115 Heidelberg, Germany

Printed by Libri Plureos GmbH
in Hamburg, Germany